PHYSICAL ACTIVITY EFFECTS ON THE ANTHROPOLOGICAL STATUS OF CHILDREN, YOUTH AND ADULTS

PHYSICAL FITNESS, DIET AND EXERCISE

Additional books in this series can be found on Nova's website
under the Series tab.

Additional e-books in this series can be found on Nova's website
under the eBooks tab.

PHYSICAL FITNESS, DIET AND EXERCISE

PHYSICAL ACTIVITY EFFECTS ON THE ANTHROPOLOGICAL STATUS OF CHILDREN, YOUTH AND ADULTS

FADILJ EMINOVIĆ
AND
MILIVOJ DOPSAJ
EDITORS

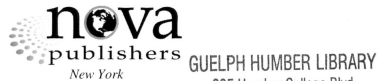

nova publishers
New York

NOTICE TO THE READER

The Publisher has taken reasonable care in the preparation of this book, but makes no expressed or implied warranty of any kind and assumes no responsibility for any errors or omissions. No liability is assumed for incidental or consequential damages in connection with or arising out of information contained in this book. The Publisher shall not be liable for any special, consequential, or exemplary damages resulting, in whole or in part, from the readers' use of, or reliance upon, this material. Any parts of this book based on government reports are so indicated and copyright is claimed for those parts to the extent applicable to compilations of such works.

Independent verification should be sought for any data, advice or recommendations contained in this book. In addition, no responsibility is assumed by the publisher for any injury and/or damage to persons or property arising from any methods, products, instructions, ideas or otherwise contained in this publication.

This publication is designed to provide accurate and authoritative information with regard to the subject matter covered herein. It is sold with the clear understanding that the Publisher is not engaged in rendering legal or any other professional services. If legal or any other expert assistance is required, the services of a competent person should be sought. FROM A DECLARATION OF PARTICIPANTS JOINTLY ADOPTED BY A COMMITTEE OF THE AMERICAN BAR ASSOCIATION AND A COMMITTEE OF PUBLISHERS.

Additional color graphics may be available in the e-book version of this book.

Library of Congress Cataloging-in-Publication Data

ISBN: 978-1-63484-782-7

Library of Congress Control Number: 2016933385

Published by Nova Science Publishers, Inc. † New York

CONTENTS

FOREWORD

*GIORGIO FERRIERO**, *MD, PhD,*
DEPARTMENT OF PHYSICAL MEDICINE AND REHABILITATION,
HAMAD MEDICAL CORPORATION, DOHA, QATAR

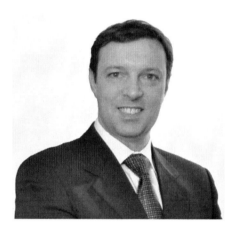

I am privileged that I had possibility to comment this important monography edited by professor Fadilj Eminović and professor Milivoj Dopsaj, since I believe that it is very important to stress the importance of practicing adequate physical activity to prevent disease with high impact on life expectancy and quality of life.

In 2010 World Health Organization has clearly established the quantity of physical activity that anyone must do according his/her age. In particular three categories are defined: younger than 18, between 19 and 65, and older than 65 years. Physical activity does not means only sport, but is a concept including all activities performed with low, medium or high energy cost.

The low level corresponds to physical activities ranging from do virtually nothing (sleep or watch television) to walk at a normal pace. During these activities the human body makes virtually no effort, consumes fewer calories and makes the slightest movement to survive.

The intermediate level of intensity (moderate) is rather to all those activities that do not require excessive effort. Among these activities is the fast walking and cycling, but also numerous fitness activities such as gymnastics, the use of minimum weights, water aerobics

---
* E mail: giorgioferriero@yahoo.it.

or low-resistance exercise bike. Even dancing is one of the physical activities of intermediate level.

The more intense level (vigorous) is that can be reached by making greater efforts, generally during any sporting activity itself (running, tennis, swimming, cycling, just to name a few). Obviously between the intense degree activities there are workouts in the gym, but also some dancing (ballet, acrobatic rock) that can lead to making high physical exertion.

Work is one of the physical activities. Sedentary work is part of the low level, while all those jobs that require some physical effort - such as shifting weights , the perform household cleaning, work the land - can be compared the same way as sport characterized by intermediate or high level of physical intensity.

However, physical activity can expose to significant risk those who practice it, especially if done with intense rhythms. For this reason national and European institutions have begun to investigate the importance of the negative effects of sport. At first they were considered the worst phenomena related to sport, such as doping and violence. Recently, attention is focused also on health issues, as sport-related trauma accidents or severe cardiovascular events. To minimize risk of accidents and cardiac incidents related to the practice of physical activity there are three forms prevention: a passive, participatory and active.

Passive prevention is to implement all those conditions of reduced risk of injury requiring no participation of people exercising, as organizing a correct competition, in adequate environment. Participatory prevention requires the person's cooperation, as using of appropriate protective equipment. Active prevention is based on education and information on human body, exercise, and sport-related injuries.

This monography deeply discusses the topic of physical activity across different ages in its fifteen chapters. Most of them are original research studies discussing specific themes about the risk related to a sedentary lifestyle, the advantages of physical activity and about its organization. My compliments are to both Editors and to each Author for the thoroughness of their valuable work, useful to update knowledge of researchers, experts and clinicians, working in the field of physical activity.

PROF. CALOGERO FOTI*, MD, FEBPRM
TOR VERGATA UNIVERSITY
PHYSICAL AND REHABILITATION MEDICINE, FULL PROFESSOR
SCHOOL OF MEDICINE, CHAIR
SCHOOL OF MOTOR SCIENCE, CHAIR
SCHOOL OF PHYSIOTHERAPY, CHAIR
PRM SCHOOL OF SPECIALIZATION, DIRECTOR
PHD ON ADVANCED SCIENCES AND TECHNOLOGIES IN
REHABILITATION MEDICINE AND SPORTS, COORDINATOR
SIMFER, VICEPRESIDENT, INTERNATIONAL AND COOPERATION
AFFAIRS DELEGATE, ROME, ITALY, EU

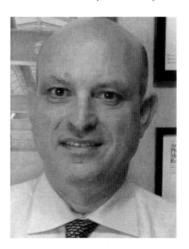

Physical activity, self-awareness, intellectual abilities, social integration, are all elements that intersect and influence each other. All this takes place regardless of the skill and agility of each of us. Exercise improves the quality of life for people of any age, gender, economic and social conditions, religious beliefs, regardless of their relationship with the environment. A skilled or disabled person, in short, lives better if doing gymnastics.

---

* E mail: foti@med.uniroma2.it.

This truth was know very well by ancient popultations.The tenth satire of *Decimus Iunius Iuvenalis*, Roman poet and rhetorician (I Century, AD), *"Mens sana in corpore sano"*, is all aimed at showing the vanity of values or goods (such as wealth, fame and honor) that men are trying, by any means, to obtain. Only the truly wise person realizes that everything is ephemeral, and sometimes even harmful. The intention of the poet, the man should aspire to only two goods: the soul's health and the health of the body.

In the book *"Effects of application of physical activity on the anthropological status of children, youth and adults"*, by Eminović Fadilj and Dopsaj Milivoj, the importance of body exercise in our life is stressed in a scientific way. All the authors are scientists that use the biomedical statistics in research to understand better the influence of physical activity in a wide range of social groups. The place of origin of the authors gives a huge universality to the contents of the book.

In the first chapter Carlo Lai, Gaia Romana Pellicano, Navkiran Kalsi, Giuseppe Massaro, Clelia Giulia Turetta, Daniela Altavilla discuss about pregnancy and mother-child relationship. Fetuses follow behavioral patterns, such as the sleep-wake cycle, which are determined by regularity of heart rate, eye movements and fetal movements. The first experiences during pregnancy promote a stronger maternal-fetal bonding and postnatal maternal-child interaction, which are crucial for the future child wellbeing

In the second chapter Ivana Milanović, Olivera M. Knezević, Miloš M. Marković, Slađana R. Rakić, Snežana Radisavljević Janić, and Dragan M. Mirkov studied the potential difference in Cardiorespiratory Fitness between schoolchildren from urban and rural areas. Monitoring and prevention of overweight and obesity in childhood in the school represents an important indicator for the public health policy in the prevention of cardiovascular and metabolic diseases and is impressive the high number of schoolchildren.

In the third chapter Tadeja Volmut, Rado Pišot, Boštjan Šimunič studied the effect of regular sport exercise on muscle contractile properties in children. The health benefits of physical exercise well beyond physical health, having a positive impact on the domains of motor skills, psychological well-being, cognitive development, social competence, and emotional maturity.

In the 4th chapter Aco Gajevic and Jelena Ivanovic describe the trend changes in physical fitness in children of elementary school age. Modern lifestyle has led to reduce motion and habitual physical activities, which have a negative influence on social health. Regarding the results obtained using comparative analysis of current testing and previous researches, the authors concluded that the National Plan does not meet the needs of the health status in children and it must be reviewed and appropriately modified.

In the 5th chapter Robert Lockie deals with the effects of linear and change of direction (COD) speed training on the sprint performance of young adults. The study interestingly stressed the concept of differences between the linear and COD speed because this sets the ground for specific trainings. Besides the analysis of the specific trainings could help the trainers to personalize the athletes' trainings.

In the 6th chapter Itaru Enomoto describes how in Japan and in many other countries socioeconomic transformation over the previous decades has induced a decline in fitness level for young adolescents. The study of Japanese female university freshmen is very interesting since it has brought out importance and positive impact of the sports experience from childhood to adolescence on physical fitness.

In the 7th chapter Fadilj Eminovic and Dragana Kljajic state that regular applied physical activity in people with Spinal Cord Injury can improve the level of functional abilities, motivation and quality of life. Applied physical exercises and sport activities are considered as a real therapy able to produce evident improvements of motor and functional abilities, to ameliorate the psychological state of the individual and to prevent systemic complications of SCI.

In the 8th chapter, Yeshayahu Hutzler describes the evolution of the two concepts of adaptation, UD (Universal Design) and UDL (Universal Design for Learning) in relation to physical activity and sports in persons with limiting conditions, such as the disabled and with health impaired.

In the chapter 9 Keith Storey focuses on the importance of recreation and integration for people with disabilities. Allow people with disabilities to participate in recreational activities in an integrated settings, is a way to let them know new people, engage new relationship, and improve their quality of life.

In the 10th chapter, Hana Válková shows the results of a pilot study based on the principles of the Special Olympics Healthy Athlete (SO HA) Program, in which 54 cross-country skiers with moderate intellectual disabilities were enrolled in order to collect data about their main health and fitness related. The author, through personal previous studies and a large amount of references, offers a comprehensive description of various interesting topics regarding physical activity and health behaviour in persons with intellectual disability, like obesity, bad eating habits and cardiovascular issues.

In the eleven chapter Milivoj Dopsaj, Marina Đorđević-Nikić, Miloš Maksimović deal with the existing relationship between physical activity and the changes in body composition in population of both genders living in Belgrade. Points of strenght are the high number of candidates, the long period of observation and data collection, the clear indication of the exclusion criteria, and the use of methods of last generation for the measurement of parameters of body composition (DSM-BIA).

In the twelve chapter Bryan McCormick points out that sedentary behavior is distinct from a lack of physical activity; physical activity and sedentary behavior can exist at the same time. Children and adolescents who begin with high levels of sedentary behavior are more likely to become highly sedentary adults, with attendant health risks.

In the 13th chapter Nevena Veljković, Sanja Glisić, Branislava Gemović, and Veljko Veljković present physical exercise as supportive therapy in cancer and HIV disease; experimental and clinical data presented in this chapter are supported by several studies.

In the 14th chapter Dragan Pavlovic showed a positive correlation between physical activity and cognitive abilities. Regular exercises reduces morbidity and mortality even in patients with chronic diseases. In older people, physical activity reduces risk of falls and cognitive decline. They considered whether the exercise in the midlife has long-lasting cognitive effects in the older age.

In the 15th chapter Evdokia Samouilidu, Sanela Pacić, Radmila Nikić, and Fadilj Eminović show interesting scientific evidences about the impact of physical activity on older people and underlines the need to facilitate access to physical activity for older people.

The book written and coordinated by Fadilj and Milivoj represents an occasion to understand better the relationship between physical activity, sports, abled and disabled people. Sports scientists, Physicians, Sports doctors, Physiatrists, Physiologists,

Physiotherapists, Psychologists, Biomechanics, are the first involved readers. They can find along the book ideas and suggestions for their professional life. Enjoy!

KALENIK ELENA NIKOLAEVNA*, PhD
CANDIDATE OF PEDAGOGICAL SCIENCES, ULYANOVSK STATE UNIVERSITY

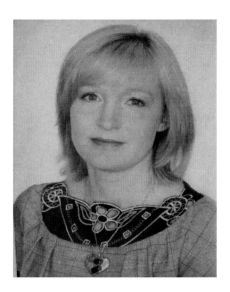

Physical activity has the large influence on human health. Physical is a sphere of social activity, aimed at preservation and strengthening of health, development of psychic and physiological abilities of a person in the process of physical activity. Today there is a question, how to efficiently solve the problem of recovery of the population. It is necessary to attract a resource of physical activity from infancy to old age, for any group of people in order to form a complete healthy lifestyle. The authors of the monograph made a test step the description of the effectiveness of physical activity.

The monograph contains material of scientific research on the effects of physical activity on the anthropological status of children, youth and adults.

Scientific group propose new research directions in the field of physical activity, from babies in the womb, to the physical culture throughout life.

The methodical manual is designed to receive the result – improving health, physical development and improving the quality of life of people.

---

* E mail: kente@mail.ru.

The special attention was made to the fact that research comprises of children, youth and adults, and all population groups obtained the results.

The work presents as a system of measures on protection and strengthening of health of schoolchildren and youth. The most acceptable teaching methods and techniques in physical activity were recommended.

The content of the monograph can be used actively in scientific research, pedagogical, psychological and other. Work with the population. The line of healthy lifestyles and the effectiveness of physical activity are traced in this monograph.

Materials of monograph create the preconditions for the decision of problems of physical activity. A number of problems, which require the further studying was revealed in the present works.

On the basis of these researches invisible necessary to develop a technology or physical activity to conduct a survey of motivation for physical activity in all age groups.

Social aspects of physical activity in people of different social status need further new researches.

The monograph is built in a logical sequence, it presents the scientific research, backed by scientific facts. This research work will be of interest to a wide range of specialists working in the sphere of physical culture, medicine, rehabilitation.

PREFACE

In the last decade a dramatic increase in overweight and obesity has been reported in both developed and underdeveloped countries. Noncommunicable diseases, as well as type 2 diabetes or obesity are one of the most common causes of long-term disability, especially cardiovascular disease (CVD) which is still the leading cause of death in the industrialized world. Accumulating evidence over the last 50 years indicates that exercise may postpone or counteract, at least partially, the debilitating consequences of CVD and prevent complications provoked by the inactive state. It has been demonstrated in coronary artery disease (CAD) patients that aerobic fitness (exercise capacity) is closely related to long-term survival.

There is now overwhelming evidence that regular physical activity has important and wide-ranging health benefits. These range from reduced risk of chronic diseases such as CVD, type 2 diabetes, hypertension and some cancers to enhanced function and preservation of function with age. Also, the beneficial effect of exercise training and exercise-based cardiac rehabilitation on symptom-free exercise capacity, cardiovascular and skeletal muscle function, quality of life, general healthy lifestyle, and reduction of depressive symptoms and psychosocial stress is nowadays well recognized.

Today, we can clearly conclude that lack of physical activity or luck of physically active lifestyle has been clearly shown to be a high overall health risk. Lack of physical activity increase the loss of muscle mass, making usual and instrumental activities of daily living much more difficult to perfom. Bone loss progress at sedentary people is much faster than in physically or exercise active people. Low level of depression is common mood state for regular physically active people. People who don't get regular physical exercise or physical activity are more likely to gain excess weight or excess body fat.

Also, we can say that thousand of deaths result each year due to lack of regular physical activity, where new scientific evidence showed to us that inactivity tends to increase with age, and it seems that women are more likely to lead inactive lifestyle, and non-Hispanic white adults are more likely to engage in physical activity than Hispanic and black adults. Official European statistical data's showed that 40% of all EU adults are physically inactive, where 17% had less than 10 minutes of walking per day, and 49% are sitting more than 4.5 hours per day.

Societal indicators of reductions in human energy expenditure and increases in sedentary behavior during the past several decades are particularly striking. By the year 2000, the human race reached a sort of historical landmark, when for the first time in human evolution the number of adults with excess weight surpassed the number of those who were underweight. Excess adiposity/body weight is now widely recognized as one of today's leading health threats. Although obesity in childhood is indicated as a complex disorder, the prevalence of overweight and obese children is continually growing globally. This has become a worrying public health concern as overweight and obesity in childhood tracks into adulthood and is associated with short- and long term adverse health outcomes.

A number of research articles in this monograph book are also presented which provide interesting and innovation practical suggestions and applications and directions for some future research. Chapter 1 investigates phenomena of the first physical movements of life recognized as fetal movements and mother's physiological states where the movement of the fetus inside womb has been recognized as a foremost indicator of fetal wellbeing. The aim of the Chapter 2 was to investigate potential differences in cardiovascular fitness between schoolchildren from urban and rural areas, with respect to their age and gender. Chapter 3 provides evidence for the 5-years regular sport exercise effect of on muscle contractile properties in children. Chapter 4 aimed to identity trend changes of physical abilities of school children aged 7 to 14 years old from 2009 to 2014 period of time. In the Chapter 5 a review on the effects of linear and change-of-direction speed training methods on the sprint performance of young adults is provided. The purpose of Chapter 6 was to clarify the relationship between sports experience and performance scores on a health-related physical fitness test among female University freshmen. Chapter 7 was aimed to determine whether the application of sports activities improves the level of the upper extremity motor abilities at people with spinal cord injury. In the Chapter 8 author provide overview about theoretical frameworks supporting learning environments information for inclusive physical education and sport practice. Chapter 9 covers the three basic approaches for the inclusion of people with disabilities in community recreation programs as well as: including the integration of existing generic programs, reverse mainstreaming, and zero exclusion model. The aim of the Chapter 10 was to give answer about relation between health and fitness characteristics of Special Olympians athletes competing as cross-country skiers. Chapter 11 investigates relations between physical activity and/or physical exercise and body composition characteristics in working-age population of both genders. Chapter 12 provides evidence based information about the effects of sedentary behavior on physiological function at humans. The evidence from numerous clinical and epidemiological studies that physical activity can reduce the risk for breast and prostate cancer was discussed in the Chapter 13. Chapter 14 provides information about connection between physical activity and cognition across the life span. Author had been concluded that across the lifespan physical activity improves attentional and executive processes, cognitive control, memory and learning, visuospatial abilities, thus improving activities of daily living and quality of life. Exercise also has the effect of preventing cognitive decline and dementia in old age. And finally, Chapter 15 examines the opinion of elderly about the impact of physical activity in some segments of the quality of life of people of the third age.

We sincerely hope that this text provides a useful scientific information and evidence based overview of a range of topics relevant to researches and individuals working within field of physical activity and exercise, sports science and health related experts.

In Belgrade, 01 November 2015   Fadilj Eminović and Milivoj Dopsaj

In: Physical Activity Effects on the Anthropological Status ...   ISBN: 978-1-63484-782-7
Editors: Fadilj Eminović and Milivoj Dopsaj   © 2016 Nova Science Publishers, Inc.

Chapter 1

THE FIRST PHYSICAL MOVEMENTS OF LIFE: FETAL MOVEMENTS, THE MOTHER'S PSYCHOLOGICAL STATES AND WELLBEING OF THE FUTURE CHILD

Carlo Lai, Gaia Romana Pellicano[*], Navkiran Kalsi, Giuseppe Massaro, Clelia Giulia Turetta and Daniela Altavilla
Department of Dynamic and Clinical Psychology, Sapienza, University of Rome, Rome, Italy

ABSTRACT

The movement of the fetus inside the womb has been recognized as a foremost indicator of fetal wellbeing. Fetal movements have a wide range of expression and the decrement of this movement is associated with numerous pathologies and poor pregnancy outcomes. An account of the fetal activity based on the mother's perception of the movements that begins between the third and fourth month of gestation, along with the technological assessment, can provide crucial information about the developing fetus. More studies report the association between maternal anxiety and depression during pregnancy and the perception of the fetal motor activity. Women who consider their lives as more stressful and report more stress about pregnancy, also report more fetal activity across gestation. Coherently, fetuses of women who perceived their pregnancy to be more pleasant and have a more positive emotional attitude toward pregnancy are less active. Moreover, mother-fetus attachment and maternal emotional regulation skills have a positive association with health practices in pregnancy and some studies reported an association between low level of prenatal attachment and high level of alexithymia. People with high alexithymia show high levels of sympathetic activity and a dissociation between subjective and physiological stress responses. In 2013, a pilot study was carried out whose aim was to investigate the relationship between mothers' emotional regulation ability, prenatal attachment and fetal movements in the first three months of pregnancy. The results of this

[*] Corresponding Author, Email: gaiapellicano@msn.com.

study showed that that the time elapsed in extensor movements by fetuses at three months of gestation was negatively associated with the emotional regulation ability of the mothers in pregnancy. The human motor activity thus has a primary relevance since the first months of life suggesting the bidirectional relationship between psychological and physical dimensions. Studying fetal body movements and their association with the maternal features could, therefore, provide a key to facilitate early intervention and optimal treatment before, during pregnancy and after birth.

Keywords: fetal movements, prenatal attachment, maternal alexithymia, child well being

INTRODUCTION

Pregnancy is a complex somatic and psychological event in a woman's life. This delicate time is essential for the development of the relationship between the mother and her fetus. A wide range of environmental and psychosocial variables have an impact on mothers' emotional experiences that could have a role on the course of pregnancy (Figueiredo and Costa, 2009; Della Vedova et al., 2008; Cranley, 1981). Mother-fetus attachment and maternal emotional regulation skills promote health practices in pregnancy (Lindgren, 2001). Since the first weeks, the fetus acquires physiological and sensorial abilities (De Vries et al., 1982; Tajani and Ianniuruberto, 1981). Fetal movements as vermicular, startle, and extension are present since the first weeks of pregnancy and their patterns become more complex and fine (Raynes-Greenow et al., 2013; Tajani and Ianniuruberto, 1981). Mothers feel such movements around 16 to 20 weeks, and this experience was believed to be essential to establish the first emotional contact with their fetuses (Mangesi and Hofmeyr, 2007). Recently, the maternal psychological state gained more relevance and it seems to be strongly associated to a series of alterations of the intrauterine milieu (DiPietro, 2012; Davis and Sandman, 2010), where maternal autonomic responsiveness is associated to motor activity and heart rate of the fetuses (DiPietro et al., 2002; Lecaneut and Jacquet, 2002; Groome et al., 2000). Current research activities are focusing on how the attachment style (Bowlby, 1973, 1980, 1982) and the levels of alexithymia (Taylor et al., 1997) are associated with the fetal movements.

FETAL DEVELOPMENT

The movement of the fetus inside the womb has been recognized as a foremost indicator of fetal wellbeing. The introduction of 2-D ultrasound in the 1970s allowed direct visualization of fetal movements in uterus gaining insights of developing fetus inside the womb. The further advancements of technology in past two decades have facilitated the in-vivo real-time observation of human fetal movements providing extensive details about the nature and emergence of these movements (Hata et al., 2010). These fetal movements have a wide range of expressions and can be categorized as sideways bending; startle reflexes; generalized movements involving complex movements of neck, trunk and limbs; twitches; jaw movements including sucking and swallowing; hand-to-face contact; stretching and rotation of the fetus (De Vries et al., 1982). These movement patterns yields important crucial information in assessing the status of the developing fetus and are considered as the fundamental index of the health of the unborn child (Milani Camporetti, 1981). Although some low-risk fetus appear to have a unique style of movement while most of the fetus show fairly consistent patterns and fluctuations in duration and frequency of movement.

The first movement patterns of the fetus develop during seventh to the fifteenth week of gestation. The initial movements are more of spontaneous which are later followed by the reflex ones. The earliest movement detected is sideways bending and trunk flexion and extension which are recorded as early as 7 weeks of gestation (Kurjak et al., 2005). It is followed by startle movements consisting of a rapid phase contraction of all limb muscles. These are attributed to the innervations and tone of muscle. The breathing and hiccups movements are generally observable from the 8 to 10 weeks of gestation (De Varies et al., 1982; Prechtl, 1989; Visser, 1992). These movements are crucial for the development of fetal lungs. But due to high inter and intra-individual differences observed, these movements are not used as an indicator of the fetal health. During 11 week of gestation opening of the jaw and complex stretch movements are reported. These movements are important for the proper development of bones and joints of the fetus. On 13 week of gestation, rhythmic sucking and swallowing movements are distinctly observable in the developing fetus. The fetus by now can swallow the amniotic fluid (Kurjak et al., 2008).

With the advancing gestation age, the movements become more complex and fine (Nijhuis, 1992). And gradually these first simple movements are replaced by different general movements. The isolated limb movements begin to appear in this duration, indicating the developing cerebral control of movement. The developing motor activity in fetus reflects the integration of nervous system activity as well as general fetal wellbeing. All the movements present in the neonates can be recorded in the fetus by about 18th week. The motor patterns become more precise and differentiable, and the child starts to actively explore the uterine environment (Mancia, 2006; De Vries et al., 1985). Around 15–18 weeks, the movements become more evident to the mothers and can now perceive these movements as baby kicks. Furthermore, with increasing of the gestational age the variations in fetal movements show a form of reaction to stimuli from the outside world or from the maternal body (Mancia, 2006).

FETAL STATE PATTERNS

In addition to the movements, fetus exhibit regular occurrence of behavior patterns like the sleep-wake cycle. These patterns are more evidently regular during the third trimester. The sleep-wake patterns of fetus although do not follow the diurnal pattern as seen in adults. Because of these quantitative and qualitative differences in the fetus as compared to the adults, fetal sleep-wake patterns are described as states. These fetal states are determined by the regularity of heart rate, eye movements and fetal movements. Thus, motor movements are affected by these states of the fetus. During awake periods and periods of Rapid Eye Movement (REM) sleep, motor activity can be observed while during the quite sleep the activity is minimal. The alterations of quiet and active periods of fetal movements have been reported as early as 21 week of gestation, though we lack evidence of regular rhythmic patterns between these states (Peirano et al., 2003). Fetal movements are continuous during early pregnancy but with increasing maturation, quite periods emerges predominantly.

FETAL SENSORY PROCESSING

The somatosensory system develops in the following chronological order: touch, smell, taste, hearing and vision (Haith, 1990). The fetus has been observed to respond to touch around the mouth as early as 8 weeks of gestation (Vanhatalo et al., 2000). Touch in utero implies contact with amniotic fluid or walls of the uterus thus the maternal movement and buoyant amniotic fluid provide stimulation to the fetus in the uterus. Nociception, the pain responses, appear around 6 weeks of gestation initially around mouth later around the trunk, arms and legs and eventually throughout the fetus (Vanhatalo et al., 2000). Proprioception, involving the perception of joint and body movements and position of the body mature by 14 to 15 weeks. Fetus may detect the aromatic substances and odours from the mother's diet around 28 weeks of gestation influencing the mother's dietary preferences (Graven et al., 2008; Cowart, 1981; Hepper, 1995). Taste buds appear in fetus as early as 7 to 8 weeks and mature by 13 to 15 weeks. But it yet unknown to what extend the fetus can experience the tastes. However, increased fetal swallowing in response to injection of a sweet substance and a decrease in response to a bitter substance has been reported (Cowart et al., 2004).

The auditory structures are mature enough for enabling the fetus to hear sounds by 24 to 25 weeks of gestation, although the internal structures are poorly developed and sensitivity to sound is still poor (Hall, 2000; Birnholz et al., 1983). The sensitivity increases rapidly during 24 to 35 weeks (Werner et al., 2011). Intra-uterine recordings demonstrate the sounds of the external environment are audible to the fetus by now (Zimmer et al., 1993). Fetus after 28 week may discriminate the maternal taped versus live voice and familiar versus novel sounds (DeCasper et al., 1980).

Formation of eyes begins during the embryonic phase of the fetus. The neurons of visual cortex are in place at 26 weeks and the visual attention, though very poor, is observed to begin at 30 to 32 weeks of gestation.

The natural sensory environment of the uterus provides rich and varied stimulations to the developing fetus and are of great significant value for the fetus. Studying these fetal movements and its surrounding environment may provide crucial information for detecting not only fetal wellbeing but also fetal compromise and facilitate early intervention and optimal treatment strategies.

FETAL MOVEMENTS AND THEIR MATERNAL PERCEPTION

A simple yet important screening method to assess the fetal wellbeing is maternal count of fetal movements.

Maternal perception of fetal movement has been used as an important screening method for fetal well-being, as decreased fetal movement is associated with a range of pregnancy pathologies and poor pregnancy outcomes.

Decreased fetal movement often precedes a stillbirth, but uterine contractions can be interpreted as a fetal movement. A single episode of extremely vigorous fetal activity can precede fetal death. The majority of the women experienced decreased, weaker, or no fetal movement at all 2 days before fetal death was diagnosed (Linde et al., 2015).

Timely intervention for decreased fetal movement results in a substantial reduction in the rate of stillbirth (Pakenham et al., 2013). Mothers should be trained to promptly report changes in fetal movement to their health care providers, using fetal movement information to evaluate possible fetal distress may lead to reductions in stillbirths (Linde et al., 2015).

A study of Hijazi et al. (2010) showed that women perceived 35.8% of 763 fetal movements seen on 14 ultrasound scans; the maternal sensitivity increased when movements involved more than one fetal body district, contacted the uterus and were of longer duration. However many studies have shown that there are contradictory evidences on whether gestational age, overweight and obesity, and placental location affect perception. This may be related to the small sample sizes of available studies and lack of clear signposts to guide mothers to classify and recognize the various movements perceived (Hijazi and East, 2009).

Pregnancy is a complex somatic and psychological event in a woman's life. Wide ranges of environmental and psychosocial variables have an impact on mother's emotional experiences that could have a role on the course of pregnancy.

Recent studies show that psychological factors and duration of the fetal movement may affect maternal perception (Hijazi and East, 2009). The subjective perception of decreased fetal movements by the mother is the most significant clinical definition (Bradford and Maude, 2014).

Apart from the above stated clinical significance, fetal movements also play an important role in facilitating the mother-fetal relationship. While the fetus begins its first movements during the first few weeks of pregnancy, mothers can feel these movements around 16 to 30 weeks and this experience allows them to establish the first emotional contact with their fetuses (Mangesi et al., 2007). These influences happen in both directions. In fact, the maternal psychological state seems to be associated to a series of complex alterations of the intrauterine milieu, where the fetus carries out fundamental steps of its development (DiPietro, 2012). The fetal movement counting seems to improve the process of maternal-fetal attachment (Mikhail et al., 1991).

ADULT AND PRENATAL ATTACHMENT

Attachment theory is a useful and influential framework for understanding personality development, relational processes, and the regulation of affect. It explains how the internalization of the different aspects of relational experience, built from early child interacting with their caregivers influences the behavior and emotion regulation in adulthood. These representations internalized Bowlby calls "internal working models" (Bowlby, 1980; Main and Goldwyn 1997; Mikulincer and Shaver, 2003; 2007).

The internal working models are based on past experience, expectations concerning the availability and the likely responses of the attachment figure to their needs and, finally, on advances related to their behavior and their own self in relation to the attachment figure in situations of distress.

In threatening situations individuals with secure attachment expect that the attachment figure, and more generally the other, will show themselves responsive to their requests for help, available to come to their rescue and able to provide appropriate responses to their needs. They will develop an image of themselves as worthy of love, a capacity to manage distress, able to tolerate separations temporary, comfort with autonomy and in forming relationships with others.

In contrast, people with insecure attachment may develop as a result of suboptimal caregiving in earlier life and are associated with later difficulties in regulating affect, poorer interpersonal functioning and negative beliefs about the self and others (Mikulincer and Shaver, 2012).

Specifically, people with avoidant attachment bonds will form a mental model of the person's attachment and the other as absent, rejecting and hostile and they will develop an image of themselves as people who are not worthy of being loved showing independent and, if necessary, they will activate defense mechanisms of denial of their need of care and affection. People who have developed a kind of anxious attachment bond will form a mental model of the attachment figure and the external reality as unpredictable, unreliable, subtly dangerous and hostile and, in parallel will form a mental model of himself as vulnerable and constantly at risk, and strongly dependent on others.

Dennett (1987) emphasizes the fact that humans are perhaps the only ones to try to understand each other in terms of mental states: thoughts, feelings, desires, and beliefs, in order to give meaning to the experience and be able to anticipate each other's actions. This ability of mentalization, that Fonagy (1991) calls "reflective function," has enhanced the understanding of the development of basic capacities for self-regulation (Slade, 2005). Mentalization integrates aspects that are at once cognitive and affective and it is the capacity to think about feeling and to feel about thinking.

The early environment and the precocious relationships give to the child the key to learn about own mental states, to understand the organization of the surrounding world and ultimately in which way the social environment has to be processed (Fonagy et al., 2002). Thus, the first interactions become essential not only for establishing a deep relationship with a specific person but also for becoming broadly able to represent the internal and external processes. The relationship between mother and child creates early symbols, whence the infant can begin to create a representation of the self, that will be, at the beginning, only as a function of the ability of the mother to make real and meaningful his experiences (Slade, 2000).

Parental reflective function appears to be associated with the attachment style; not only is it more likely that parents with a high reflective ability promote secure attachment in their children, also in cases where their own childhood experiences were negative, but that is precisely the secure attachment to be a key precursor of a solid reflective ability (Fonagy et al., 1996).

Moreover, when the child has not yet been born, the parental thinking about him/her is an especially demanding but important process that lays the basis for future adequate representation and successive secure attachment. The respective abilities of mentalization of both parents meet halfway and together produce a possible internal organization of another yet unborn person.

The particular connection that parents develop towards the fetus during pregnancy is called "prenatal attachment." Winnicott introducing the concept of "primary maternal preoccupation" described the importance of the investment affection of the mother to the fetus. The quality of the bond prenatal parents-baby is considered very important for the subsequent development of the attachment relationship and psychic development of children (Winnicott, 1958; 1969).

In 1981, Cranley theorizes the creation of the attachment bond from the earliest stages of pregnancy, calling it "maternal-fetal attachment."

It would be the quality of the prenatal affective investment that would influence the processes of pregnancy, the subsequent parent-child attachment bond and infant mental development.

The deep symbiosis between the mother and the fetus makes that psychosocial, emotional and effective factors linked to the mother's experiences during pregnancy will inevitably fall on the mother-child relationship and on attachment, creating memory traces that will remain intact in the psyche of the child and then the adult (Cranley, 1981; 1992).

Seimyr and colleagues (2009) showed how aspects of prenatal attachment, the experiences of pregnancy and the experiences of fetal movements, are related to maternal depressive mood. Mothers with slight depressive symptoms were somewhat less positive about the pregnancy but showed more attention to the fetal movements.

A study carried out by Teixeira and colleagues (2009), measuring anxiety and depression in pregnant women at 3-month intervals, showed that anxiety follows a U pattern during pregnancy, which peaks in the 1st and 3rd trimesters, while depression decreases throughout the whole gestation. In another study mother's depression predicted a worse emotional involvement before childbirth, while mother's anxiety predicted a worse emotional involvement with the infant after childbirth (Figueiredo and Costa, 2009). These results suggest that maternal anxiety and depression during pregnancy could impact fetal development (DiPietro et al., 2002), affecting also the ability to image, represent, fantasize on internal states of future newborn and the relationship with her/him. (Benoit et al., 1997; Huth-Bocks et al., 2004; Siddiqui and Hagglof, 2000; Siddiqui et al., 2000).

ATTACHMENT AND ALEXITHYMIA

Davis and Sandman (2010) describe the "programming" as the prenatal period during which the fetus receives several influences that can have a long-lasting or permanent effect in terms of health outcomes, depending on the type of influence, its timing and the developmental stage of the organs. Birth phenotypes should, therefore, reflect the fetal adaptation to such exposures that contribute to the shaping of the physiological functions (Gluckman and Hanson, 2004). Davis and Sandman (2010) found out that while high levels of cortisol in mothers at late gestation were associated with faster cognitive development and higher development scores in the one year old baby, exposure to high concentration of cortisol in early gestation was on the contrary associated with a slower development rate and lower scores at the end of the first year.

Cortisol levels are directly affected by autonomic responses, and maternal autonomic responsiveness has been associated to motor activity and heart rate of the fetuses (Lecanuet and Jacquet, 2002). In particular, fetuses of women who consider their lives as more stressful, and report more stress about pregnancy are more active across gestation, while fetuses of women who perceived their pregnancy to be more pleasant and have a more positive emotional attitude toward pregnancy are less active (DiPietro et al., 2002).

Alexithymia is a deficit of emotional regulation characterized by difficulty recognizing emotions, difficult to verbalize emotions and externally oriented thinking (Taylor et al., 1999). In the last decades, Alexithymia has not been anymore considered as a specific disorder nor as a stable single personality trait, but as a multivariate expression of personality, linked to a cognitive and affective style which includes also lack of empathy (Goleman, 1995;

Parker et al., 2001) and difficulty distinguishing between emotional states and physical sensations (Taylor et al., 1997). Alexithymia can also vary on a continuum ranging from normal to pathological (Parker et al., 2008). Relational difficulties (including social avoidance, hostility and lack of empathy) characterize the interpersonal background of individuals with high level Alexithymia (Berenbaum et al., 1998; Meganck et al., 2009; Spitzer et al., 2005). It has also been suggested that alexithymic subjects are more prone to using negative coping strategies, such as avoidance and distancing, to avoid highly emotional situations (Corcos and Speranza, 2003). Moreover, conflicts seem to be more present in the interpersonal relationships of alexithymic individuals than in those of non-alexithymic individuals (Sturgeon, 2004; Pérusse et al., 2012). This is probably due to the lower ability to control physiological arousal associated with emotions.

Attachment experiences in early childhood also influence the development of emotional schemas, imagination, and other cognitive skills involved in affect regulation. This process is mediated by the "emotional tuning" of the caregiver with the baby and its positive outcome is the development of the "reflective function," which involves the ability to differentiate the internal from the outer reality (Cassidy, 1994; Fonagy and Target, 1997; Asen and Fonagy, 2012). The ability to regulate one's emotional responses towards others and the environment, is acquired in meaningful relationships and is therefore related to the quality of the experience of child's attachment with the caregivers (Bowlby, 1980). The process of emotional development progresses towards the verbalization and desomatization of emotional responses. This happens due to the caregiver ability to provide adequate care and to act as a "mirror" for the baby, who learns to manage the emotions also due to the game experiences with significant adults (Krystal, 1988).

Alexithymia has also been associated with insecure attachment styles (avoidant/dismissing, preoccupied or fearful) (Troisi et al., 2001; Tayor and Bagby, 2004). This may account for the low level of social support that has been found among alexithymic individuals (Posse et al., 2002; Kojima et al., 2003) and, given the impact on health (Berkman, 1995; Maunder and Hunter, 2001), for the subsequent link between Alexithymia and diseases (and their course) (Lumley et al., 1996; Picardi et al., 2003).

Many studies also showed that the ability of emotional regulation is associated with a lower activation of hypothalamus-pituitary-adrenal axis and with a decreased autonomic arousal. Martin and Phil (1996) demonstrated that people with high alexithymia show high levels of sympathetic activity and a dissociation between subjective and physiological stress responses.

Bogdanov and colleagues (2013) also proved that high alexithymia is linked to increased autonomic arousal at the onset of emotional stimulation.

A study (Vedova et al., 2008) reported an association between low level of prenatal attachment and high level of alexithymia. This is particularly important in the light of the fact that mother-fetus attachment and maternal emotional regulation skills have a positive association with health practices in pregnancy (Lindgren, 2001).

A PILOT RESEARCH

Given the state of the art described above, including the involvement of alexithymia, prenatal attachment, autonomic responses on the mother's side, and development and motor activity on the fetus's side, it is quite surprising that before 2013 no studies had been carried out about the relationship between the emotional regulation in the mothers and the motility of their fetuses.

In 2013, a pilot study was carried out whose aim was to investigate the relationship between mothers' emotional regulation ability, prenatal attachment and fetal movements in the first three months of pregnancy. This is the time of pregnancy when the fetus begins to move and can become very active. However the mothers still cannot feel such movements, while they experience the first peak of anxiety and the highest levels of depression (Teixeira et al., 2009), two conditions that put to the test the ability of emotional regulation. The hypothesis of the pilot study was that higher ability of emotional regulation and a higher secure prenatal attachment would have been predictive of lesser fetal motor activity.

The sample was composed by Italian pregnant women on the first trimester of pregnancy, recruited at the 'Life' Medical Center in Frosinone, since October 2012 until July 2013. All women were in good general health assessed by a gynecologist. Fetal ultrasound scans of about 300 seconds duration (on the side profile of fetus) were recorded on CDs during the routine gynecological check at the 12th week of gestation. Therefore, frame by frame video coding was carried out on the first 180 seconds of each scan on the following behavioral classes: right and left arm; right and left leg; right and left hand.

Each behavioral class had the following comprehensive and mutually exclusive behaviors: extension (any movement that increases the width of the angle of the articulation), flexion (any movement that decreases the width of the angle of the articulation), no movement (absence of movement), and no codable (the specific body district of fetus was not visible).

One trained observer blinded for hypotheses coded frame-by-frame the fetal movements. The coding was carried out using the Observer Video Pro© software, version 5.0 (© Noldus Information Technology 2012, The Netherlands) following the operative definitions. A complete and continuous coding list with the timing (start and end time for each behavior) of the movements was compiled for each fetus. The 30% of the sample was codified by a second observer in order to test the inter - observer reliability. The Pearson r were higher than 0.72 ($p < 0.00001$) and lower than 0.88 ($p < 0.00001$).

All participants underwent the psychological assessment. The Toronto 20 item-Toronto Alexithymia Scale (TAS-20) (Bagby et al., 1994a, 1994b) and the Prenatal Attachment Inventory (PAI) (Muller, 1993) were administered.

Statistical analysis showed that the main finding of the study was that the time elapsed in extensor movements by fetuses at three months of gestation was negatively associated with the ability of emotional regulation of the mothers in pregnancy.

Specifically higher levels of externally-oriented thinking were associated with the extensor movements of fetuses. Externally-oriented thinking reflects a cognitive style of avoiding introspective thought (Henry et al., 2006) and a mechanism to protect people from intensive affective responses to challenges or distress (Davydov et al., 2010). Coherently the prenatal attachment toward the fetus was negatively associated with the extensor movements, however, this association was not significant.

Previous studies reported that psychological measures of the mothers were significantly related to fetal response at 24-36 weeks of gestation, as heart rate and motor activity (DiPietro, 2012; Field et al. 2005; DiPietro et al., 2002).

To the best of our knowledge, the present is the first study showing this relation as early as the first trimester of pregnancy. It could be argued that the maternal psychological dimensions can influence the fetal motor activity through hormonal metabolism. A previous study demonstrated that the fetuses of mothers with higher levels of cortisol were more active than the fetuses of mothers with lower cortisol levels (DiPietro et al., 2009). Moreover, an interesting study reported that maternal distress can affect fetal motor activity. However, in these findings, the reported rapidity of the onset of fetal responsiveness to maternal physiological alterations seems to exceed the temporal response curve of products of the hypothalamic-pituitary-adrenal axis, making less plausible the hormonal hypothesis (DiPietro, 2012). Moreover, another study failed to identify an association between cortisol levels of the mothers and maternal stress (Voegtline et al., 2013). Considering these findings, it seems that the response to the maternal distress cannot be related only to the hormonal exchange in the placental barrier. An alternative interpretation is that the fetus can be affected by the maternal autonomic response, such as more tone, vasodilatation and neuroendocrine release and responds with different behaviors (DiPietro, 2012; Novak, 2004). This interpretation is sustained also by a comparative study where the stimulation associated with contractions can affect the early behavioral organization (Robertson et al., 1996).

As already discussed above, many studies showed that the inability of emotional regulation in adults is associated with increased autonomic arousal (Bogdanov et al., 2013; Fukunishi et al., 1999). This evidence could explain how in the present study the higher value of alexithymia in the mother could affect the fetal motor activity: the higher difficulty of emotional regulation in the mothers could increase their autonomic arousal that could increase the fetal movements.

Another finding of the study was that the externally oriented thinking and the difficulties to identify the emotions were associated with the attachment toward the fetus. This result suggests that the reduction of the ability of emotional regulation interferes with the maternal mental representation of the future child and with the attachment towards the fetus. In addition, the attachment toward the fetus was negatively associated with the extensor movements of the fetuses despite the effect was less clear.

A possible interpretation of the findings of the present study is that as early as three months fetuses could perform more extensor movements with mothers with reduced attention toward their children and less oriented toward their own feelings and emotions. This mechanism could have the evolutionistic effect to redirect the maternal attention on the fetus (Saastad et al., 2012; Peat et al., 2012; Berbey et al., 2001).

CONCLUSION

In conclusion, the data show a clear association between the maternal emotional ability as well as the prenatal attachment and the extensor movements of the fetus as early as three months. This phenomenon could represent an evolutionistic solution that increases the chances for the fetus to receive maternal attention and care. This research was a pilot study and then the sample must be increased in order to show more stable and clear effect. However, the data of this study suggest that the human motor activity has a primary relevance since the first months of life and show the bidirectional relationship between psychological and physical dimensions.

It is, therefore, possible to conclude that the first experiences that occur during pregnancy promote a stronger maternal-fetal bonding and postnatal maternal-child interaction, enhancing broadly the future child wellbeing.

REFERENCES

Asen, E. and Fonagy, P. (2012). Mentalization based Therapeutic Interventions for Families. *Journal of Family Therapy, 34*(4), 347-370.

Bagby, R. M., Parker, J. D. A. and Taylor, G. J. (1994[a]). The twenty item Toronto alexithymia scale I. Item selection and cross validation of the factor structure. *Journal of Psychosomatic Research, 38*, 23–32.

Bagby, R. M., Taylor, G. J. and Parker, J. D. A. (1994[b]). The twenty item Toronto alexithymia scale II. Convergent, discriminant, and concurrent validity. *Journal of Psychosomatic Research, 38*, 33–40.

Berbey, R., Manduley, A. and Vigil-De Gracia, P. (2001). Counting fetal movements as a universal test for fetal wellbeing. *International Journal of Gynecology and Obstetrics, 74*, 293-5.

Berenbaum, H., Davis, R. and McGrew, J. (1998). Alexithymia and the interpretation of hostile-provoking situations. *Psychotherapy and psychosomatics, 67*(4-5), 254-258.

Berkman, L. F. (1995). The role of social relations in health promotion. *Psychosomatic medicine, 57*(3), 245-254.

Birnholz, J. C. and Benacerraf, B. R. (1983). The development of human fetal hearing. *Science, 222*(4623), 516-518.

Bogdanov, V. B., Bogdanova, O. V., Gorlov, D. S., Gorgo, Y. P., Dirckx, J. J., Makarchuk, M. Y., Schoenen, J. and Critchley, H. (2013). Alexithymia and Empathy Predict Changes in Autonomic Arousal During Affective Stimulation. *Cognitive and Behavioral Neurology, 26*, 121-132.

Bowlby, J. (1980). *Attachment and loss* (Vol. 3). Basic books.

Bradford, B. and Maude, R. (2014). Fetal response to maternal hunger and satiation – novel finding from a qualitative descriptive study of maternal perception of fetal movements. *BMC Pregnancy Childbirth, 26*, 14:288.

Cassid, J. (1994). Emotional regulation: Influences of attachment relationships. *Monographs of the Society for research in child development, 59(2-3)*, 228-249.

Corcos, M. and Speranza, M. (2003). *Psychopathologie de l'alexithymie.* Dunod.

Cowart, B. J., Beauchamp, G. K. and Mennella, J. A. (2004). Development of taste and smell in the neonate. *Fetal, Neonatal Physiology, 2*, 1819-1827.

Cowart, BJ (1981). Development of taste perception in humans: sensitivity and preference Throughout the life span. *Psychological bulletin, 90* (1), 43.

Cranley M. (1981) Development of a tool for the measurement of maternal attachment during pregnancy. *Nursing Research. 30*, 281–284.

Cranley M. (1992). Response to "a critical review of prenatal attachment research." Scholarly *Inquiry for Nursing Practice, 6*, 23–26.

Davis, E. P. and Sandman, C. A. (2010). The timing of prenatal exposure to maternal cortisol and psychosocial stress is associated with human infant cognitive development. *Child development*, *81*, 131-148.

Davydov, D. M., Stewart, R., Ritchie, K. and Chaudieu, I. (2010). Resilience and mental health. *Clinical Psychology Review*, *30*, 479-495.

De Vries, J. I. P., Visser, G. H. A. and Prechtl, H. F. R. (1985). The emergence of fetal behaviour: II Quantitative aspects. *Early Human Development*, *12*, 99-120.

De Vries, J. I., Visser, G. H. and Prechtl, H. F. (1982). The emergence of fetal behaviour: I. Qualitative aspects. *Early Human Development*, *7*, 301-322.

DeCasper, A. J. and Fifer, W. P. (1980). Of human bonding: Newborns prefer their mothers' voices. *Science*, *208*(4448), 1174-1176.

Dennett D.C. (1987). *The intentional stance*. Cambridge, MA: MIT Press.

DiPietro, J. A. (2012). Maternal stress in pregnancy: considerations for fetal development. *Journal of Adolescent Health*, *51*, S3-S8.

DiPietro, J. A., Costigan, K. A., Kivlighan, K. T., Chen, P. and Laudenslager, M. L. (2011). Maternal salivary cortisol differs by fetal sex during the second half of pregnancy. *Psychoneuroendocrinology*, *36*, 588–591.

DiPietro, J. A., Hilton, S. C., Hawkins, M., Costigan, K. A. and Pressman, E. K. (2002). Maternal stress and affect influence fetal neurobehavioral development. *Developmental Psychology*, *38*, 659-668.

Field, T., Diego, M. and Hernandez-Reif, M. (2010). Prenatal Depression Effects and Interventions: A Review. *Infant Behavior and Development*, *33*, 409–418.

Figueiredo, B. and Costa, R. (2009). Mother's stress, mood and emotional involvement with the infant: 3 months before and 3 months after childbirth. *Archives of Women's Mental Health*, *12*, 143-153.

Fonagy P. (1991). L'approccio evolutivo per la comprensione del transfert nel trattamento di pazienti con distubi borderline della personalità. [he evolutionary approach to the understanding of transference in the treatment of patients with borderline personality distubi] In: *Zabonati A., Migone P. and Maschietto G. (a cura di), La validazione scientifica delle psicoterapie psicoanalitiche.* [The scientific validation of psychoanalytic psychotherapies.] Mestre (VE): IPAR, 1993.

Fonagy P., Leigh T., Steele M., Steele H., Kennedy R., Mattoon G., Target M. and Gerber A. (1996). The relation of attachment status, psychiatric classification, and response to psychotherapy. *Journal of Consulting and Clinical Psychology, 64*, 22-31.

Fonagy, P. and Target, M. (1997). Attachment and reflective function: Their role in self-organization. *Development and psychopathology*, *9*(4), 679-700.

Fonagy, P., Gergely, G., Jurist, E. and Target, M. (2002). *Affect regulation. Mentalization, and the Development of the Self,* New York: Other Press LLC.

Fukunishi, I., Sei, H., Morita, Y. and Rahe, R. H., (1999). Sympathetic activity in alexithymics with mother's low care. *Journal of Psychosomatic Research*, *46*, 579–589.

Gluckman, P. D. and Hanson, M. A. (2004). Living with the past: evolution, development, and patterns of disease. *Science, 305*, 1733-1736.

Goleman, D. (1995). *Emotional intelligence*. New York: Bantam Books.

Graven, S. N. and Browne, J. V. (2008). Sensory development in the fetus, neonate, and infant: introduction and overview. *Newborn and Infant Nursing Reviews*, *8*(4), 169-172.

Haith, M. M. (1990). Progress in the understanding of sensory and perceptual processes in early infancy. *Merrill-Palmer Quarterly*, 1-26.

Hall 3rd, J. W. (2000). Development of the ear and hearing. *Journal of perinatology: official journal of the California Perinatal Association*, 20(8 Pt 2), S12-20.

Hata, T., Dai, S.-Y. and Marumo, G. (2010). Ultrasound for evaluation of fetal neurobehavioural development: from 2-D to 4-D ultrasound. *Infant and Child Development*, 19, 99–118.

Henry, J. D., Phillips, L. H., Maylor, E. A., Hosie, J. A., Milne, A. B. and Meyer, C. (2006). A new conceptualization of alexithymia in the general adult population: implications for research involving older adults. *Journal of Psychosomatic Research*, 60, 535-543.

Hepper, P. G. (1995). Human fetal olfactory learning. *The International journal of prenatal and perinatal psychology and medicine*, 7(2), 147-151.

Hijazi, Z. R, Callan, S. E. and East, C. E. (2010). Maternal perception of foetal movement compared with movement detected by real-time ultrasound: an exploratory study. *Australian and New Zealand Journal of Obstetrics and Gynaecology*, 50, 144-7.

Hijazi, Z. R. and East, C. E. (2009). Factors affecting maternal perception of fetal movement. *Obstetrical and Gynecological Survey*, 64, 489-97.

Joukamaa, M., Kokkonen, P., Veijola, J., Läksy, K., Karvonen, J. T., Jokelainen, J. and Järvelin, M. R. (2003). Social situation of expectant mothers and alexithymia 31 years later in their offspring: a prospective study. *Psychosomatic Medicine*, 65(2), 307-312.

Kojima, M., Senda, Y., Nagaya, T., Tokudome, S. and Furukawa, T. A. (2003). Alexithymia, depression and social support among Japanese workers. *Psychotherapy and Psychosomatics*, 72(6), 307-314.

Kokkonen, P., Veijola, J., Karvonen, J. T., Läksy, K., Jokelainen, J., Järvelin, M. R. and Joukamaa, M. (2003). Ability to speak at the age of 1 year and alexithymia 30 years later. *Journal of psychosomatic research*, 54(5), 491-495.

Krystal, H. and Krystal, J. H. (1988). *Integration and self-healing: Affect, trauma, alexithymia*. Analytic Press, Inc.

Kurjak, A., Pooh, R. K., Merce, L. T., Carrera, J. M., Salihagic-Kadic, A., Andonotopo, W. (2005). Structural and functional early human development assessed by three-dimensional and four-dimensional sonography. *Fertility and Sterility*, 84, 1285–1299.

Kurjak, A., Tikvica, A., Stanojevic, M., Miskovic, B., Ahmed, B., Azumendi, G. and Renzo, G. C. D. (2008). The assessment of fetal neurobehavior by three-dimensional and four-dimensional ultrasound. *Journal of Maternal-Fetal and Neonatal Medicine*, 21, 675-684.

Lecanuet, J. P. and Jacquet, A. Y. (2002). Fetal responsiveness to maternal passive swinging in low heart rate variability state: effects of stimulation direction and duration. *Developmental psychobiology*, 40, 57-67.

Linde, A., Pettersson, K. and Rådestad, I. (2015). Women's experiences of fetal movements before the confirmation of fetal death-contractions misinterpreted as fetal movement. *Birth*. Feb 23. doi: 10.1111/birt.12151.

Lindgren, K. (2001). Relationships among maternal–fetal attachment, prenatal depression, and health practices in pregnancy. *Research in Nursing and Health*, 24, 203-217.

Lumley, M. A., Stettner, L. and Wehmer, F. (1996). How are alexithymia and physical illness linked? A review and critique of pathways. *Journal of psychosomatic research*, 41(6), 505-518.

Main, M., Goldwyn, R. (1997). *Adult attachment interview scoring and classification system*. University of California at Bekeley.

Mancia, M. (2006). Funzioni integrative del cervello e origine dello psichismo fetale: riflessioni teoriche e cliniche. [Integrative functions of the brain and the origin of fetal psyche: theoretical and clinical considerations.] In G. B. La Sala, V. Iori, F. Monti e P. Fagandini (Eds), *La "normale" complessità del venire al mondo [The "normal" complexities of coming into the world]* (pp. 207-220). Milano: Edizioni Guerini.

Mangesi, L., Hofmeyr, G. J. and Smith, V. (2007). *Foetal movement counting for assessment of fetal wellbeing*. The Cochrane Library.

Martin, J. B. and Pihl, R. O. (1986). Influence of alexithymic characteristics on physiological and subjective stress responses in normal individuals. *Psychotherapy and Psychosomatics, 45*, 66-77.

Maunder, R. G. and Hunter, J. J. (2001). Attachment and psychosomatic medicine: developmental contributions to stress and disease. *Psychosomatic medicine, 63*(4), 556-567.

Meganck, R., Vanheule, S., Inslegers, R. and Desmet, M. (2009). Alexithymia and interpersonal problems: A study of natural language use. *Personality and Individual Differences, 47*(8), 990-995.

Mikhail, M. S., Freda, M. C, Merkatz, R. B., Poliziotto, R., Mazloom, E. and Merkatz, I. R. (1991). The effect of fetal movement counting on maternal attachment to fetus. *American Journal of Obstetrics and Gynecology, 165*, 988-91.

Mikulincer, M. and Shaver, P.R. (2003). The Attachment behavioural system in adulthood: Activation, dynamics, and interpersonal processes. In Zanna, M. P., *Advances in Experimental Social Psychology*. Accademy Press, New York.

Mikulincer, M. and Shaver, P.R. (2007). *Attachment in adulthood: Structure, dynamics, and change*. New York, NY: Guilford Press.

Mikulincer, M. and Shaver, P. R. (2012). Adult attachment orientations and relationship processes. *Journal of Family Theory and Review, 4*(4), 259-274.

Milani Comparetti, A. (1981). Interpretazioni funzionali dei movimenti fetali. In *Età evolutiva*, 10, 88-92.

Muller, M. E. (1993). Development of the prenatal attachment inventory. *Western Journal of Nursing Research, 15*, 199-215.

Nijhuis, J. G. (1992). *Fetal behaviour: Developmental and perinatal aspects*. Oxford University Press, USA.

Novak, K. (2004). Epigenetics changes in cancer cells. *Medscape general medicine, 6*, 17.

Pakenham, S., Copeland, A. and Farine, D. (2013) Kick-starting action: Canadian women's understanding of fetal movement guidelines. *Journal of Obstetrics and Gynaecology Canada, 35*, 111-8.

Parker, J. D., Keefer, K. V., Taylor, G. J. and Bagby, R. M. (2008). Latent structure of the alexithymia construct: a taxometric investigation. *Psychological Assessment, 20*(4), 385.

Parker, J. D., Taylor, G. J. and Bagby, R. M. (2001). The relationship between emotional intelligence and alexithymia. *Personality and Individual differences,30*(1), 107-115.

Peat, A. M., Stacey, T., Cronin, R. and McCowan, L. M. (2012). Maternal knowledge of fetal movements in late pregnancy. *Australian and New Zealand Journal of Obstetrics and Gynaecology, 52*, 445-9.

Peirano, P., Algarín, C. and Uauy, R. (2003). Sleep-wake states and their regulatory mechanisms throughout early human development. *The Journal of Pediatrics, 143*(4), 70-79.

Pérusse, F., Boucher, S. and Fernet, M. (2012). Observation of couple interactions: Alexithymia and communication behaviors. *Personality and Individual Differences*, *53*(8), 1017-1022.

Picardi, A., Pasquini, P., Cattaruzza, M. S., Gaetano, P., Melchi, C. F., Baliva, G. and Biondi, M. (2003). Stressful life events, social support, attachment security and alexithymia in vitiligo. *Psychotherapy and Psychosomatics*, *72*(3), 150-158.

Posse, M., Hällström, T. and Backenroth-Ohsako, G. (2002). Alexithymia, social support, psycho-social stress and mental health in a female population. *Nordic Journal of Psychiatry*, *56*(5), 329-334.

Prechtl, H. F. (1989). Fetal behavior. In: Hill, A. and Volpe, J. J., editors. *Fetal neurology.* New York: Raven Press; pp 1–16.

Robertson, S. S., Johnson, S. L., Bacher, L. F., Wood, J. R., Wong, C. H., Robinson, S. R., Smotherman, W. P. and Nathanielsz, P. W. (1996). Contractile activity of the uterus prior to labor alters the temporal organization of spontaneous motor activity in the fetal sheep. *Developmental Psychobiology, 29*, 667-683.

Saastad, E., Winje, B. A., Israel, P. and Frøen, J. F. (2012). Fetal movement counting— maternal concern and experiences: a multicenter, randomized, controlled trial. *Birth*, *39*, 10-20.

Seimyr, L., Sjögren, B., Welles-Nyström, B. and Nissen, E. (2009). Antenatal maternal depressive mood and parental-fetal attachment at the end of pregnancy. *Archives of Women's Mental Health, 12*, 269-79.

Slade, A. (2000). The development and organization of attachment: Implications for psychoanalysis. *Journal of the American Psychoanalytic Association*, *48*(4), 1147-1174.

Slade, A., Cohen, L. J., Sadler, L. S. and Miller, M. (2009). The psychology and psychopathology of pregnancy. *Handbook of infant mental health, 3*, 22-39.

Spitzer, C., Siebel-Jürges, U., Barnow, S., Grabe, H. J. and Freyberger, H. J. (2005). Alexithymia and interpersonal problems. *Psychotherapy and Psychosomatics*, *74*(4), 240-246.

Sturgeon, C.L., (2004). *Typology of violence and alexithymia, empathy, perfectionism, and substance abuse in federal offenders.*

Taylor, G. J, Bagby, M. R. and Parker, J. D. A. (1999). *Disorders of Affect Regulation: Alexithymia in Medical and Psychiatric Illness.* Cambridge: Cambridge University Press.

Taylor, G. J. and Bagby, R. M. (2004). New trends in alexithymia research. *Psychotherapy and psychosomatics*, *73*(2), 68-77.

Taylor, G. J., Bagby, R. M. and Parker, J. D. A. (1997). The development and regulation of affects. *Disorders of Affect Regulation*, 7-25.

Teixeira, C., Figueiredo, B., Conde, A., Pacheco, A. and Costa, R. (2009). Anxiety and depression during pregnancy in women and men. *Journal of affective disorders*, *119*, 142-148.

Troisi, A., D'Argenio, A., Peracchio, F. and Petti, P. (2001). Insecure attachment and alexithymia in young men with mood symptoms. *The Journal of nervous and mental disease*, *189*(5), 311-316.

Vanhatalo, S. and van Nieuwenhuizen, O. (2000). Fetal pain? *Brain and Development, 22*(3), 145-150.

Vedova, A. M. D., Dabrassi, F. and Imbasciati, A. (2008). Assessing prenatal attachment in a sample of Italian women. *Journal of Reproductive and Infant Psychology, 26*, 86-98.

Visser, G. H. (1992). The second trimester. In: Nijhuis, J. G., editor. *Fetal behavior: Developmental and perinatal aspects.* Oxford: Oxford University Press. pp 17–26.

Voegtline, K. M., Costigan, K. A., Kivlighan, K. T., Laudenslager, M. L., Henderson, J. L. and DiPietro, J. A. (2013). Concurrent levels of maternal salivary cortisol are unrelated to self-reported psychological measures in low-risk pregnant women. *Archives of Women's Mental Health*, *16*, 101-108.

Werner, L., Fay, R. R. and Popper, A. (Eds.). (2011). *Human auditory development* (Vol. 42). Springer Science and Business Media.

Winnicott, D. W. (1958). *Dalla pediatria alla psicoanalisi.* (From pediatrics to psychoanalysis.) Tr. It. Martinelli, Firenze 1975.

Winnicott, D. W. (1969). *Colloqui con i genitori.* (Interviews with parents.). Tr. It. Raffaello Cortina Editore, Milano.

Zimmer, E. Z., Fifer, W. P., Kim, Y. I., Rey, H. R., Chao, C. R. and Myers, M. M. (1993). Response of the premature fetus to stimulation by speech sounds. *Early human development*, *33*(3), 207-215.

In: Physical Activity Effects on the Anthropological Status ...   ISBN: 978-1-63484-782-7
Editors: Fadilj Eminović and Milivoj Dopsaj   © 2016 Nova Science Publishers, Inc.

Chapter 2

POTENTIAL URBAN–RURAL DIFFERENCES IN CARDIORESPIRATORY FITNESS AND BMI IN SERBIAN SCHOOLCHILDREN

Ivana Milanović[1], Olivera M. Knezevic[2],
Miloš M. Marković[1], Slađana R. Rakić[1],
Snežana Radisavljević Janić[1] and Dragan M. Mirkov[1,]·

[1]University of Belgrade, Faculty of sport and Physical Education,
Belgrade, Serbia
[2]University of Belgrade, Institute for Medical Research,
Belgrade, Serbia

ABSTRACT

Cardiorespiratory fitness (CRF) represents an essential health-related physical fitness component most frequently assessed by Shuttle-run test (SRT). The aim of this study was to investigate potential differences in CRF between schoolchildren from urban and rural areas, with respect to their age and gender. Data for this part of study were derived from a broad national cross-sectional school-based study aimed to evaluate physical fitness and overweight/obesity prevalence.

The study consisted of two parts: the pilot study that was conducted in national capital and vicinity and the national study that included schoolchildren from territory of Republic of Serbia. For the purpose of the pilot study, 2230 schoolchildren (boys n = 1163, girls n =1067, age 9 to 14 years) from urban (3) and rural primary schools (4) were included in the study. Afterwards, the study was expanded on the territory of the Republic of Serbia. For that purpose, 11607 primary schoolchildren (boys n = 5913 and girls n = 5694, age 9 to 14 years) from urban (n = 44) and rural schools (n = 54) were included in the study. All measurements were conducted during regular physical education classes. In addition to time in SRT, basic anthropometric measures were taken (body height (BH), body weight (BW) and body mass index (BMI)). Age, gender and school location interaction associated differences in SRT were examined.

---

* Corresponding author: Dragan M. Mirkov, E-mail: dragan.mirkov@fsfv.bg.ac.rs.

Schoolchildren living in the urban area of the national capital had significantly higher BH and BW than their rural peers (there was no difference in BMI between these groups). Regarding the SRT, it was gender- and age-dependent (p < 0.001). Rural schoolchildren had longer time on SRT than urban only in 3rd and 4th- grade (p < 0.001), while in higher grades no difference was observed. The results from the national study showed that urban schoolchildren from Republic of Serbia had higher BH, BW and BMI than their rural peers. Boys had better results in SRT which increased with age (p < 0.001). SRT data revealed that 3rd- grade schoolchildren (regardless of gender) from rural schools achieved better results than their urban peers, contrary to the results from 6th- and 7th- graders.

Urban-rural differences in BMI were observed only for schoolchildren participating in the national study. Schoolchildren from rural area of the national capital generally had better cardiorespiratory fitness than their peers from urban area of the national capital, but those differences were mostly age and gender associated. The national study yielded results that were only partly similar to the results from the pilot study. CRF was strongly influenced by age and gender, while area of residence had small impact on CRF. Rural schoolchildren had better CRF in lower grades however due to potential influence of factors other than the area of residence (participation in organized physical activity, life-style, eating habits) urban schoolchildren had better levels of CRF in higher grades.

Keywords: aerobic fitness, endurance, schoolchildren, urban, rural

INTRODUCTION

Cardiorespiratory fitness (CRF; also known as aerobic fitness) or maximal aerobic power is operationalized either as peak oxygen consumption (in laboratory tests) or time/distance covered (in field test) (Mora et al., 2003; Ortega, Ruiz, Mesa, Gutierrez and Sjostrom, 2007; Sallis et al., 1997). CRF represents an essential health-related physical fitness component that is related with better "cardiovascular profile" in childhood and adolescence and in later life as well (Mora, et al., 2003; Ortega, et al., 2007; Sallis, et al., 1997; Twisk, Kemper and van Mechelen, 2002). CRF is also considered as an important predictor of success in a number of daily living and sport activities (Armstrong, Tomkinson and Ekelund, 2011; Haskell et al., 2007).

There is a positive relationship between low level of CRF and increased risk for developing cardiovascular diseases in early childhood, adolescence and later in life (Anderssen et al., 2007; Boreham et al., 2002b; Eisenmann, Wickel, Welk and Blair, 2005) and over a past few decades, poor CRF and increasing obesity became one of the main reasons of decreased life expectancy (Olshansky et al., 2005). The results obtained from *The European Youth Heart Study* (EYHS) conducted on schoolchildren from Sweden and Estonia showed that higher body fat percentage had negative impact on cardiovascular capacity (Ruiz, Ortega, et al., 2006). In addition, several longitudinal studies showed that lower level of CRF during childhood and adolescence in combination with certain risk factors could lead to obesity and development of serious cardiovascular conditions (Boreham and Riddoch, 2001; Boreham et al., 2002a; Hasselstrom, Hansen, Froberg and Andersen, 2002; Twisk, et al., 2002).

In addition to obesity, a variety of factors (e.g., genetics, physical activity level, life-style etc.) has been shown to have influence on CRF (Armstrong, et al., 2011). Further, it has been proved that maturation is significantly affecting CRF since a linear increase has been observed between the age of seven and seventeen (Malina, Bouchard and Bar-Or, 2004). Finally, although number of studies have shown that age-related rise in CRF is gender-independent (i.e., equal in both girls and boys) (Milanović, Radisavljević Janić and Mirkov, 2013; Olds, Tomkinson, Léger and Cazorla, 2006; M. S. Tremblay et al., 2010; M.S. Tremblay et al.), it should be noted that boys have had higher levels of CRF than girls (Olds, et al., 2006; M. S. Tremblay, et al., 2010; M.S. Tremblay, et al.). A linear increase in CRF has been observed between the age of 7 and 17. In particular, from the ages of 9 to 14 years, boys and girls experienced a continuous and a rather large increase in CRF, with different trend in boys vs. girls. Boys experienced a gradual increase in CRF from the ages of 9 to 14 years and by the end of this period the increase in CRF is three-folded (Malina, et al., 2004). However, the increase in CRF that was observed in girls was only two-folded, reaching its peak at the age of 12, after which it gradually declined. Difference in CRF between boys and girls was present across all ages (Lazarević, Radisavljević Janić, Milanović and Lazarević, 2011; Malina, et al., 2004).

It has been shown that CRF along with other components of physical fitness, particularly muscular fitness and body fat could have combined and cumulative effect on cardiorespiratory health in youth. These components represent an indicator of good cardiovascular health and therefore are recommended to be used in PE classes for the purpose of health monitoring of schoolchildren and youth (Ruiz, Rizzo, et al., 2006). Such monitoring could have a significant role in prevention of overweight and obesity and therefore decrease a risk of developing some serious health conditions (Carnethon, Gulati and Greenland, 2005; Moreno et al., 2006; Ortega, Ruiz, Castillo and Sjostrom, 2008; Plowman et al., 2006). A lack of physical activity and unhealthy food habits became typical characteristics of a life style of children and adolescents across the world, contributing to increase in number of obese and overweight children (Hills, King and Armstrong, 2007; Jurak, Radisavljević Janić, Milanović, Strel and Kovac, 2012; Murnan, Price, Telljohann, Dake and Boardley, 2006). Childhood obesity could be one of the causes leading not only to some psychological issues (lack of self-confidence, shame, depression etc.) but to cardiovascular and metabolic diseases (particularly diabetes type 2) as well (Burke et al., 2005; Janic et al., 2014; Lazarević, et al., 2011; Ribeiro et al., 2003; Schwartz and Puhl, 2003; Sjoberg, Nilsson and Leppert, 2005).

In addition of biological factors, a number of studies have pointed that the area of residence might also have significant influence on CRF (Albarwani D Phil, Al-Hashmi, Al-Abri, Jaju and Hassan, 2009; Chen, Unnithan, Kennedy and Yeh, 2008; Dollman, Norton and Tucker, 2002; Karkera, Swaminathan, Pais, Vishal and Rai, 2014; Kriemler et al., 2008). Although the area of residence could be described as urban or rural, definitions of urban and rural areas are inconsistent and they vary across geographical areas and countries depending on their national standards (Hall, Kaufman and Ricketts, 2006). These definitions are usually based on variables such as distance from trading centres and cut off population sizes of 100 000, 50 000, and 10 000 inhabitants (Tsimeas, Tsiokanos, Koutedakis, Tsigilis and Kellis, 2005). Several studies have investigated whether growing-up and living in urban, suburban or rural areas and area-specific life-style could have impact on CRF and overall physical activity of children and youth (Chen, et al., 2008; Karkera, et al., 2014; Özdirenç, Özcan, Akin and Gelecek, 2005). Namely, variables related to lifestyle [media use (T. N. Robinson, 1999); nutritional habits such as not consuming breakfast, eating at fast food restaurants, food frequency (Rampersaud, Pereira, Girard, Adams and Metzl, 2005), sleep duration (Reilly et al., 2005)], educational and economic features of the geographic context are commonly highlighted as having an important impact on public health (Chen, et al., 2008).

Area of residence is a factor that influences lifestyle, especially opportunities for physical activity (PA) and in turn CRF and public health policy (Joens-Matre et al., 2008; Machado-Rodrigues et al., 2011). Currently available data relating area of residence (i.e., urbanization) to PA, sedentary behaviour and CRF indicate somewhat variable and inconsistent results within and among specific countries and regions (Albarwani D Phil, et al., 2009; Dollman, et al., 2002; Karkera, et al., 2014; Mota, Gomes, Almeida, Ribeiro and Santos, 2007). It has been found that children and youth from rural communities were more likely to be classified as physically fit, particularly in CRF, than their age-matched peers from urban areas (Chen, et al., 2008; Karkera, et al., 2014; Özdirenç, et al., 2005). As shown by Dolman et al. (Dollman, et al., 2002) Australian children from rural areas had higher CRF than their urban peers. The results from Spain, Switzerland and Oman have also shown that children and adolescents with rural place of residence had higher CRF than their urban peers (Albarwani D Phil, et al., 2009; Kriemler, et al., 2008). In contrast to these findings, the results from the United States (US) have shown that urban US children had higher levels of cardiorespiratory fitness when compared to those living in rural areas (McMurray, Harrell, Bangdiwala and Deng, 1999).

However, research dealing with the potential influence of area of residence on CRF of Serbian youth is rather limited. Since that depression in the national economic conditions have led to apparent increase of inequalities between urban and rural communities, it could be assumed that social inequalities would be particularly pronounced regarding health and educational resources (Machado-Rodrigues et al., 2014). Having in mind aforementioned problem, we aimed to investigate potential differences in CRF between schoolchildren from urban and rural areas, with respect to their age and gender. For that purpose, a pilot study was conducted on primary schoolchildren living within the city and the vicinity of the national capital. Afterwards, a broad national cross-sectional school-based study was conducted, including primary schoolchildren living within the rural and urban areas across the Republic of Serbia.

METHODS

Participants

This study is a part of a large national project, aimed to follow up physical fitness and PA of schoolchildren from Serbia during their elementary school education. The study consisted of two parts: the pilot study that was conducted in national capital and vicinity and the national study that included schoolchildren from territory of Republic of Serbia.

Pilot Study

The pilot study included schoolchildren from the national capital of Serbia (city of Belgrade) and vicinity. Specifically, 2230 schoolchildren (boys n = 1163 and girls n = 1067, age 9 to 14 years) who at the time of the study attended primary schools (7) within the city (n = 3) and the vicinity of the national capital (n = 4) were included. The criterion for school selection was made according to their geographical location. Schools that were selected were assigned to one of two groups of schools. The first group consisted of schools located in strict city centre (urban schools), while the second group included schools from rural areas of Belgrade (rural schools; Figure 1). All data for the pilot study were collected during the winter semester of 2011/12 school year. All selected schools agreed to participate in the study. Schoolchildren were included in the study only if they had regular participation in physical education classes, while the exclusion criteria were chronic diseases and recent musculoskeletal injuries.

National Study

The second part of this study was the national study conducted on the territory of the Republic of Serbia. Data for this part of study were derived from a broad national cross-sectional school-based study that evaluated physical fitness and overweight/obesity prevalence. For the purpose of the national study, 11607 schoolchildren (boys n = 5913 and girls n = 5694, age 9 to 14 years) who at the time of the study attended primary schools on territory of the Republic of Serbia were included in the study. There are approximately 1300 primary schools in Serbia, and according to their geographical location, they are divided into 18 school districts. The schools included in the study were randomly selected from all school districts in Republic Serbia. According to their geographical location (Figure 2) the selected schools (n = 98) were divided into either urban (n = 44) or rural schools (n = 54). It should be noted that the definition of rural and urban varies across geographical areas and countries depending on their national standards (Hall, et al., 2006). The criterion used in this study to describe an urban area was >10 000 inhabitants, and 10 000 inhabitants for a rural area.

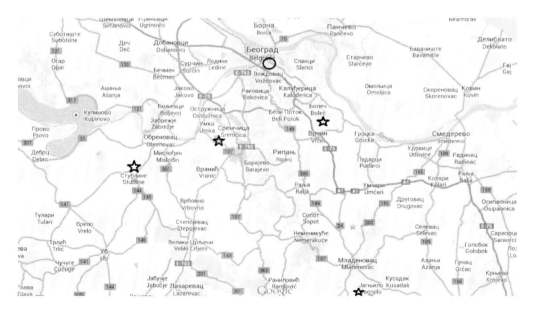

Figure 1. Map of City of Belgrade with geographical location of schools selected to participate in the study (* - selected schools from rural areas; O - strict city center and location of "urban" schools).

Data Collection

All data for the national study were collected during the spring semester of 2012/13 school year.

The schools that were selected agreed to participate in the study. The inclusion criterion was the identical to those in the pilot study. Only schoolchildren who reported regular participation in physical education classes and no chronic diseases and recent musculoskeletal injuries were selected to participate. Both pilot and national study were approved by the University Ethics Committee and an institutionally approved informed consent was signed by the parents of all schoolchildren participating in this study.

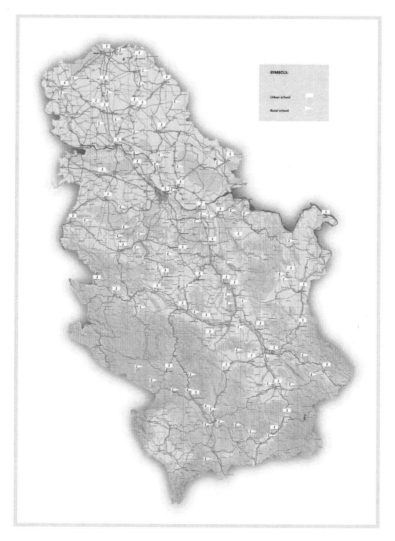

Figure 2. Map of Republic of Serbia with geographical location of schools selected to participate in the study. Square flags represent urban areas, while triangle flags represent rural areas. Number inside the flags denotes number of schools selected from particular area.

Testing Procedures

Testing procedure was identical both in the pilot study and the national study. It consisted of anthropometric measures and the estimation of cardiorespiratory fitness.

Anthropometric Measures

Participants were evaluated during school physical education classes by physical education teachers specially trained for this type of data collection. Prior to warm-up, standard anthropometric measurements were taken. Body height (BH) was measured to the nearest 0.1 cm using a Seca Stadiometer 208 (Seca, Hamburg, Germany). The subjects were barefoot, minimally dressed (shorts and T-shirts), and the head was positioned using the Frankfurt method (Frankfurt plane parallel to the floor). Body weight (BW) was measured to the nearest 0.1 kg using a pre-calibrated portable weighting scale (Tanita Inner Scan BC 532). Afterwards, a standardized 15-minute warm-up procedure was performed and followed by detailed explanation and quality demonstration of Shuttle-run test.

Cardiorespiratory Fitness

Among a number of field methods used to assess CRF, one of the commonly used and quite simple to conduct is the Shuttle run test (SRT). Validity and reliability of SRT for determining CRF was evaluated in a number of studies (Léger, Mercier, Gadoury and Lambert, 1988; Ruiz, Rizzo, et al., 2006). In addition, it has been reported that reliability of SRT when used to assess CRF in youth was also high (≥ 0.89) (C. A. Boreham, Paliczka and Nichols, 1990; Liu, Plowman and Looney, 1992; Mahar et al., 1997). Regarding the feasibility of SRT, this test is simply to conduct and it allows for simultaneous testing of a group of subjects, without any special requirements and therefore is suitable for use in physical education class. It should be mentioned that by using specific equation maximum oxygen consumption (VO_{2max}) can be indirectly calculated from the results obtained from SRT (Leger et al., 1984). The equation ($VO_{2max} = 31.025 + 3.238 \times S - 3.248 \times A + 0.1536 \times S \times A$) takes into account the subject's age (A) and final velocity (S) (S = 8 + 0.5 x last stage completed).

Shuttle run was conducted according to a standardized procedure (Léger, et al., 1988). Specifically, SRT is a multi-stage test that involves running continuously between two points that are 20 meters apart from side to side. These runs are synchronized with a pre-recorded audio tape, CD or computer software, which plays beeps at set intervals. As the test proceeds, the interval between each successive beep decreases, forcing the subjects to increase their speed over the course of the test, until it is impossible to keep in sync with the recording (or, in rare occasions, until the subject completes the test). Children were instructed to keep up with the cadence for as long as possible. Initial speed was 8.5 km/h (20 m in 9 s) which corresponds to slow pace running (or fast walking). After each minute, the speed was increased for 0.5 km/h. When subjects were unable to keep with the pace, the achieved time was recorded in seconds (with stop-watch) that represented directly measured variable.

Statistical Analysis

Descriptive statistics (mean, standard deviation and confidence intervals) was calculated for all variables (BH, BM, BMI and total time in SRT). To analyse data from the pilot study, separate three-factor ANOVAs were used to explore potential differences in anthropometric variables and CRF between boys and girls (factor "gender") of different age (factor "age") who attended either urban or rural schools (factor "school location"). Where significant main effect of factor or their interactions were found post-hoc analysis (t-test with Bonfferroni) was performed. The identical statistical procedures were applied for the analysis of data obtained from the national study. The level of significance was set to $p < 0.05$. Finally, the effects size was estimated via partial eta squared and according to Cohen, it was considered as either small (0.01), medium (0.06) or large (0.138) (Pallant, 2010). All data were analysed using SPSS 18.0 (SPSS Inc. Chicago, IL).

RESULTS

Pilot Study

Descriptive statistics for anthropometric measures (BH, BW and BMI) as well as the result from SRT obtained from national capital and vicinity are presented in Figure 3, Figure 4 and Figure 5. Schoolchildren from urban schools were significantly higher than schoolchildren from rural schools ($p < 0.05$), regardless of age (Figure 3). In addition, although the obtained results showed that boys were in general taller than girls ($p < 0.001$), the post-hoc analysis revealed that boys attending 7th and 8th grade boys were taller than the age (grade) – matched girls ($p < 0.01$).

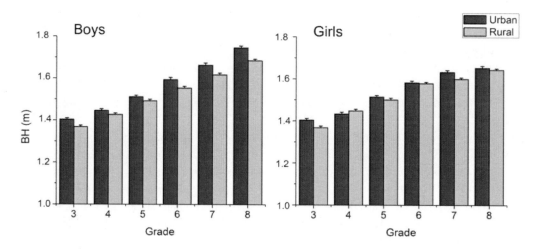

Figure 3. Body height (BH) data obtained from the pilot study - boys and girls by age and school location. Data presented as Mean (SD).

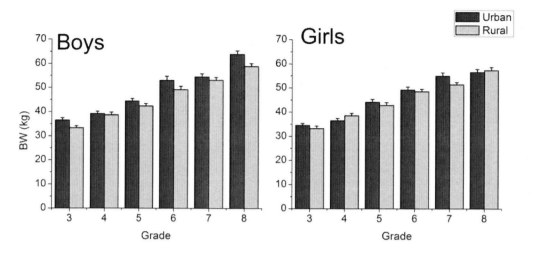

Figure 4. Body weight (BW) data obtained from the pilot study - boys and girls by age and school location. Data presented as Mean (SD).

Regarding the BW results (Figure 4), both boys and girls from urban schools had significantly larger BW than schoolchildren from rural schools (p < 0.001), particularly for 3rd (p < 0.05), 6th (p < 0.001) and 7th graders (p < 0.001). Although boys had larger BW than girls (p < 0.001), it should be mentioned that only in 8th grade boys had significantly larger BW than age-matched girls (p < 0.001).

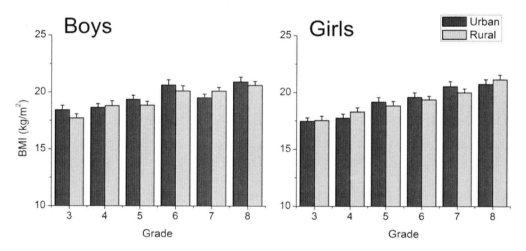

Figure 5. Body mass index (BMI) data obtained from the pilot study - boys and girls by age and school location. Data presented as Mean (SD).

Finally, regarding the BMI (Figure 5), it increased with age significantly (p < 0.01), however that increase was similar both in urban and rural schoolchildren, regardless of gender.

The results of three-factor ANOVA performed on time achieved in SRT are presented in Table 1.

Table 1. Results of ANOVA performed on Shuttle-run test data obtained from the pilot study

Factors	F value	Eta Squared
Gender	218.58**	.090
Age	44.43**	.091
School location	8.66*	.004
Gender × Age	14.74**	.032
Gender × School location	4.08*	.002
Age × School location	4.36**	.010
Gender × Age × School location	1.74	.004

F value – derived from ANOVA, Eta squared – effect size, **-main effect of factor or factor interaction significant at $p < 0.01$, *-main effect of factor or factor interaction significant at $p < 0.05$.

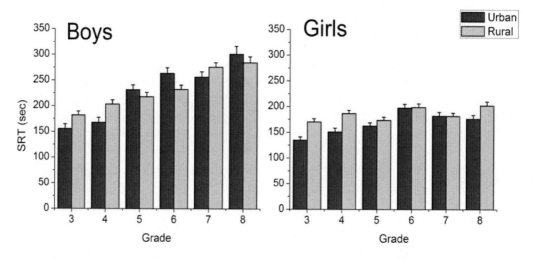

Figure 6. The results of the SRT obtained from the pilot study - boys and girls by age and school location. Data presented as Mean (SD).

The ANOVA revealed that all main effects of factors and their interactions were significant, with the exception of "Gender × Age × School location" interaction. Descriptive data for SRT, for rural and urban boys (left panel) and girls (right panel), with respect to their age (grade) are presented in Figure 6. The results indicate that boys, regardless of place of residence, had better results than girls, across all age categories ($p < 0.001$). In addition, there was an age-associated increase in SRT time ($p < 0.001$) in both boys and girls, regardless of the place of residence and therefore, school location. Such age-associated increase was particularly pronounced in boys, who had better results than girls in all grades ($p < 0.001$), except in 3rd and 4th grade. Of particular interest for the main aim of this study could be the results obtained from comparison of schoolchildren from urban and rural areas. Specifically, rural schoolchildren achieved overall better results on SRT than their peers from schools located at urban area ($p < 0.001$), regardless of gender and age. When gender was taken into account, both boys and girls from rural schools had better results on SRT than their urban peers. However, when the age was taken into account, the results of post-hoc analysis revealed that schoolchildren from rural schools achieved better results (i.e., had longer time on SRT) than their urban peers only in 3rd and 4th grade (p < 0.001), while in higher grades such difference was diminished and no difference was found. Although the observed effect sizes suggest that factors "gender" and "age" have the largest impact on the recorded differences (medium effect size $\eta > 0.06$), the factor "School location" had small influence ($\eta > 0.01$).

National Study

Descriptive statistics for anthropometric measures (BH, BW and BMI) as well as the result from SRT obtained from schoolchildren from Serbia are presented in Figure 7, Figure 8 and Figure 9. Schoolchildren from urban schools were significantly higher than schoolchildren from rural schools (p < 0.05), regardless of age (Figure 7). In addition, although the obtained results showed that boys were in general taller than girls (p < 0.001), the post-hoc analysis revealed that girls attending 4th and 5th grade were taller than age (grade) – matched boys (p < 0.05), while 7th and 8th grade boys were taller than the girls (p < 0.01).

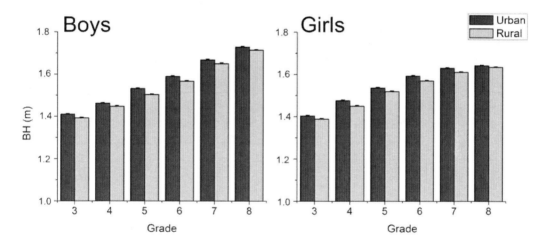

Figure 7. Body height (BH) data obtained from the national study - boys and girls by age and school location. Data presented as Mean (SD).

Regarding the BW results (Figure 8), schoolchildren from urban schools had significantly larger BW than schoolchildren from rural schools (p < 0.001), particularly for 3rd (p < 0.05), 5th (p < 0.001) and 6th graders (p < 0.001). Although boys had larger BW than girls (p < 0.001), it should be mentioned that only boys from 7th and 8th grade had significantly larger BW than age-matched girls (p < 0.001).

Finally, regarding the BMI (Figure 9), significant difference between urban and rural schoolchildren was found only in 5th grade, being larger for urban schoolchildren (p < 0.05). Boys had larger BMI than girls, regardless of their age (p < 0.01).

The results of three-factor ANOVA performed on time achieved in SRT are presented in Table 2.

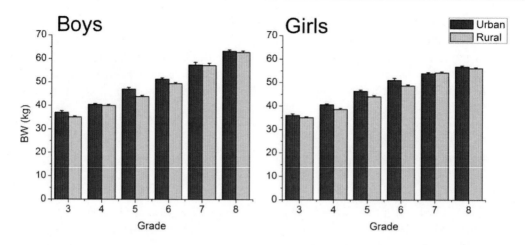

Figure 8. Body weight (BW) data obtained from the national study - boys and girls by age and school location. Data presented as Mean (SD).

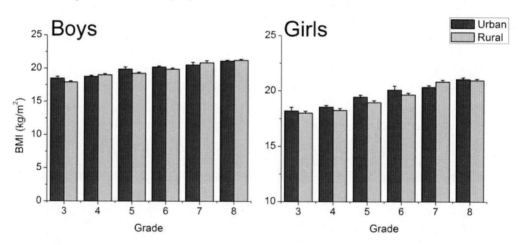

Figure 9. Body mass index (BMI) data obtained from the national study - boys and girls by age and school location. Data presented as Mean (SD).

Table 2. Results of ANOVA performed on Shuttle-run data obtained from the national study

Factors	F value	Eta Squared
Gender	1036.83**	0.08
Age	136.56**	0.06
School location	6.76*	0.00
Gender × Age	37.61**	0.02
Gender × School location	0.837	0.00
Age × School location	3.91**	0.00
Gender × Age × School location	0.49	0.00

F value – derived from ANOVA, Eta squared – effect size, **-main effect of factor or factor interaction significant at $p < 0.01$, *-main effect of factor or factor interaction significant at $p < 0.05$.

In general, all main effects of factors and their interactions were significant, with the exception of "Gender × School location" and "Gender × Age × School location" interactions. Descriptive statistics for SRT data is presented in Figure 10, for boys (left panel) and girls (right panel) respectively. The results indicate that boys, regardless of school location, had better results than girls, across all age categories ($p < 0.001$). In addition, there was an age-associated increase in SRT time ($p < 0.001$) in both boys and girls, regardless of the place of residence and therefore, school location. Such age-associated increase was particularly pronounced in boys, who had better results than girls, across all age categories ($p < 0.001$). Of particular interest for the main aim of this study could be the results obtained from comparison of schoolchildren from urban and rural areas. Specifically, regardless of gender and age, urban schoolchildren achieved overall better results on SRT than their peers from schools located at rural areas ($p < 0.001$). Further, the results of post-hoc analysis revealed that 3rd - grade schoolchildren (regardless of gender) from rural schools achieved better results (Figure 4) than their urban peers, contrary to the results from 6th - and 7th graders. Although the observed effect sizes suggest that factors "gender" and "age" have the largest impact on the recorded differences (medium effect size $\eta > 0.06$), the factor "school location" had small influence ($\eta < 0.01$).

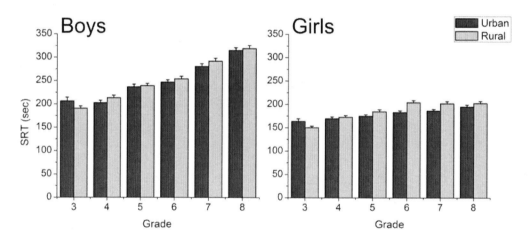

Figure 10. The results of the SRT obtained from the national study - boys and girls by age and school location. Data presented as Mean (SD).

DISCUSSION

This study is a part of a large national project, aimed to follow up physical fitness of schoolchildren from Serbia during their elementary school education. The study consisted of two parts: the pilot study that was conducted in national capital and vicinity and the national study that included schoolchildren from territory of Republic of Serbia. Before discussing the main findings of this study, some important methodological issues have to be emphasized. Firstly, it should be noted that the present study was a cross-sectional one and, therefore, could potentially affect the main outcome of the study. Secondly, factors such as age, gender, morphology and level of physical activity, could also affect CRF (Nedeljkovic, Mirkov, Kukolj, Ugarkovic and Jaric, 2007; A. M. Nevill and Holder, 2000).

Pilot Study

The aim of this study was to explore potential differences in CRF between primary schoolchildren living within the city and the vicinity of the national capital (urban and rural area of Belgrade). It should be noted that tested subjects represent the population of schoolchildren living in two contrasting areas of the national capital, providing equally proportionate sample of boys and girls not only within each age group, but also between genders, comparable to the number of participants in most of similar studies (Nedeljkovic, et al., 2007; A. Nevill, Tsiotra, Tsimeas and Koutedakis, 2009; Tsimeas, et al., 2005).

As expected, boys had better results than girls in all tested variables, regardless of the grade (i.e., age) or school location. The only exception was BMI, which appeared to be similar between the genders, at all ages. This finding is somewhat surprising since the results from our previous study, conducted on representative sample of 9-14 year schoolchildren from Belgrade, showed that a higher BMI has been observed in boys than in girls in all age groups (S Radisavljević Janić, Milanović, Živković and Mirkov, 2013). Moreover, the similar trend was recorded in Portugal (Sardinha et al., 2011), Slovenia (Kovac, Jurak and Leskosek, 2012), and Finland (Vuorela, Saha and Salo, 2011).

The gender-related difference in CRF increased with maturation, since it was particularly pronounced in higher-grades (5th to 8th) and these findings are generally in line with the previous studies investigating CRF (Malina, et al., 2004; Milanović, et al., 2013; Ortega, et al., 2008). Furthermore, age-related increase in both anthropometric measures and CRF was particularly pronounced in boys, where a linear increase has been observed, while in girls it reached plateau at the age of 12. The obtained findings are in line with the previously published results (Carson, Iannotti, Pickett and Janssen, 2011; Chen, et al., 2008; Karkera, et al., 2014; Özdirenç, et al., 2005) and the potential explanation of these findings could originate from difference in the amount of time boys and girls spend involved in organized physical activity. When compared to boys, girls appear to be less involved in organized physical activity during leisure time, particularly in the early post-pubertal years, which correspondence to higher school grades (Klomsten, Marsh and Skaalvik, 2005; Milanović and Radisavljević Janić, 2011; Pasic et al., 2014; S. Radisavljević Janić, Milanović and Lazarević, 2012). These findings have been confirmed by results from our previous study where 53.3% of girls who attend schools in Belgrade and vicinity do not participate in any type of physical activity (Živković, Stamenković and Marković, 2013).

The findings related to the main aim of the pilot study i.e., the comparison of urban schoolchildren and their age-matched peers from rural schools revealed higher levels of CRF in rural schoolchildren than in urban schoolchildren. Moreover, difference between urban and rural schoolchildren was observed in both genders, but it was particularly prominent in girls. However, those differences were limited only to schoolchildren in 3rd and 4th grade, while in the higher grades (5th to 8th grade) those differences have diminished so that rural and urban schoolchildren had similar levels of CRF. According to the findings from the earlier studies, in higher grades it could have been expected that due to differences between urban and rural life-style (Eiben and Mascie-Taylor, 2004; Pfister and Reeg, 2006) boys and girls from urban areas have higher levels of CRF than their rural peers. Namely, as reported by Karkera and associates (Karkera, et al., 2014) urban schoolchildren were less involved in regular physical activity (95 minutes/day) than their peers from rural schools who spent significantly more time being physically active (150 minutes/day). This could be explained by the fact that living in urban area provides a variety of opportunities for participation in organized physical activity. In contrast to that, children in rural areas have limited options for participation in organized physical activity. In addition, the observed differences between urban and rural schoolchildren could be attributed to life style, cultural influence, socio-economic status, etc. (Eiben and Mascie-Taylor, 2004).

This pilot study revealed that schoolchildren who live in urban and rural areas differ in CRF and that those differences are mostly age and gender associated. The rural schoolchildren achieved better results in CRF than their urban peers, but that was dominant in lower grades. Moreover, difference between urban and rural schoolchildren was particularly prominent in girls. In addition, the obtained results partially support previous findings regarding the differences in CRF between boys and girls across the ages.

The main limitation of the pilot study was that schoolchildren from relatively small number of schools located in the center and the vicinity of the national capital were included in the study.

National Study

To confirm the findings obtained from the pilot study, broad national cross-sectional school-based study was conducted including primary schoolchildren living within the rural and urban areas across the Republic of Serbia. Schools (118) were randomly selected from all school districts of Serbia since differences in life style could be particularly pronounced in provincial urban and rural areas. Similar to the aim of pilot study, the aim of this study was to explore potential differences in CRF between primary schoolchildren with respect to gender, age and area of residence (urban and rural).

The results obtained from the sample of schoolchildren from Serbia were to some extent similar to the results from the pilot study. Boys were taller and heavier than girls, regardless of their age or school location, however, unlike in the pilot study, boys participating in the national study had larger BMI than girls. Nonetheless, the findings regarding the anthropometric variables that were obtained in the national study are generally in line with the previous studies investigating similar problems (Jurak, Milanović, Radisavljević Janić, Soric and kovac, 2015; Kovac, et al., 2012; Malina, et al., 2004; S. Radisavljević Janić, et al., 2012; Sardinha, et al., 2011; Vuorela, et al., 2011). These findings are also in line with the results from our previous study on representative sample of 9-14 year schoolchildren from Serbia where, besides higher BW and higher BMI, a higher prevalence of overweight has been observed in boys (27.0%) than in girls (22.4%), in all age groups (Milanović and Radisavljević Janić, 2014; S Radisavljević Janić, et al., 2013). A possible reason for higher BMI and possibly higher prevalence of overweight and obesity in boys than in girls from Serbia might be that boys spend more time in sedentary activities (watching television and specially playing computer games; (Ho and Lee, 2001)) than girls. In addition, girls are more sensitive to pubertal physiological and physical changes than boys (Klomsten, Skaalvik and Espnes, 2004) and under larger influence of the cultural ideal of thinness that is strongly present in Western cultures (Blyth, Simmons and Zakin, 1985). Finally, other factors such as change in dietary patterns in recent decades, including an increased consumption of soft drinks, candies and junk food also have large influence on body composition of schoolchildren (French, Story and Jeffery, 2001; Hills, Andersen and Byrne, 2011). In the recent decades physical activity patterns in adolescents have changed as a result of increase in time spent watching television and playing computer games (French, et al., 2001; J. P. Robinson and Godbey, 1997). Demographic trends have shown that children and adults in the countries in transition, Serbia included, have already adopted the Western model of urban lifestyle, i.e., a sedentary lifestyle and food rich in fats, meat products and snacks, regardless of the place of residence (urban or rural) of schoolchildren.

Regarding CRF, the obtained findings indicated that in all age groups boys have better CRF than girls, which is similar to findings from other countries (Olds, et al., 2006; M.S. Tremblay, et al., 2010). Olds and associates (Olds, et al., 2006) have analyzed 109 studies from 37 countries and noted that differences in cardiorespiratory fitness between boys and girls are consistent across a wide range of countries with different social, political, and economic systems, and they concluded that those differences are probably biological rather than social in origin. Indeed, as aforementioned, a linear increase in CRF has been observed between the age of 7 and 17. In particular, from the ages of 9 to 14 years, boys and girls experience a continuous and a rather large increase in CRF, with different trend in boys vs. girls. Namely, boys experienced a gradual increase in CRF from the ages of 9 to 14 years and by the end of this period the increase in CRF is three-folded (Lazarević, et al., 2011; Malina, et al., 2004). However, the increase in CRF that was observed in girls was only two-folded, reaching its peak at the age of 12, after which it gradually declined. Although biological factors primarily contribute to these differences, other factors, like time spent in physical activity could also be an important one that contributes to difference between the genders (Eiben and Mascie-Taylor, 2004; Pfister and Reeg, 2006). Namely, when compared to boys, girls appear to be less involved in organized physical activity during leisure time, particularly in the early post-pubertal years (Klomsten, et al., 2005; Milanović and Radisavljević Janić, 2011; Živković, et al., 2013) and that could be a possible explanation for the results obtained at this age.

Regarding the findings originating from the comparison of CRF between schoolchildren living in the urban and rural areas they were only partially similar to those obtained in the pilot study. In particular, urban schoolchildren achieved overall better results on SRT than their peers from schools located at rural areas, regardless of gender. It has been found that children and youth from rural communities were more likely to be classified as physically fit, particularly in CRF, than their age-matched peers from urban areas (Chen, et al., 2008; Karkera, et al., 2014; Özdirenç, et al., 2005). However, when factor "Age" was taken into account, the results revealed that in lower grades rural schoolchildren had better CRF than urban schoolchildren, while in higher grades those differences change in favor of schoolchildren from urban schools. Karkera et al. (Karkera, et al., 2014) also reported that rural schoolchildren spent significantly more time being physically active through regular physical activity than their peers from urban schools, thus having better CRF. However, the effect of "Age" on the observed differences could be attributed to the fact that the activity habits associated with school physical education and lifestyle can differ between children and adolescents, and it is interesting to further explore whether the relationship between place of residence and cardiorespiratory fitness differ between children and adolescents. Although a number of factors could have contributed to the observed differences, an important one could be the difference between urban and rural life-style (Eiben and Mascie-Taylor, 2004; Pfister and Reeg, 2006). Differences between urban and rural schoolchildren that were observed in higher grades could be potentially explained by the fact that living in urban area provides a variety of opportunities for participation in organized physical activity. It has been shown that starting with a sixth grade (approximately 12 years of age) boys who live in urban areas usually begin with participation in sport or other types of organized physical activity (soccer, basketball, handball, volleyball, martial arts etc.) which may contribute to improvement in their CRF (Machado-Rodrigues, et al., 2014). However, when compared to boys, girls appear to be less involved in organized physical activity during leisure time, particularly in the early post-pubertal years (Klomsten, et al., 2005; Milanović and Radisavljević Janić, 2011; Živković, et al., 2013) and that could be a possible explanation for the results obtained at this age. This is supported by findings of Živković et al. (Živković, et al., 2013) where 62.8% boys from urban schools reported participation in organized physical activity. In contrast to that, children in rural areas have limited options for participation in organized physical activity which could be a potential reason for the observed lower level of CRF than in their peers from urban schools. In addition, the observed differences between urban and rural schoolchildren could be attributed to life style, cultural influence, socio-economic status, etc. (Eiben and Mascie-Taylor, 2004). Although there is no direct evidence for these assumptions, a number of published studies exploring the same problem founded that the aforementioned factors significantly contribute to differences in CRF between urban and rural schoolchildren (Davison and Lawson, 2006; Joens-Matre, et al., 2008).

Limitations

Due to the cross-sectional design of the conducted study, we cannot infer that our observed associations reflect a causal relationship. Nevertheless since there were no significant differences between age-matched boys and girls from urban and rural areas, we could speculate that the obtained differences in CRF mainly originated from the place of residence. Another limitation is the lack of direct information on socio-economic factors, which might vary regardless of the place of residence. Therefore, the future study on CRF should be analyzed along with the analysis of life style habits of schoolchildren, living conditions, socio-economic differences and other potentially contributing factors. Differences in maturation, especially among children and adolescents, might influence the physical fitness results; the lack of information about the sexual maturation status of the study sample is another limitation. Finally, someone could argue that determination of precise parameters used to assess CRF requires sophisticated apparatus and technical expertise. Nevertheless, a number of simple performance tests have been developed to estimate aerobic fitness of children and adolescents, among which SRT has been the most reliable, valid and widely used by scientists, teachers and coaches being the 20-m shuttle run test (SRT) (Artero et al., 2012; Ruiz et al., 2011). Having this all in mind, we believe that the present study provides a valid set of data, while the most often used and a relatively simple SRT provides an opportunity to compare our findings with the findings of previous studies. In addition, since this is the first national study exploring the potential differences in CRF between urban and rural schoolchildren, the obtained findings provide novel and important information regarding the potential influence of place of residence on CRF of schoolchildren.

CONCLUSION

The results of this study revealed urban-rural differences in BMI of schoolchildren participating in the national study, but not among the schoolchildren living in the national capital and the vicinity. Although the findings obtained from schoolchildren from the national capital and vicinity indicate that schoolchildren who live in urban and rural areas differ in CRF, those differences were mostly age and gender associated. Rural schoolchildren generally had better cardiorespiratory fitness than their urban peers, but that difference was observed in lower grades and it was particularly prominent in girls. The national study, conducted on a broad sample of urban and rural schoolchildren yielded results that were only partly similar to the results from the pilot study. Again, CRF was strongly influenced by age and gender, while area of residence had small impact on CRF. Rural schoolchildren had better CRF in lower grades however due to potential influence of factors other than the area of residence (participation in organized physical activity, life-style, eating habits, socio-economic status, etc.) urban schoolchildren had better levels of CRF in higher grades.

ACKNOWLEDGMENTS

This study was supported in part by the grants from Serbian Ministry of Education, Science and Technological Development (#47015, #175037 and #175012).

REFERENCES

Albarwani D Phil, S., Al-Hashmi, K., Al-Abri, M., Jaju, D. and Hassan, M. O. (2009). Effects of overweight and leisure-time activities on aerobic fitness in urban and rural adolescents. *Metab Syndr Relat D, 7*(4), 369-374.

Anderssen, S. A., Cooper, A. R., Riddoch, C., Sardinha, L. B., Harro, M., Brage, S. and Andersen, L. B. (2007). Low cardiorespiratory fitness is a strong predictor for clustering of cardiovascular disease risk factors in children independent of country, age and sex. *Eur J Cardiov Prev R, 14*(4), 526-531.

Armstrong, N., Tomkinson, G. and Ekelund, U. (2011). Aerobic fitness and its relationship to sport, exercise training and habitual physical activity during youth. *Br J Sport Med, 45*(11), 849-858.

Artero, E. G., Lee, D., Lavie, C. J., España-Romero, V., Sui, X., Church, T. S. and Blair, S. N. (2012). Effects of muscular strength on cardiovascular risk factors and prognosis. *J Cardiopulm Rehabil, 32*(6), 351-358.

Blyth, D. A., Simmons, R. G. and Zakin, D. F. (1985). Satisfaction with body image for early adolescent females: The impact of pubertal timing within different school environments. *J Youth Adolesc, 14*(3), 207-225.

Boreham, C. A., Paliczka, V. J. and Nichols, A. K. (1990). A comparison of the PWC170 and 20-MST tests of aerobic fitness in adolescent schoolchildren. *J Sports Med Phys Fitness, 30*(1), 19-23.

Boreham, C. and Riddoch, C. (2001). The physical activity, fitness and health of children. *J Sports Sci, 19*(12), 915-929.

Boreham, C., Twisk, J., Neville, C., Savage, M., Murray, L. and Gallagher, A. (2002a). Associations between physical fitness and activity patterns during adolescence and cardiovascular risk factors in young adulthood: the Northern Ireland Young Hearts Project. *Int J Sports Med, 23*, S22-26.

Boreham, C., Twisk, J., Neville, C., Savage, M., Murray, L. and Gallagher, A. (2002b). Associations between physical fitness and activity patterns during adolescence and cardiovascular risk factors in young adulthood: the Northern Ireland Young Hearts Project. *Int J Sports Med, 23 (S1)*, 22-26.

Burke, V., Beilin, L. J., Simmer, K., Oddy, W. H., Blake, K. V., Doherty, D., Kendall, G. E., Newnham, J. P., Landau, L. I. and Stanley, F. J. (2005). Predictors of body mass index and associations with cardiovascular risk factors in Australian children: a prospective cohort study. *Int J Obes (Lond), 29*(1), 15-23.

Carnethon, M. R., Gulati, M. and Greenland, P. (2005). Prevalence and cardiovascular disease correlates of low cardiorespiratory fitness in adolescents and adults. *JAMA, 294*(23), 2981-2988.

Carson, V., Iannotti, R. J., Pickett, W. and Janssen, I. (2011). Urban and rural differences in sedentary behavior among American and Canadian youth. *Health Place, 17*(4), 920-928.

Chen, J. L., Unnithan, V., Kennedy, C. and Yeh, C. H. (2008). Correlates of physical fitness and activity in Taiwanese children. *Int Nurs Rev, 55*(1), 81-88.

Davison, K. K. and Lawson, C. T. (2006). Do attributes in the physical environment influence children's physical activity? A review of the literature. *Int J Behav Nutr Phy, 3*(1), 19.

Dollman, J., Norton, K. and Tucker, G. (2002). Anthropometry, fitness and physical activity of urban and rural South Australian children. *Pediatr Exerc Sci, 14*(3), 297-312.

Eiben, O. G. and Mascie-Taylor, C. G. N. (2004). Children's growth and socio-economic status in Hungary. *Econ Hum Biolog, 2*(2), 295-320.

Eisenmann, J. C., Wickel, E. E., Welk, G. J. and Blair, S. N. (2005). Relationship between adolescent fitness and fatness and cardiovascular disease risk factors in adulthood: the Aerobics Center Longitudinal Study (ACLS). *Am Heart J, 149*(1), 46-53.

French, S. A., Story, M. and Jeffery, R. W. (2001). Environmental influences on eating and physical activity. *Annu Rev Publ Health, 22*(1), 309-335.

Hall, S. A., Kaufman, J. S. and Ricketts, T. C. (2006). Defining urban and rural areas in U.S. epidemiologic studies. *J Urban Health, 83*(2), 162-175.

Haskell, W. L., Lee, I. M., Pate, R. R., Powell, K. E., Blair, S. N., Franklin, B. A., Macera, C. A., Heath, G. W., Thompson, P. D. and Bauman, A. (2007). Physical activity and public health: updated recommendation for adults from the American College of Sports Medicine and the American Heart Association. *Med Sci Sport Exer, 39*(8), 1423-1434.

Hasselstrom, H., Hansen, S. E., Froberg, K. and Andersen, L. B. (2002). Physical fitness and physical activity during adolescence as predictors of cardiovascular disease risk in young adulthood. Danish Youth and Sports Study. An eight-year follow-up study. *Int J Sports Med, 23*(Suppl 1), S27-31.

Hills, A. P., Andersen, L. B. and Byrne, N. M. (2011). Physical activity and obesity in children. *Br J Sports Med, 45*(11), 866-870.

Hills, A. P., King, N. A. and Armstrong, T. P. (2007). The contribution of physical activity and sedentary behaviours to the growth and development of children and adolescents: implications for overweight and obesity. *Sports Med, 37*(6), 533-545.

Ho, S. M. Y. and Lee, T. M. C. (2001). Computer usage and its relationship with adolescent lifestyle in Hong Kong. *J Adolescent Health, 29*(4), 258-266.

Janic, S. R., Jurak, G., Milanovic, I., Lazarevic, D., Kovac, M. and Novak, D. (2014). Physical self-concept of adolescents in Western Balkan countries: a pilot study. *Percept Mot Skills, 119*(2), 629-649. doi: 10.2466/08.PMS.119c23z7.

Joens-Matre, R. R., Welk, G. J., Calabro, M. A., Russell, D. W., Nicklay, E. and Hensley, L. D. (2008). Rural–urban differences in physical activity, physical fitness, and overweight prevalence of children. *J Rural Health, 24*(1), 49-54.

Jurak, G., Milanović, I., Radisavljević Janić, S., Soric, M. and kovac, M. (2015). Some indicators of fatness and motor fitness in Slovenian and Serbian children. *Int. J. Morphol.*, accepted for publishing.

Jurak, G., Radisavljević Janić, S., Milanović, I., Strel, J. and Kovac, M. (2012). Physical fitness of 12-year-old girls from capitals of Serbia and Slovenia. *Acta Universitatis Carolinae Kinanthropologica, 48*(1), 42-49.

Karkera, A., Swaminathan, N., Pais, S. M. J., Vishal, K. and Rai, S. (2014). Physical fitness and activity levels among urban school children and their rural counterparts. *Indian J Pediatr, 81*(4), 356-361.

Klomsten, A. T., Marsh, H. W. and Skaalvik, E. M. (2005). Adolescents' perceptions of masculine and feminine values in sport and physical education: A study of gender differences. *Sex roles, 52*(9-10), 625-636.

Klomsten, A. T., Skaalvik, E. M. and Espnes, G. A. (2004). Physical self-concept and sports: Do gender differences still exist? *Sex roles, 50*(1-2), 119-127.

Kovac, M., Jurak, G. and Leskosek, B. (2012). The prevalence of excess weight and obesity in Slovenian children and adolescents from 1991 to 2011. *Anthropological Notebooks, 18*(1), 91103.

Kriemler, S., Manser-Wenger, S., Zahner, L., Braun-Fahrlander, C., Schindler, C. and Puder, J. J. (2008). Reduced cardiorespiratory fitness, low physical activity and an urban environment are independently associated with increased cardiovascular risk in children. *Diabetologia, 51*(8), 1408-1415.

Lazarević, D., Radisavljević Janić, S., Milanović, I. and Lazarević, Lj. B. (2011). Physical self-concept of normal-weight and overweight adolescents: Gender specificities. *Zbornik Instituta za pedagoska istrazivanja, 43*(2), 347-365.

Léger, L. A., Mercier, D., Gadoury, C. and Lambert, J. (1988). The multistage 20 metre shuttle run test for aerobic fitness. *J Sport Sci, 6*(2), 93.

Liu, N. Y., Plowman, S. A. and Looney, M. A. (1992). The reliability and validity of the 20-meter shuttle test in American students 12 to 15 years old. *Res Q Exerc Sport, 63*(4), 360-365.

Machado-Rodrigues, A. M., Coelho-e-Silva, M. J., Mota, J., Cumming, S. P., Riddoch, C. and Malina, R. M. (2011). Correlates of aerobic fitness in urban and rural Portuguese adolescents. *Ann Hum Biol, 38*(4), 479-484.

Machado-Rodrigues, A. M., Coelho-E-Silva, M. J., Mota, J., Padez, C., Martins, R. A., Cumming, S. P., Riddoch, C. and Malina, R. M. (2014). Urban–rural contrasts in fitness, physical activity, and sedentary behaviour in adolescents. *Health Promot Intl, 29*(1), 118-129.

Mahar, M. T., Rowe, D. A., Parker, C. R., Mahar, F. J., Dawson, D. M. and Holt, J. E. (1997). Criterion-referenced and norm-referenced agreement between the mile run/walk and PACER. *Measurement in Physical Education and Exercise Science, 1*(4), 245-258.

Malina, R. M., Bouchard, C. and Bar-Or, O. (2004). *Growth, Maturation and Physical Activity*. (Second Edition ed.): Human Kinetics. USA.

McMurray, R. G., Harrell, J. S., Bangdiwala, S. I. and Deng, S. (1999). Cardiovascular disease risk factors and obesity of rural and urban elementary school children. *J Rural Health, 15*(4), 365-374.

Milanović, I. and Radisavljević Janić, S. (2011). *Elementary school pupils' involvement in sports in Serbia*. Paper presented at the Proceedings book of 6th FIEP european congress: Physical Education in the 21st century–Pupils' competencies.

Milanović, I. and Radisavljević Janić, S. (2014). *Praćenje fizičkih sposobnosti učenika osnovne škole u nastavi fizičkog vaspitanja*: Fakultet sporta i fizičkog vaspitanja. [Monitoring the physical abilities of primary school students in physical education: Faculty of Sport and Physical Education.] Beograd, Srbija.

Milanović, I., Radisavljević Janić, S. and Mirkov, D. M. (2013). Cardiorespiratory fitness of schoolchildren in elementary schools in Belgrade. *Journal of The International Federation of Physical Education, 83*(Special Edition - Article III), 230-232.

Mora, S., Redberg, R. F., Cui, Y., Whiteman, M. K., Flaws, J. A., Sharrett, A. R. and Blumenthal, R. S. (2003). Ability of exercise testing to predict cardiovascular and all-cause death in asymptomatic women: a 20-year follow-up of the lipid research clinics prevalence study. *JAMA, 290*(12), 1600-1607.

Moreno, L. A., Mesana, M. I., Gonzalez-Gross, M., Gil, C. M., Fleta, J., Warnberg, J., Ruiz, J. R., Sarria, A., Marcos, A. and Bueno, M. (2006). Anthropometric body fat composition reference values in Spanish adolescents. The AVENA Study. *Eur J Clin Nutr, 60*(2), 191-196.

Mota, J., Gomes, H., Almeida, M., Ribeiro, J. C. and Santos, M. P. (2007). Leisure time physical activity, screen time, social background, and environmental variables in adolescents. *Pediatr Exerc Sci, 19*, 279- 290.

Murnan, J., Price, J. H., Telljohann, S. K., Dake, J. A. and Boardley, D. (2006). Parents' perceptions of curricular issues affecting children's weight in elementary schools. *J School Health, 76*(10), 502-511.

Nedeljkovic, A., Mirkov, D. M., Kukolj, M., Ugarkovic, D. and Jaric, S. (2007). Effect of maturation on the relationship between physical performance and body size. *J Strength Cond Res, 21*(1), 245-250.

Nevill, A. M. and Holder, R. L. (2000). Modelling health-related performance indices. *Ann Hum Biol, 27*(6), 543-559.

Nevill, A., Tsiotra, G., Tsimeas, P. and Koutedakis, Y. (2009). Allometric associations between body size, shape, and physical performance of Greek children. [Comparative Study]. *Pediatr Exerc Sci, 21*(2), 220-232.

Olds, T., Tomkinson, G., Léger, L. and Cazorla, G. (2006). Worldwide variation in the performance of children and adolescents: an analysis of 109 studies of the 20-m shuttle run test in 37 countries. *J Sport Sci, 24*(10), 1025-1038.

Olshansky, S. J., Passaro, D. J., Hershow, R. C., Layden, J., Carnes, B. A., Brody, J., Hayflick, L., Butler, R. N., Allison, D. B. and Ludwig, D. S. (2005). A potential decline in life expectancy in the United States in the 21st century. *New Engl J Med, 352*(11), 1138-1145.

Ortega, F. B., Ruiz, J. R., Castillo, M. J. and Sjostrom, M. (2008). Physical fitness in childhood and adolescence: a powerful marker of health. *Int J Obes (Lond), 32*(1), 1-11.

Ortega, F. B., Ruiz, J. R., Mesa, J. L., Gutierrez, A. and Sjostrom, M. (2007). Cardiovascular fitness in adolescents: the influence of sexual maturation status-the AVENA and EYHS studies. *Am J Hum Biol, 19*(6), 801-808.

Özdirenç, M., Özcan, A., Akin, F. and Gelecek, N. (2005). Physical fitness in rural children compared with urban children in Turkey. *Pediatr Int, 47*(1), 26-31.

Pallant, J. (2010). *SPSS survival manual: A step by step guide to data analysis using SPSS*: McGraw-Hill International.

Pasic, M., Milanovic, I., Radisavljevic Janic, S., Jurak, R. J., Soric, M. and Mirkov, D. M. (2014). Physical activity levels and energy expenditure in urban Serbian adolescents--a preliminary study. *Nutr Hosp, 30*(5), 1044-1053.

Pfister, G. and Reeg, A. (2006). Fitness as 'social heritage': a study of elementary school pupils in Berlin. *Eur Phys Educ Rew, 12*(1), 5-29.

Plowman, S. A., Sterling, C. L., Corbin, C. B., Meredith, M. D., Welk, G. J. and Morrow Jr, J. R. (2006). The history of FITNESSGRAM® ESSGRAM. *Journal of Physical Activity and Health, 3*(2), S5-S20.

Radisavljević Janić, S, Milanović, I., Živković, M. and Mirkov, D. M. (2013). Prevalence of overweight and obesity among Belgrade youth: A study in a representative sample of 9–14-year-old children and adolescents. *Anthropological Notebooks XIX/III*, 71-80.

Radisavljević Janić, S., Milanović, I. and Lazarević, D. (2012). Fizička aktivnost adolescenata: uzrasne i polne razlike. *Nastava i vaspitanje*(1), 183-194.

Rampersaud, G. C., Pereira, M. A., Girard, B. L., Adams, J. and Metzl, J. D. (2005). Breakfast habits, nutritional status, body weight, and academic performance in children and adolescents. *J Am Diet Assoc, 105*(5), 743-760.

Reilly, J. J., Armstrong, J., Dorosty, A. R., Emmett, P. M., Ness, A., Rogers, I., Steer, C. and Sherriff, A. (2005). Early life risk factors for obesity in childhood: cohort study. *BMJ*.

Ribeiro, J., Guerra, S., Pinto, A., Oliveira, J., Duarte, J. and Mota, J. (2003). Overweight and obesity in children and adolescents: relationship with blood pressure, and physical activity. *Ann Hum Biol, 30*(2), 203-213.

Robinson, J. P. and Godbey, G. (1997). Time for Life: The Surprising Ways Americans Use Their Time. University Park PA: Pennsylvania State University.

Robinson, T. N. (1999). Reducing children's television viewing to prevent obesity: a randomized controlled trial. *JAMA, 282*(16), 1561-1567.

Ruiz, J. R., Castro-Piñero, J., España-Romero, V., Artero, E. G., Ortega, F. B., Cuenca, M. M., Jimenez-Pavón, D., Chillón, P., Girela-Rejón, M. J. and Mora, J. (2011). Field-based fitness assessment in young people: the ALPHA health-related fitness test battery for children and adolescents. *Br J Sport Med, 45*(6), 518-524.

Ruiz, J. R., Ortega, F. B., Gutierrez, A., Meusel, D., Sjöström, M. and Castillo, M. J. (2006). Health-related fitness assessment in childhood and adolescence: a European approach based on the AVENA, EYHS and HELENA studies. *J Public Health, 14*(5), 269-277.

Ruiz, J. R., Rizzo, N. S., Hurtig-Wennlöf, A., Ortega, F. B., Wärnberg, J. and Sjöström, M. (2006). Relations of total physical activity and intensity to fitness and fatness in children: the European Youth Heart Study. *Am J Clin Nutr, 84*(2), 299.

Sallis, J. F., McKenzie, T. L., Alcaraz, J. E., Kolody, B., Faucette, N. and Hovell, M. F. (1997). The effects of a 2-year physical education program (SPARK) on physical activity and fitness in elementary school students. Sports, Play and Active Recreation for Kids. *Am J Public Health, 87*(8), 1328-1334.

Sardinha, L. B., Santos, R., Vale, S., Silva, A. M., Ferreira, J. P., Raimundo, A. M., Moreira, H., Baptista, F. and Mota, J. (2011). Prevalence of overweight and obesity among Portuguese youth: A study in a representative sample of 10–18-year-old children and adolescents. *Int J Pediatr Obes, 6*(2Part2), e124-e128.

Schwartz, M. B. and Puhl, R. (2003). Childhood obesity: a societal problem to solve. *Obes Rev, 4*(1), 57-71.

Sjoberg, R. L., Nilsson, K. W. and Leppert, J. (2005). Obesity, shame, and depression in school-aged children: a population-based study. *Pediatrics, 116*(3), e389-392.

Tremblay, M. S., Shields, M., Laviolette, M., Craig, C. L., Janssen, I. and Connor Gorber, S. (2010). Fitness of Canadian children and youth: results from the 2007-2009 Canadian Health Measures Survey. *Health Rep, 21*(1), 7-20.

Tremblay, M.S., Shields, M., Laviolette, M., Craig, C.L., Janssen, I. and Connor Gorber, S. (2010). Fitness of Canadian children and youth: Results from the 2007-2009. *Health Rep, 21*(1), 7-20.

Tsimeas, P. D., Tsiokanos, A. L., Koutedakis, Y., Tsigilis, N. and Kellis, S. (2005). Does living in urban or rural settings affect aspects of physical fitness in children? An allometric approach. [Research Support, Non-U.S. Gov't]. *Br J Sport Med, 39*(9), 671-674.

Twisk, J. W., Kemper, H. C. and van Mechelen, W. (2002). The relationship between physical fitness and physical activity during adolescence and cardiovascular disease risk factors at adult age. The Amsterdam Growth and Health Longitudinal Study. *Int J Sports Med, 23* (Suppl 1), S8-14.

Vuorela, N., Saha, M. T. and Salo, M. K. (2011). Change in prevalence of overweight and obesity in Finnish children–comparison between 1974 and 2001. *Acta paediatrica, 100*(1), 109-115.

Živković, M., Stamenković, M. and Marković, M. (2013). Angažovanost dece u sportu na teritoriji grada Beograda. *Journal of the Antropological Society of Serbia, 48*, 129-136.

In: Physical Activity Effects on the Anthropological Status ...   ISBN: 978-1-63484-782-7
Editors: Fadilj Eminović and Milivoj Dopsaj   © 2016 Nova Science Publishers, Inc.

Chapter 3

THE EFFECT OF REGULAR SPORT EXERCISE ON MUSCLE CONTRACTILE PROPERTIES IN CHILDREN

Tadeja Volmut, Rado Pišot and Boštjan Šimunič[*]
University of Primorska, Science and Research Centre,
Koper, Slovenia

ABSTRACT

Regular physical exercise is important in many aspects of child health. There is limited 5-year or longer longitudinal studies on the effects of regular physical exercise on child health. Furthermore, there is no longitudinal study that on a yearly basis explored the skeletal muscle phenotype shift. Since 2011 tensiomyography has been proposed for non-invasive assessment of skeletal muscle contractile properties, and several studies have emerged for estimating its phenotype, therefore, this is the first one done in children. Therefore, we presented longitudinal data on contraction time (Tc) for two skeletal muscles (vastus lateralis – VL, and biceps femoris – BF) and sprinting velocity in 90 children (51% boys, aged 9-14 years) divided in two groups: (i) sporters, the ones regularly involved in organised sport activities (62%), and (ii) non-sporters, the ones that were not involved in any organised sport activity. We have found higher sprinting velocities in the groups of sporters for boys (from 12 to 14 years) and girls (from 9 to 14 years). We have also found preserved Tc in BF after the age of 12 years, while in non-sporters Tc BF increased. To confirm the link between Tc BF and sprinting velocity we found negative correlation in boys (r = -0.33; P < 0.05) and in girls (r = -0.46; P < 0.05); however, only after 14 years of age. To conclude, regular physical exercise has an effect on both sexes, predominantly on contractile properties of non-postural skeletal muscles that can be evident also in sprinting velocity.

Keywords: tensiomyography, physical activity, sprint, skeletal muscle, twitch

---

[*] Garibadlijeva 1, 6000 Koper, Slovenia, Email: bostjan.simunic@zrs.upr.si.

INTRODUCTION

As a result of global health trends, there is a growing interest in children's physical exercise. Physical exercise is important to many aspects of child health and development, where in children, the lack of physical activity is a risk factor for high blood pressure, weight gain, excess body fat, bad cholesterol, respiratory difficulties, cardiovascular diseases, and bone health problems (Janz et al., 2001; Reilly et al., 2006). Moreover, the health benefits of physical exercise extend well beyond physical health, having a positive impact on the domains of motor skills, psychological well-being, cognitive development, social competence, and emotional maturity (Hinkley et al., 2008).

Skeletal muscle is indispensable for locomotion where contractile speed and force of the muscle are important for muscle function. Muscle function and especially the speed of muscle contraction is largely determined by fibre type composition, where there are numerous data of growth and exercise related skeletal muscle composition proportions on adults and adolescents, few cross-sectional data on two months to 11-year old children's skeletal muscle composition (Bell, MacDougal, Billeter and Howald, 1980; Dahlström, Liljedahl, Gierup, Kaijser and Jansson, 1997; Kriketos et al., 1997; Lexell, Sjöström, Nordlund and Taylor, 1992; Lundberg, Eriksson and Mellgren, 1979; Österlund, Thornell and Eriksson, 2011), but only one longitudinal study that followed changes from childhood to adulthood (Glenmark, Hedberg and Jansson, 1992). Furthermore, only three studies followed the same skeletal muscle – vastus lateralis that allows us for the establishing developmental trends (Bell et al., 1980; Dahlström et al., 1997; Glenmark et al., 1992), and there is no data on physical exercise specific developmental trends.

The major reason for the above mentioned lack of studies is in invasiveness of procedures that are regularly used. Muscle composition is determined after invasive biopsies of muscle tissue. Furthermore, this consideration is even less ethical when one aim to obtain developmental or physical exercise specific trends in more than one muscle that is important to make conclusions on coherent posture, functional symmetries or coordinated motor development.

All these issues could be overcome by using non-invasive and selective method named Tensiomyography – TMG (Valenčič, 1990; Valenčič and Knez, 1997) that allows for indirect myosin heavy chain type I (MHC-I) estimation (Šimunič et al., 2011). Additionally, TMG amplitude gives us an important insight on muscle atrophic processes (Pišot et al., 2008), specifically on the muscle tone change prior an atrophy on anatomical level actually take place (Šimunič et al., 2008). MHC-I composition is determined using multiple linear model of contraction time (Tc), delay/latency time (Td), and half-relaxation time (Tr) calculated from TMG-response. Although the same labels are used for contractile times as in standard torque/force twitch responses, there is no correlation between TMG and torque twitch response contractile times (Koren et al., 2015). Figure 1 presents the principles of TMG assessment with the definition of contractile parameters.

Therefore, the objectives of our study were (i) to age-related and sex-related trends of Tc in vastus lateralis (VL) and biceps femoris (BF) in the groups of children that are involved in regular organised sport activities to those that are not; ii) for both groups to report maximal sprinting velocity and correlate sprinting velocity to tensiomyographic contraction time.

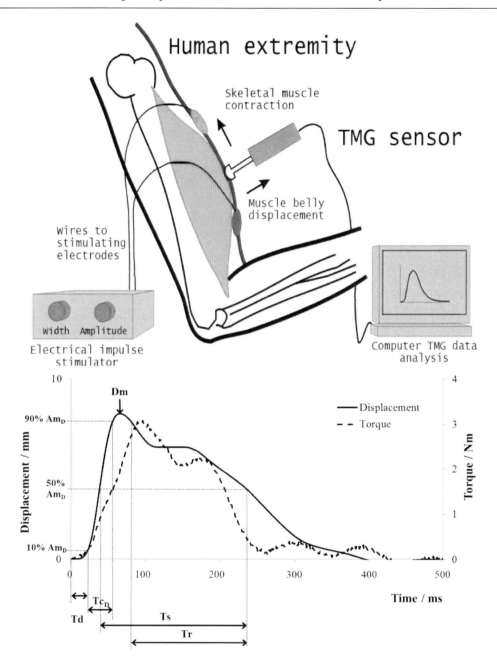

Figure 1. Principle of TMG assessment (upper graph). When twitch electrical impulse triggers muscle contraction a displacement sensor detects muscle belly displacement (adopted from Dahmane et al., 2001). A tensiomyographic twitch response (lower graph) is described by contractile parameters (Delay time – Td; Contraction time – Tc; Sustain time – Ts, Half-relaxation time – Tr; and Maximal displacement – Dm) that has nothing or little in common in comparison to the same parameters estimated from simultaneously assessed torque twitch response (Koren et al., 2015).

METHODS

Participants

The children (9 ± 0.5 years; n = 257) were initially included in the 5-year longitudinal study. None of the children had any history of neuromuscular disorders. Children were recruited from four randomly selected primary schools in three of the most populated regions of Slovenia. From those children, 90 were selected for this analysis, those who were involved in regular organized sport activities (more than 3 times per week) and those were not included in any regular sport activity during whole 5 years (Table 1). All participants and their parents were fully informed about the procedures and parents gave their written consents to participate in the study. All procedures conformed to the 1964 Declaration of Helsinki and were approved by the National Medical Ethics Committee of the Republic of Slovenia.

Table 1. Longitudinal descriptive anthropometric data of 90 children included in the study

	Age/years	Body height/cm		Body mass/kg	
		SPORT	NO SPORT	SPORT	NO SPORT
Boys (N = 46) $N_{NOSPORT}$ = 17 N_{SPORT} = 29	9.1 ± 0.5	140.9 ± 7.2	136.8 ± 5.3*	35.6 ± 7.7	34.2 ± 6.9
	9.9 ± 0.5	144.6 ± 7.6	140.6 ± 5.7	38.6 ± 8.9	37.4 ± 7.8
	10.6 ± 0.5	148.8 ± 7.9	145.1 ± 5.9	40.4 ± 9.5	38.9 ± 8.5
	12.0 ± 0.5	157.5 ± 8.7	154.2 ± 6.1	48.7 ± 10.7	48.1 ± 10.8
	12.9 ± 0.5	163.7 ± 9.1	160.4 ± 6.4	54.3 ± 12.3	53.5 ± 10.9
	13.6 ± 0.5	168.3 ± 9.0	165.7 ± 6.3	57.9 ± 12.1	56.1 ± 11.4
Girls (N = 44) $N_{NOSPORT}$ = 17 N_{SPORT} = 27	9.1 ± 0.5	142.1 ± 7.7	137.4 ± 6.1*	34.4 ± 6.9	30.7 ± 7.4
	9.9 ± 0.5	146.1 ± 8.1	141.0 ± 5.8*	37.9 ± 8.0	33.9 ± 8.0
	10.6 ± 0.5	151.0 ± 7.7	145.6 ± 6.6*	39.4 ± 8.1	35.7 ± 8.5
	12.0 ± 0.5	161.0 ± 6.8	155.9 ± 6.7*	48.1 ± 7.9	44.1 ± 11.1
	12.9 ± 0.5	165.0 ± 6.3	159.7 ± 5.8*	52.4 ± 8.4	49.5 ± 11.3
	13.6 ± 0.5	167.0 ± 5.8	160.5 ± 8.5*	54.2 ± 8.2	49.5 ± 10.0

SPORT – Group involved in regular sport activity; NO SPORT – Group not involved in organized any sport activity; * – significantly different from SPORT group at $P < 0.05$.

Study Design

We performed six longitudinal measurements on children who progressed from the third to the eighth primary school grade. Follow-up measurements took place yearly. At every measurement, we followed the same procedure. One week before each measurement, we notified each school and asked them to follow a specific protocol; no major physical or sport activity should be performed 2 days before the measurement and all children had to be available for the measurements. In each child, we first measured body height and mass, followed by TMG measurements and a short questionnaire.

Testing Procedures

Tensiomyographic Assessments

TMG measurements were done in the VL and BF and took approximately 10 minutes. In all cases, TMG was performed on the muscles of the dominant leg. The measurements on the VL were performed supine at 30° knee flexion, where 0° represents an extended joint. The measurements on the BF were performed prone at 5° knee flexion.

Foam pads were used for leg support and straps were used to assure isometric conditions. All muscles were relaxed before and after the measurement (twitch contraction). The oscillations of the muscle belly in response to an electrically-induced twitch were recorded on the skin surface using a sensitive displacement sensor (TMG–BMC, Slovenia). The sensor was set perpendicular to the skin overlying the muscle belly: in VL at 30% of femur length above the patella on the lateral side; in BF at the midpoint of the line between the fibula head and the ischial tuberosity.

To elicit a twitch contraction we applied a single 1-ms pulse through the self-adhesive cathode and anode that were placed 5 cm distally and 5 cm proximally to the measuring point, respectively. The stimulation current at the start was just above the contraction threshold and was then gradually increased until the response amplitude did not increase further. If needed, the measuring point, sensor inclination, and electrode positions were adjusted to obtain the maximal response amplitude. Two maximal twitch responses were recorded and saved. Those children who found electric stimulation disturbing were not forced to undergo the measurement.

From every twitch response the maximal displacement amplitude (Dm), and contraction time (Tc) were calculated as proposed by Valenčič (1990), Valenčič and Knez (1997). The Dm (in mm) was defined as the peak amplitude in the displacement-time curve of the TMG twitch response. Contraction time (in ms) was the time between 10% and 90% Dm. The average value of these parameters extracted from two twitch responses was used for further analysis.

Sport Participation Assessment

A short questionnaire was used to obtain information about the out-of-school sport participation of the children. Boys and girls were divided into two groups; sporters (SPORT) and nosporters (NONSPORT). Sporters were members of sport clubs with at least three hours per week of organized exercise (e.g., football, basketball, volleyball, handball, athletics – jumps, sprints, and throws, etc.), consistent over the 5 years. Children that were not members of sport clubs during a 5-year period and did not perform regular organized exercise were nosporters. Following these criteria 17 boys and 17 girls were nosporters and 29 boys and 27 girls were sporters. A comparison was performed for VL and BF muscles. Furthermore, we extrapolated our data in both groups with TMG data in the adult population (Šimunič, 2012), sprinters (Praprotnik et al., 2001), dancers (Zagorc et al., 2010), volleyball players (Rodríguez Ruiz et al., 2011), football players (Rey et al., 2012) and sport gymnasts (Šimunič and Samardžija Pavletič, 2015).

Maximal Sprinting Velocity

Was measured in a gym, using wireless photocells (Brower Timing Systems Ltd., USA) over 7 meter distance, and 15 meters of flying start. All children passed 15 minutes of standardized warm up, with two warm-up sprints. Afterwards children passed three test sprints, where the one with highest sprinting velocity was taken for further analysis.

Statistics

All data are expressed as means ± standard deviation. For all variables the hypothesis of a normal distribution was tested with visual inspection and the Shapiro-Wilk's test. The effects of sport on sprinting velocity a 3-way repeated measures analysis of variance was used with age (6) as within factor and gender (2) and sport (2) as between factor. The effect of sport on the Tc of the VL and BF a three-way repeated measures analysis of variance was used, with age (6) and muscle (2) as within factors and sport (2) as between factor. We excluded 3-way interactions in the analysis. The correlation between Tc and sprinting velocity was performed using Pearson correlation coefficient. Statistical significance was accepted at P < .05 level.

RESULTS

The growth of children was normal, following general trends reported by Rogol, Clark and Roemmich (2000). Both boys and girls showed a progressive increase in body height (P < .001) and body mass (P < .001). The age x sex interactions for body height (P < .001) and body mass (P = .028) are reflected by a larger increase in body height and body mass in boys than girls in the 5-year period (Table 1).

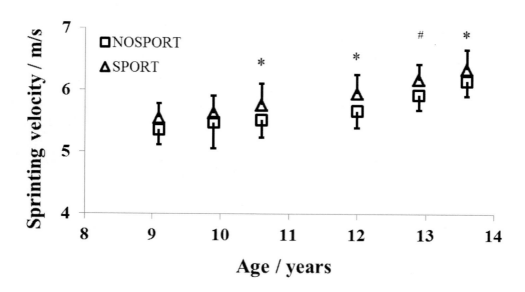

Figure 2. (Continued).

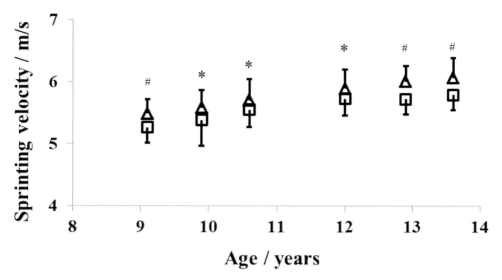

* – significantly different between both groups at P < 0.05; # – significantly different between both groups at P < 0.01.

Figure 2. Sprinting velocity in boys (upper graph) and girls (lower graph): differences between sporters (SPORT) and nonsporters (NO SPORT).

Sprinting velocity increased with age (P < 0.001) in boys and girls (Figure 2), with no interaction age x sex effect. Boys' sporters have higher sprinting velocity from age of 10.6 years than non-sporters, while girls' sporters have higher sprinting velocity from age of 9.1 years than non-sporters.

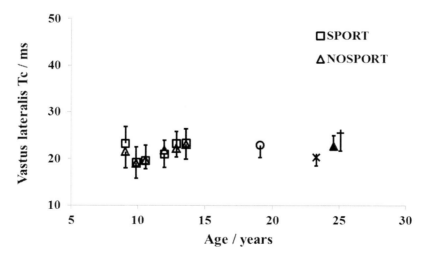

Figure 3. (Continued).

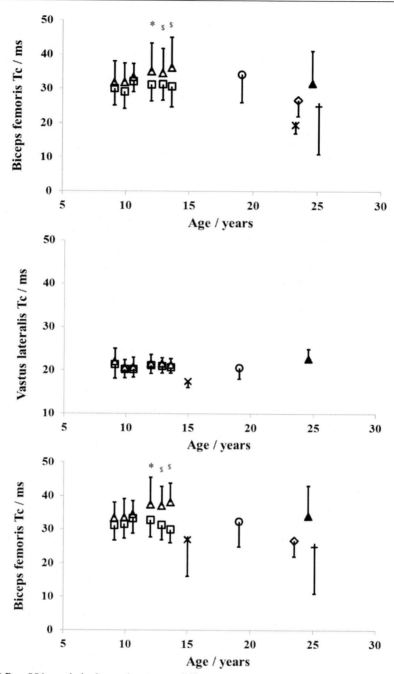

* P < .05; $ P < .001: statistical sport/non sport differences.

Figure 3. Age and sport-participation effects on contraction time (Tc) in the vastus lateralis muscle (A, B) and biceps femoris muscle (C, D) of boys (A, C) and girls (B, D). For comparison, published data of adult boys: non-athletes '▲' (Šimunič, 2012), sprinters '*' (Praprotnik et al., 2001), dancers 'o' (Zagorc et al., 2010), volleyball players '+' (Rodríguez Ruiz et al., 2011), and football players '◊' (Rey et al., 2012) are also shown. And for girls, published data of adult girls: non-athletes '▲' (Šimunič, 2012), sport gymnasts '*' (Šimunič and Samardžija Pavletič, 2015), dancers 'o' (Zagorc et al., 2010) are also shown.

A three-way ANOVA revealed an effect of age (P = .004; η^2 = .086), muscle (P < .001; η^2 = .914), age x sport (P = .011; η^2 = .074), and muscle x sport interactions (P = .002; η^2 = .209) on Tc. Post hoc analysis revealed that in the BF Tc was longer in non-sporters than sporters older than 12 years. For comparison with other populations we have also illustrated data of others in adult non-athletes, sprinters, dancers, volleyball players, and football players (Šimunič, 2012; Praprotnik et al., 2001; Zagorc et al., 2010; Ruiz Rodriguez et al., 2011; Rey et al., 2012).

We have found significant correlation between sprinting velocity and BF Tc only at the age of 13.6 years (Figure 4; in boys r = -0.33; in girls r = -0.46; both P < 0.05); although at an early age also a non-significant negative correlation exists. There was no correlation between sprinting velocity and VL Tc.

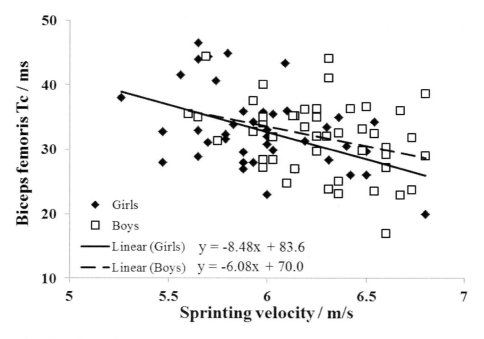

Figure 4. A linear correlation between sprinting velocity and biceps femoris contraction time (Tc) at the age of 13.6 years.

DISCUSSION

Our longitudinal study contributed an insight into children's skeletal muscle development, focusing on skeletal muscle composition. Using a non-invasive TMG, we assessed muscle composition related contractile parameter (Tc) in two skeletal muscles. Although there were initially 263 children included in the study, a representative subsample of 90 children (34%) were selected for this study and all 90 were present in all six measurements. Skeletal muscle composition is very difficult, if not even ethically impossible, to measure in healthy children. Therefore, using a non-invasive approach we presented age- and gender-related longitudinal trends in Tc in two skeletal muscles.

The main finding of our study is that Tc, a TMG parameter linearly related to MHC-1 proportion (Šimunič et al., 2011), increases with age in BF from 12 years. The magnitude of the increase differed between both muscles, where in VL no significant increase was found. Furthermore, higher BF Tc increase was evident in girls more than in boys. A similar situation was seen in adult track and field sprinters where sport participation resulted in an increased proportion of type 2c fibres in the BF, which was also associated with a reduction in Tc (19.5 vs. 30.25ms, in sprinters vs. sedentary) (Dahmane et al., 2006). It could be that the load on weight bearing muscles from normal daily physical activities in children is already relatively high in non-sporters and that in particular the non-weight bearing muscles get challenged more during sport participation. If so, this may explain the larger adaptation to regular exercise in the BF than the VL. When we compare this with specific adult populations we see that fast-explosive sports (e.g., sprints, gymnastics, volley-ballers) have faster BF Tc; however, in the trend line in further children Tc development. It thus appears that participating in sport as a child may result in a faster profile of the BF and better baseline for further sport participation.

We also found that sprinting velocity increases with age and that this increase differs between sporters and non-sporters. While in boys difference occurs after the age of 10.6 years, in girls difference occurs in all age span, starting from 9 years. For both genders, sporters have higher sprinting velocity. Boys achieve higher sprinting velocity than girls after the age of 12 years in both groups.

Interestingly, we found a negative correlation between Tc and sprinting velocity only in BF muscle and only after 13.6 years of age. However, this study has showed no correlation between VL Tc and sprinting velocity, which is quite logical since the fact that VL muscle is not the core muscle for achieving the maximal sprinting velocity. Negative correlation between BF Tc and sprinting velocity found only at age of 13.6 years is comparable in both sexes (boys: -0.33; females: -0.46) and is significantly lower than in adult male professional sprinters -0.6 (Praprotnik et al., 2002). This could be explained with less mastered sprinting technique in children in comparison to professional sprinters. The role of BF (and other hamstring muscles) is to perform hip extension that is the primary joint movement during sprinting. Due to its important role grouping with high physical loads the muscle is regularly reported as the most injured muscle in various sports that require sprinting such as soccer (Arnason et al., 2004), rugby (Brooks et al., 2006), track and field (Askling et al., 2007). For hamstring injuries in sprinting sports, the location of the injury is most commonly in the long head of the BF muscle (Askling et al., 2007; Verrall et al., 2003; Connell et al., 2004; Slavotinek et al., 2002) and the reason is that the BF muscle is required to exert more force, relative to the other two hamstring muscles, during a lengthening muscle contraction (Dolman et al., 2014).

CONCLUSION

This study has demonstrated that children that are regularly participating in sport activities at 9 to 13.6 years of age have shorter BF Tc, but not VL Tc, and have higher sprinting velocity. Furthermore, sprinting velocity has been found to correlate to BF Tc; however, only at 13.6 years of age.

STUDY LIMITATIONS

The multiple linear model for estimating the VL MHC-1 proportion from three mechanical (TMG) three twitch parameters (Equation 1; Šimunič et al., 2011) was developed on 27 participants aged between 20 and 83 years. Here we used it to examine our sample of children from 9.1 to 13.6 years of age. Although this approach has not been validated in children, there are no obvious reasons to believe that it would not equally well apply to muscles of children.

REFERENCES

Arnason, A, Sigurdsson, S. B., Gudmundsson, A., Holme, I., Engebretsen, L. and Bahr, R. (2004). Risk factors for injuries in football. *American Journal of Sports Medicine, 32(1S),* 5S–16S.

Askling, C. M., Tengvar, M., Saartok, T. and Thorstensson, A. (2007). Acute first-time hamstring strains during high speed running: a longitudinal study using clinical and magnetic resonance imaging findings. *American Journal of Sports Medicine, 35(2),* 197–206.

Bell, R. D., MacDougal, J. D., Billeter, R. and Howald, H. (1980). Muscle fibre types and morphometric analysis of skeletal muscle in six-year-old children. *Medicine and Science in Sports and Exercise, 12(1),* 28–31.

Brooks, J. H., Fuller, C. W., Kemp, S. P. and Reddin, D. B. (2006). Incidence, risk and prevention of hamsting injury in professional rugby union. *American Journal of Sports Medicine, 34(8),* 1297–1306.

Connell, D. A., Schneider-Kolsky, M. E., Hoving, J. L., Malara, F., Buchbinder, R., Koulouris, G., Burke, F. and Bass, C. (2004). Longitudanal study comparing sonographic and MRI assessment of acute and healing hamstring injuries. *American Journal of Roentgenology, 183(4),* 975–984.

Dahlström, M., Liljedahl, M. E., Gierup, J., Kaijser, L. and Jansson, E. (1997). High proportion of type I fibres in thigh muscle of young dancers. *Acta Physiologica Scandinavica, 160(1),* 49–55.

Dahmane, R., Djordjević, S. and Smerdu, V. (2006). Adaptive potential of human biceps femoris muscle demonstrated by histochemical, immunohistochemical and mechanomyographical methods. *Medical and Biological Engineering and Computing, 44(11),* 999–1006.

Dolman, B., Verrall, G. and Reid, I. (2014). Physical principles demonstrate that the biceps femoris muscle relative to the other hamstring muscles exerts the most force: implications for hamstring muscle strain injuries. *Muscles Ligaments Tendons Journal, 4(3),* 371–377.

Glenmark, B., Hedberg, G. and Jansson, E. (1992). Changes in muscle fibre type from adolescence to adulthood in women and men. *Acta Physiologica Scandinavica, 146(2),* 251–259.

Hinkley, T., Crawford, D., Salmon, J., Okely, A. D. and Hesketh, K. (2008). Preschool children and physical activity: A review of correlates. *American Journal of Preventive Medicine, 34(5),* 435–441.

Janz, K. F., Burns, T. L., Torner, J. C., Levy, S. M., Paulos, R., Willing, M. C. and Warren, J. J. (2001). Physical activity and bone measures in young children: The Iowa bone development study. *Pediatrics, 107(6)*, 1387.

Koren, K., Šimunič, B., Rejc, E., Lazzer, S. and Pišot, R. (2015). Differences between skeletal muscle contractile parameters estimated from transversal tensiomyographic and longitudinal torque twitch response. *Kinesiology, 47(1)*, 19–26.

Kriketos, A. D., Baur, L. A., O'Connor, J., Carey, D., King, S., Caterson, I. D. and Storlien, L. H. (1997). Muscle fibre type composition in infant and adult populations and relationships with obesity. *International Journal of Obesity and Related Metabolic Disorders, 21(9)*, 796–801.

Lexell, J., Sjöström, M., Nordlund, A. S. and Taylor, C. C. (1992). Growth and development of human muscle: a quantitative morphological study of whole vastus lateralis from childhood to adult age. *Muscle and Nerve, 15(3)*, 404–409.

Lundberg, A., Eriksson, B. O. and Mellgren, G. (1979). Metabolic substrates, muscle fibre composition and size in late walking and normal children. *European Journal of Pediatrics, 130(2)*, 79–92.

Österlund, C., Thornell, L. E. and Eriksson, P. O. (2011). Differences in fibre type composition between human masseter and biceps muscles in young and adults reveal unique masseter fibre type growth pattern. *The Anatomical Record (Hoboken), 294(7)*, 1158–1169.

Pišot, R., Narici, M. V., Šimunič, B., De Boer, M., Seynnes, O., Jurdana, M., Biolo, G. and Mekjavić, I. B. (2008). Whole muscle contractile parameters and thickness loss during 35-day bed rest. *European Journal of Applied Physiology, 104(2)*, 409–414.

Praprotnik, U., Valenčič, V., Čoh, M. and Šimunič, B. (2001). Maximum running velocity is related to contraction time of muscle biceps femoris. In B. Donne and N. J. Mahoney (Eds.), Proceedings of the International Sports Medicine Conference (pp. 189–190). Dublin, Ireland: Trinity College Dublin.

Reilly, J. J., Kelly, L., Montgomery, C., Williamson, A., Fisher, A., McColl, J. H., Lo Conte, R., Paton, J. Y. and Grant, S. (2006). Physical activity to prevent obesity in young children: Cluster randomised controlled trial. *British Medical Journal, 333(7577)*, 1041–1043.

Rey, E., Lago-Peñas, C., Lago-Ballesteros, J. and Casáis, L. (2012). The effect of recovery strategies on contractile properties using tensiomyography and perceived muscle soreness in professional soccer players. *The Journal of Strength and Conditioning Research, 26(11)*, 3081–3088.

Rodríguez Ruiz, D., Quiroga Escudero, M. E., Rodríguez Matoso, D., Sarmiento Montesdeoca, S., Losa Reyna, J., de Saá Guerra, Y, Bautista, G. P. and García Manso, J. M. (2011). The tensiomyography used for evaluating high level beach volleyball players. *Revista Brasileira de Medicina do Esporte, 18(2)*, 95–99.

Slavotinek, J. P., Verrall, G. M. and Fon, G. T. (2002). Hamstring injury in athletes: the association between MR measurements of the extent of muscle injury and the amount of time lost from competition. *American Journal of Roentgenology, 179*, 1621–1628.

Šimunič, B., Degens, H., Rittweger, J., Narici, M. V., Mekjavić, I. B. and Pišot, R. (2011). Noninvasive estimation of myosin heavy chain composition in human skeletal muscle. *Medicine and Science in Sports and Exercise, 43(9)*, 1619–1625.

Šimunič, B. (2012). Between-day reliability of a method for non-invasive estimation of muscle composition. *Journal of Electromyography and Kinesiology, 22(4)*, 527–530.

Šimunič, B., Rittweger, J., Cankar, G., Jurdana, M., Volmut, T., Šetina, T., Mekjavić, I. B. and Pišot, R. (2008). Changes in body composition, muscle stiffness and postural stability occurring in healthy young men submitted to a 35-day bed rest. *Slovenian Journal of Public Health, 47(2)*, 60–71.

Šimunič, B. and Samardžija Pavletič, M. (2015). Sport-related differences in contractile parameters: a gymnasts have shortest contraction time in brachial muscles and vastus lateralis. In M. Samardžija Pavletič and M. Bučar Pajek (Eds.). Book of abstracts and book of proceedings (pp. 53). Ljubljana, Slovenia, Slovenian Gymnastics Federation.

Valenčič, V. (1990). Direct measurement of the skeletal muscle tonus. In: D. Popovič (Ed.), Advances in external control of human extremities (pp. 102–108). Beograd: Nauka.

Valenčič, V. and Knez, N. (1997). Measuring of skeletal muscles' dynamic properties. *Artificial Organs, 21(3)*, 240–242.

Verrall, G. M., Slavotinek, J. P., Barnes, P. G. and Fon, G. T. (2003). Diagnostic and prognostic value of clinical findings in 83 athletes with posterior thigh injury. Comparison of clinical findings with magnetic resonance imaging documentation of hamstring muscle strain. *American Journal of Sports Medicine, 31(6)*, 69–973.

Zagorc, M., Šimunič, B., Pišot, R. and Oreb, G. (2010). A comparison of contractile parameters among twelve skeletal muscles of inter-dance couples. *Kinesiology, 16(3)*, 57–65.

In: Physical Activity Effects on the Anthropological Status …   ISBN: 978-1-63484-782-7
Editors: Fadilj Eminović and Milivoj Dopsaj   © 2016 Nova Science Publishers, Inc.

Chapter 4

TREND CHANGES IN PHYSICAL FITNESS IN CHILDREN OF ELEMENTARY SCHOOL AGE – TRANSVERSAL MODEL

Jelena Ivanović and Aco Gajević[*]
Serbian Institute for Sport and Sports Medicine, Belgrade, Serbia

ABSTRACT

The growing concern in society for the health of children and young people has directed the work of research scientists towards identifying the condition and state of development for physical abilities. This is aimed at achieving better, i.e., top level results in sport, but also to the function of assessing health, improving the quality of physical education, and increasing motivation among young people where involvement in physical activity is concerned. This may be especially useful given the lifestyle trends prevalent in so-called developed countries. The primary aim is to identify trends in terms of changes concerning physical abilities among children, with a view to reestablishing and improving the system that's in place, as well as monitoring methods in our schools. This paper presents a comparative study of the transversal type involving children aged 7 to 14, extracted from the population of elementary school pupils. The total sample of examinees was 839 pupils (424 boys and 415 girls) measured in 2014, and 878 students (456 boys and 422 girls) measured in 2009. All students were measured using a Eurofit Test Battery with the same procedures and equipment as prescribed by the Commission for Sport Development of the Council of Europe. On a general level, ANOVA linear regression analysis determined the statistically significant difference for the level of the male and female sample between the observed subsamples with respect to trend changes in all studied characteristics at the level of $F = 208.178$, $p = 0.000$ and $F = 197.900$, $p = 0.000$ in the examinees measured in 2009, and at the level of $F = 222.865$, $p = 0.000$ and $F = 179.934$, $p = 0.000$ in the examinees measured in 2014. At the level of the total sample in the function of age testing and trend changes, the results showed a tendency of change for the observed characteristics of physical fitness in relation to the initial stratum in both samples (boys and girls) measured in 2009. Regarding the results obtained using a comparative analysis of current testing and previous research, at a general level it can be

---

[*] Corresponding Author Email: aco.gajevic@rzsport.gov.rs.

concluded that children from our primary schools are still recording results which indicate that physical fitness does not adequately follow physical development.

Keywords: children of primary school age, physical fitness, Eurofit test battery

INTRODUCTION

The more frequent presence of obesity in children, as well as the question of (un)suitable physical activity, is to a large extent a result of the modern lifestyle, i.e., fewer opportunities or requirements for walking and motion, as well as poorer health conditions, including those that relate to nutrition. Mechanically adopting a sedentary lifestyle due to industrial development and the influence of science and technology has detracted not only from the engagement of the larger muscle groups, but it has also resulted in minimum levels of stimulus for providing the normal function of the vital systems. The modern lifestyle among both the urban and rural populations, has brought about a characteristic phenomenon, one which is manifested by reduced motion and habitual activities. This phenomenon, defined as hypokinesis, brings with it many disadvantages. The main characteristics can be recognised in terms of the specific, negative adaptation of the human body, mainly with regard to diminished physical abilities, i.e., to a diminished level of physical-working capabilities among individuals (Booth, 2000; Vuori, 2004; Wilsgaard et al., 2005). This diminished level of physical ability, coupled with poor posture among children, can mean that physical education classes in schools often involve the only exercise children get.

Based on numerous pieces of research (WHO, 2013), under the influence of these factors and increased levels of pollution, health conditions in general and in children can be characterised by a significant increase in so-called chronic-noncommunicable conditions and diseases of the modern civilisation – high blood pressure, cardiovascular diseases, diabetes, osteoporosis, and so on. These increases are mainly caused by a greater number of instances where individuals are overweight, and in some countries this problem has reached epidemic proportions. The hypokinesis phenomenon, the poor nutrition that causes obesity, and high levels of stress involving nervous tension and physical and social exhaustion, are the primary causes of a phenomenon defined as a the "triple syndrome," which is cited as the most common cause of health problems and death in the modern human (Vuori, 2004; Tomkinson, 2007; Kallings et al., 2008).

Physical ability is defined as the ability of a human to perform a physical act (each body motion as a result of muscle activity and which, as a consequence, involves greater energy consumption in the human body) and is positively connected with health quality and longevity. In developed countries, the issue of this (low) level of physical ability as a consequence of the modern lifestyle has been raised on both the national and global level. From the aspect of general social benefits, good levels of physical ability, which brings with it a positive influence on health, also possesses enormous social and economic potential. Good health (as in a state of physical, psychological, and social prosperity) contributes in the following ways:

- It becomes easier to achieve pedagogic goals and sports results in children;
- An increase in positive indicators when it comes to the general workforce, our armed forces, and those of an age to reproduce.
- A decrease in expenditure on medical treatment.

In this sense, the physical ability of an individual, in all its developmental stages, from childhood to old age, is a factor contributing to success and quality life and work, and as such it must be thought of as both a personal and species-wide social issue.

The subject of this study is to explore the space of the basic motor, or physical abilities in children of school age (7 to 14 years) in the Municipality of Čukarica, measured in 2014.

The primary aim, based on a conducted pilot survey in children of school age in the Belgrade Municipality of Čukarica, is to gain an insight into the situation and to identify trends for changes related to physical abilities among children, in order to reestablish and improve the system in place, and the monitoring methods in our schools.

METHODS

Participants

The research presents a comparative study of the transversal type involving children aged 7 to 14, extracted from the population of elementary school children in the Belgrade Municipality of Čukarica.

The first group of examinees, measured in 2014, consisted of a sample which was extracted from a population of pupils from five elementary schools. The total sample of examinees was 839 students (424 boys and 415 girls). Thus defined, the sample was distributed among eight subsamples in boys and eight subsamples in girls. The criteria for the distribution of subsamples were years of age, with rounding to ±6 months, which provided the following subsamples in both genders: 7, 8, 9, 10, 11, 12, 13 and 14 years.

The second group consisted of pupils from the Municipality of Čukarica extracted from five elementary schools. The sample of this group, measured in 2009, consisted of 878 students (456 boys and 422 girls) and was distributed in the same manner as the sample from 2014.

The study involved only healthy pupils. Criteria for absence from testing were identical to those for exemption from physical education classes. In addition, the analysis results excluded all pupils who, for some reason, had not completed all the tests (illness, injury, etc).

The survey was conducted within a project monitoring physical fitness in children of school age in the Republic of Serbia (the proposed aim of which was to help bring about a general interest in sport; no. 01-3635, from 21.7.2010, Gajević 2010), and which was conducted by means of cooperation between the Institute for Sport and Sports Medicine of the Republic of Serbia, the Ministry of Education and the Ministry of Youth and Sports, on the basis of Memorandum of Understanding no. 01-265 45P-02-218/09-11, from 02.2.2009, which was signed by the Director of the Institute, the Minister of Youth and Sports and the Minister of Education.

Testing Procedure

All students were measured using a Eurofit Test Battery, as well as the same procedures and equipment prescribed by the Commission for Sport Development of the Council of Europe (Council of Europe, 1993). Data collection involved physical fitness testing and anthropometric measurements.

Muscular endurance is the ability of a muscle group to execute repeated contractions over time or to maintain a maximal voluntary contraction for a prolonged period of time. The endurance strength (functional strength) of the upper body was measured using a Bent Arm Hang Test (BAH), which determines the maximum length of time a subject can remain suspended by the arms from a bar.

Trunk strength (i.e., abdominal muscular endurance) was assessed using a Sit-Ups Test (SUP) completed within half a minute. The total number of completed sit-ups performed within 30 s was counted.

Handgrip strength refers to the maximal isometric force that can be generated mainly by the hand and a forehand muscle (upper limb) involved in performing the handgrip, and was assessed with a Handgrip Test (HGR).

Lower limb explosive strength was assessed using a Standing Broad Jump Test (SBJ). The explosive strength developed by the legs from a standing position was recorded as the maximum horizontal distance covered by jumping with the feet together.

Mobility of the trunk and hips was assessed using the Sit-and-Reach Test (SAR), which is a reflection of overall flexibility. Flexibility was measured in the sitting position with feet placed flat against a box and the fingertips placed on the edge of the top plate. The subject attempted to reach forward as far as possible, keeping his or her knees straight, without jerking and with hands stretched out. The maximum distance reached with the fingers when bending forward while sitting on the floor was recorded.

Speed testing covered the assessment of speed of movement/agility and speed of limb movement. Speed of movement/agility was assessed using a 10x5m Shuttle Run Test (SHR). This test assessed the subjects' speed of movement, agility and coordination in an integrated fashion. The subjects run back and forth five times along a 10-m track at the highest speed possible. Therefore, the test permitted measurement not only of speed of displacement, but also of agility and coordination.

The Plate Tapping Test (PLT) assessed the speed and coordination of limb movement. Two discs are placed with their centres 60 cm apart on the table. The subject moved the preferred hand back and forth between the discs, and over the hand in the middle, as quickly as possible. This action was repeated for 25 full cycles (50 taps).

The Flamingo Balance Test assessed the ability to balance successfully on one leg. The subject stood on a beam (a metal beam 50cm long, 5cm high, and 3cm wide) with shoes removed. The number of falls in 60 s of balancing was recorded.

Statistics

All the results were processed with the application of descriptive statistics and the tendency for changes in observed characteristics in the function of age was afterwards defined by applying the linear regression method, using the general equation: $y = ab^x$ (Hair et al.,

1998). All statistical analysis was accomplished by applying the SPSS for Windows software package, Release 16.0 (Copyright © SPSS Inc., 1989–2002).

RESULTS

Trend Change of Monitored Characteristics Compared According to Years of Testing

Tables 1 and 2 show mean values of observed characteristics and the results of the defined functions of the linear regression equation regarding the age for estimating the observed characteristics of physical fitness in male and female pupils.

Trend Change

ANOVA linear regression analysis determined the statistically significant difference at the level of the male sample between the observed subsamples with respect to trend changes in all studied characteristics at the level of $F = 208.178$, $p = 0.000$ in the examinees measured in 2009 and at the level of $F = 222.865$, $p = 0.000$ in the examinees measured in 2014.

Table 3 shows the results of ANOVA linear regression analysis on the partial level for all the observed indicators of physical abilities in relation to the measurements from 2009 and 2014 in male students. ANOVA linear regression analysis determined general statistically significant difference at the level of the female sample between the observed subsample in regard to trend changes, in all examined characteristics at the level of $F = 197.900$, $p = 0.000$, in female examinees measured in 2009 and at the level of $F = 179.934$, $p = 0.000$ in female examinees measured in 2014.

Table 4 shows the results of ANOVA linear regression analysis on the partial level for all the observed indicators of physical abilities in relation to measurements in 2009 and 2014 for female pupils.

The results showed that the trend for change in the Flamingo Balance Test (Table 3, 4 and Graph 1) showed a statistically significant growth of body balance in girls measured in 2014 and in boys measured in 2009 as follows:

- In boys measured in 2009 – 0.38 attempts at establishing balance in 60 seconds of negative growth annually, compared to the period of eight years, at the level of significance $p = 0.010$,
- In boys measured in 2014 – 0.55 attempts at establishing balance in 60 seconds of positive growth annually, compared to the period of eight years, at the level of significance $p = 0.237$,
- In girls measured in 2009 – 0.49 attempts at establishing balance in 60 seconds of negative growth annually compared to the period of eight years, at the level of significance $p = 0.628$,
- In girls measured in 2014 – 1.22 attempts at establishing balance in 60 seconds of positive growth annually, compared to the period of eight years, at the level of significance $p = 0.024$.

Table 1. Results of the defined functions of the linear regression equation in males

		7 years (N = 117)	8 years (N = 109)	9 years (N = 117)	10 years (N = 107)	11 years (N = 106)	12 years (N = 108)	13 years (N = 111)	14 years (N = 105)
FLB (n)	2014	11.67	16.96	16.43	15.88	15.56	18.00	16.66	15.55
		$y = 0.357x + 14.23$; with estimating reliability at the level of 21.93% $R^2 = 0.2193$							
	2009	15.82	21.49	16.95	16.97	17.54	17.14	14.34	13.18
		$y = 0.632x + 19.52$; with estimating reliability at the level of 39.31% $R^2 = 0.3931$							
PLT (s/25n)	2014	19.787	16.510	16.356	14.196	13.570	12.482	12.029	11.180
		$y = 1.129x + 19.59$; with estimating reliability at the level of 93.08% $R^2 = 0.9308$							
	2009	21.321	17.369	16.098	16.981	13.354	12.751	11.981	10.977
		$y = 1.345x + 21.15$; with estimating reliability at the level of 90.86% $R^2 = 0.9086$							
SAR (cm)	2014	14.34	13.20	13.54	11.50	14.22	10.61	13.32	18.92
		$y = 0.316x + 12.28$; with estimating reliability at the level of 9.85% $R^2 = 0.0985$							
	2009	14.02	15.54	15.33	15.22	13.68	15.49	15.26	17.73
		$y = 0.280x + 14.02$; with estimating reliability at the level of 32.09% $R^2 = 0.3209$							
SBJ (cm)	2014	110.20	117.72	128.02	139.45	147.52	153.10	190.03	191.63
		$y = 12.08x + 92.84$; with estimating reliability at the level of 94.18% $R^2 = 0.9418$							
	2009	103.61	121.51	127.03	135.52	148.07	166.47	174.70	188.13
		$y = 11.76x + 92.67$; with estimating reliability at the level of 98.79% $R^2 = 0.9879$							
HGR (kg)	2014	14.70	14.61	16.60	19.07	22.93	25.99	34.70	39.61
		$y = 3.653x + 7.088$; with estimating reliability at the level of 91.10% $R^2 = 0.9110$							
	2009	14.27	16.66	20.87	22.81	25.61	30.28	34.21	41.61
		$y = 3.692x + 9.174$; with estimating reliability at the level of 96.97% $R^2 = 0.9697$							
SUP (n/30s)	2014	14.13	16.84	15.26	18.84	21.10	22.43	22.57	24.59
		$y = 1.495x + 12.73$; with estimating reliability at the level of 93.21% $R^2 = 0.9321$							
	2009	13.18	16.78	19.10	19.50	22.36	23.56	23.77	24.45
		$y = 1.548x + 13.36$; with estimating reliability at the level of 92.16% $R^2 = 0.9216$							
BAH (s)	2014	3.900	3.932	7.309	5.994	10.184	8.529	15.291	24.845
		$y = 2.515x + 1.319$; with estimating reliability at the level of 76.37% $R^2 = 0.7637$							
	2009	4.009	8.208	7.693	8.466	8.170	12.446	15.296	21.043
		$y = 2.007x + 1.632$; with estimating reliability at the level of 83.57% $R^2 = 0.8357$							
SHR (s)	2014	23.433	23.010	22.171	20.849	20.286	20.763	19.126	18.969
		$y = 0.660x + 24.04$; with estimating reliability at the level of 93.82% $R^2 = 0.9382$							
	2009	26.550	25.554	23.762	23.338	21.682	22.282	20.694	20.646
		$y = 0.853x + 26.90$; with estimating reliability at the level of 93.07% $R^2 = 0.9307$							

Table 2. Results of the defined functions of the linear regression equation in female

		7 years (N = 114)	8 years (N = 110)	9 years (N = 119)	10 years (N = 106)	11 years (N = 111)	12 years (N = 95)	13 years (N = 92)	14 years (N = 90)
FLB (n)	2014	9.24	12.90	17.43	17.09	14.21	13.57	17.95	17.75
		$y = 0.837x + 11.24$; with estimating reliability at the level of 44.10% $R^2 = 0.4410$							
	2009	19.80	21.48	19.80	17.96	18.91	17.67	15.17	16.36
		$y = 0.727x + 21.66$; with estimating reliability at the level of 76.61% $R^2 = 0.7661$							
PLT (s/25n)	2014	19.886	16.845	15.747	14.667	13.916	12.190	12.539	11.905
		$y = 1.057x + 19.47$; with estimating reliability at the level of 90.32% $R^2 = 0.9032$							
	2009	20.666	17.548	20.666	14.522	13.939	12.678	12.250	11.920
		$y = 1.336x + 21.53$; with estimating reliability at the level of 81.27% $R^2 = 0.8127$							
SAR (cm)	2014	17.64	17.73	17.67	16.99	19.61	18.67	22.26	21.51
		$y = 0.6596x + 16.044$; with estimating reliability at the level of 68.40% $R^2 = 0.6840$							
	2009	19.61	19.10	19.61	18.02	19.26	20.37	21.89	24.22
		$y = 0.5926x + 17.592$; with estimating reliability at the level of 55.51% $R^2 = 0.5551$							
SBJ (cm)	2014	101.61	110.17	117.25	132.38	134.93	138.27	149.26	150.35
		$y = 7.169x + 97.01$; with estimating reliability at the level of 96.33% $R^2 = 0.9633$							
	2009	101.18	105.17	101.18	123.92	133.69	146.13	152.31	146.62
		$y = 8.314x + 88.86$; with estimating reliability at the level of 89.29% $R^2 = 0.8929$							
HGR (kg)	2014	12.38	13.23	14.80	18.17	21.41	24.45	30.19	29.62
		$y = 2.828x + 7.801$; with estimating reliability at the level of 96.00% $R^2 = 0.9600$							
	2009	13.98	14.92	13.98	21.92	23.30	27.39	28.81	32.38
		$y = 2.855x + 9.237$; with estimating reliability at the level of 94.19% $R^2 = 0.9419$							
SUP (n/30s)	2014	13.41	15.76	14.00	17.56	19.91	19.17	20.45	20.48
		$y = 1.080x + 12.73$; with estimating reliability at the level of 84.38% $R^2 = 0.8438$							
	2009	14.66	15.48	14.66	17.73	19.39	19.65	20.41	21.30
		$y = 1.044x + 13.20$; with estimating reliability at the level of 91.65% $R^2 = 0.9165$							
BAH (s)	2014	2.805	2.528	5.183	5.727	5.555	3.220	7.271	7.508
		$y = 0.602x + 2.265$; with estimating reliability at the level of 57.65% $R^2 = 0.5765$							
	2009	2.823	4.454	2.823	5.976	5.194	6.933	6.344	6.624
		$y = 0.566x + 2.596$; with estimating reliability at the level of 71.85% $R^2 = 0.7185$							
SHR (s)	2014	25.112	24.064	23.995	22.380	22.605	21.153	20.368	20.603
		$y = 0.694x + 25.66$; with estimating reliability at the level of 94.34% $R^2 = 0.9434$							
	2009	26.666	26.519	26.666	24.741	23.807	22.802	22.654	22.750
		$y = 0.705x + 27.75$; with estimating reliability at the level of 89.70% $R^2 = 0.8970$							

Table 3. Results of linear regression analysis regarding the observed characteristics in male pupils in relation to year of measurement

	2009		2014	
	t value	p sig.	t value	p sig.
Flamingo Balance (n)	-2.576	0.010	1.184	0.237
Plate Tapping (s/25n)	-1.964	0.050	-4.517	0.000
Sit-and-Reach (cm)	-1.024	0.306	-1.777	0.076
Standing Broad Jump (cm)	5.184	0.000	3.348	0.001
Handgrip (kg)	0.387	0.699	-0.802	0.423
Sit-Ups (n/30s)	3.758	0.000	2.306	0.022
Bent Arm Hang (s)	-0.081	0.936	1.947	0.052
Shuttle Run (s)	-1.700	0.090	-1.340	0.181

Table 4. Results of linear regression analysis regarding the observed characteristics in female students in relation to year of measurement

	2009		2014	
	t value	p sig.	t value	p sig.
Flamingo Balance (n)	-0.485	0.628	2.260	0.024
Plate Tapping (s/25n)	-4.929	0.000	-4.503	0.000
Sit-and-Reach (cm)	0.252	0.801	0.743	0.458
Standing Broad Jump (cm)	0.404	0.687	0.142	0.887
Handgrip (kg)	3.698	0.000	3.053	0.002
Sit-Ups (n/30s)	-0.254	0.800	1.600	0.110
Bent Arm Hang (s)	1.095	0.274	2.961	0.003
Shuttle Run (s)	0.296	0.767	-1.443	0.150

The results showed that the trend for change in the Plate Tapping Test (Table 3, 4 and Graph 1) had statistically significant growth in speed of movement as follows:

- In boys measured in 2009 – 1.48 s needed for performing 25 regular cycles of growth, on an annual basis compared to the period of eight years, at the level of significance $p = 0.050$,
- In boys measured in 2014 – 1.23 s needed for performing 25 regular cycles of growth, on an annual basis compared to the period of eight years, at the level of significance $p = 0.000$,
- In girls measured in 2009 – 1.25 s needed for performing 25 regular cycles of growth, on an annual basis compared to the period of eight years $p = 0.000$,
- In girls measured in 2014 – 1.14 s needed for performing 25 regular cycles of growth, on an annual basis compared to the period of eight years, at the level of significance $p = 0.000$.

The results showed that the trend for change in the Sit-and-Reach Test (Table 3, 4 and Graph 1) revealed no statistically significant growth in hip joint flexibility as follows:

- In boys measured in 2009 – 0.53 cm of growth, on an annual basis compared to the period of eight years, at the level of significance p = 0.306,
- In boys measured in 2014 – 0.65 cm of growth, on an annual basis compared to the period of eight years, at the level of significance p = 0.076,
- In girls measured in 2009 – 0.66 cm of growth, on an annual basis compared to the period of eight years, at the level of significance p = 0.801,
- In girls measured in 2014 – 0.55 cm of growth, on an annual basis compared to the period of eight years, at the level of significance p = 0.458.

The results showed that the trend for change in the Standing Broad Jump Test (Table 3, 4 and Graph 1) revealed statistically significant growth in leg muscles explosive force only in boys, as follows:

- In boys measured in 2009 – 12.07 cm of positive growth, on an annual basis compared to the period of eight years, at the significance level p = 0.000,
- In boys measured in 2014 – 11.63 cm of positive growth, on an annual basis compared to the period of eight years, at the significance level p = 0.001,
- In girls measured in 2009 – 6.49 cm of positive growth, on an annual basis compared to the period of eight years, at the significance level p = 0.687,
- In girls measured in 2014 – 6.96 cm of positive growth, on an annual basis compared to the period of eight years, at the significance level p = 0.887.

The results showed that the trend for change in the Handgrip Test (Table 3, 4 and Graph 1) revealed statistically significant growth in dominant hand isometric force only in girls, as follows:

- In boys measured in 2009 – 3.91 kg of positive growth of muscle force, on an annual basis compared to the period of eight years, at the level of significance p = 0.699,
- In boys measured in 2014 – 3.56 kg of positive growth of muscle force, on an annual basis compared to the period of eight years, at the level of significance p = 0.423,
- In girls measured in 2009 – 2.63 kg of positive growth of muscle force, on an annual basis compared to the period of eight years, at the level of significance p = 0.000,
- In girls measured in 2014 – 2.46 kg of positive growth of muscle force, on an annual basis compared to the period of eight years, at the level of significance p = 0.002.

The results showed that the trend for change in the Sit-Ups Test (Table 3, 4 and Graph 1) revealed statistically significant growth in repetitive trunk force and hip flexors force only in boys, as follows:

- In boys measured in 2009 – growth of 1.61 raising the upper body into the sitting position from the prone position, which is achieved in 30 seconds, on an annual basis, compared to the period of eight years, at the level of significance p = 0.000,
- In boys measured in 2014 – growth of 1.49 raising the upper body into the sitting position from the prone position, which is achieved in 30 seconds, on an annual basis, compared to the period of eight years, at the level of significance p = 0.022,

- In girls measured in 2009 – growth of 0.95 raising the upper body into the sitting position from the prone position, which is achieved in 30 seconds, on an annual basis, compared to the period of eight years, at the level of significance $p = 0.800$,
- In girls measured in 2014 – growth of 1.01 raising the upper body into the sitting position from the prone position, which is achieved in 30 seconds, on an annual basis, compared to the period of eight years, at the level of significance $p = 0.110$.

The results showed that the trend for change in the Bent Arm Hang Test (Table 3, 4 and Graph 1) revealed statistically significant growth in static hand muscle force and shoulder girdle force only in girls, as follows:

- In boys measured in 2009 – 2.43 s of growth on an annual basis compared to the period of eight years, at the level of significance $p = 0.936$,
- In boys measured in 2014 – 2.99 s of growth on an annual basis compared to the period of eight years, at the level of significance $p = 0.052$,
- In girls measured in 2009 – 0.54 s of growth on an annual basis compared to the period of eight years, at the level of significance $p = 0.274$,
- In girls measured in 2014 – 0.67 s of growth on an annual basis compared to the period of eight years, at the level of significance $p = 0.003$.

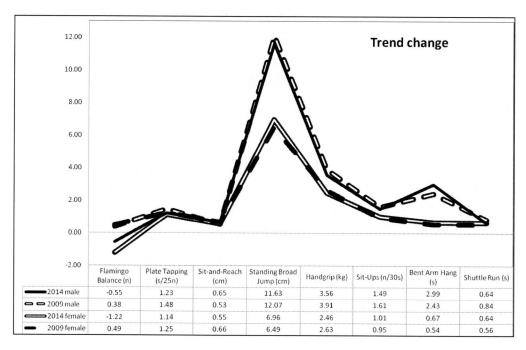

	Flamingo Balance (n)	Plate Tapping (s/25n)	Sit-and-Reach (cm)	Standing Broad Jump (cm)	Handgrip (kg)	Sit-Ups (n/30s)	Bent Arm Hang (s)	Shuttle Run (s)
2014 male	-0.55	1.23	0.65	11.63	3.56	1.49	2.99	0.64
2009 male	0.38	1.48	0.53	12.07	3.91	1.61	2.43	0.84
2014 female	-1.22	1.14	0.55	6.96	2.46	1.01	0.67	0.64
2009 female	0.49	1.25	0.66	6.49	2.63	0.95	0.54	0.56

Graph 1. Trend changes in observed characteristics.

The results showed that the trend for change in the Shuttle Run Test (Table 3, 4 and Graph 1) revealed no statistically significant growth in static hand muscle force and shoulder girdle force only in girls, as follows:

- In boys measured in 2009 – 0.84 s of growth on an annual basis compared to the period of eight years, at the level of significance p = 0.090,
- In boys measured in 2014 – 0.64 s of growth on an annual basis compared to the period of eight years, at the level of significance p = 0.181,
- In girls measured in 2009 – 0.56 s of growth on an annual basis compared to the period of eight years, at the level of significance p = 0.767,
- In girls measured in 2014 – 0.64 s of growth on an annual basis compared to the period of eight years, at the level of significance p = 0.150.

DISCUSSION

Today, data related to physical abilities among children and young people is collected worldwide, by means of various systems. It is considered and scientifically proven (Sauka et al., 2011; Keane et al., 2010; Ivanović et al., 2013) that the level of physical fitness is an excellent indicator of health among children and adolescents, and that continuously monitoring and controlling levels of physical fitness should be considered a public health priority.

In the existing System for monitoring the status of physical development and physical abilities in children of school age in the Republic of Serbia (7 to 14 years of age) which has been conducted by means of a continuous scientific and operational project in the Institute for Sport and Sports Medicine of the Republic of Serbia, data obtained in recent years has established a tendency for growth in certain morphological indicators, and a consistent decline for certain physical capabilities (Gajević, 2009). In other words – the same negative trend has become established here as in the other parts of the world (Westerstahl et al., 2003; Vuori, 2004; Serbescu et al, 2006; Tomkinson, 2007). The results of extensive research in Slovenia, with the "Longitudinal comparison of the development of certain physical characteristics and motor abilities in two generations of children and the young population, aged 7 to 18, in Slovenian primary and secondary schools in the period from 1990-2001 and 1997-2008" (Strel et al., 2009), show that body weight among students has increased by 4%, and the amount of subcutaneously fat by 13%. Negative changes were detected in motor efficiency: in terms of muscular endurance in the area of the shoulders and hands, results have declined by 15%, and in terms of flexibility by 15%. On the other hand, in comparison with the results of other international studies, the Slovenian research revealed a positive trend for trunk muscle endurance of 6% (a result of the so-called "cult of beautiful bodies" espoused as a result of television and other media, and promoting home exercise and the use of various new devices designed for the purpose). It was concluded that, in addition to adequate professional and technical conditions for engaging in sports and physical activities in Slovenia, it is still necessary to improve and promote an active lifestyle, to increase physical activity and promote healthy eating habits at the global and state level. Also, Slovenian scientists believe that the extremely rapid increase in negative effects on levels of fitness among young Slovenes could be halted if two hours instead of the formerly recommended one hour of physical activity were practiced each day, adapted to the needs and interests of the various children involved. (Strel et al., 2009).

Certainly the importance of the Eurofit Test Battery lies mainly in its ability to assess health status and physical ability among children of school age (Michaud et al., 1999; Deforche et al., 2003; Ekblom et al., 2005; Eminović and Gajević, 2011; Sauka et al., 2011), which is its main function. As already stated in the introduction, the question of rising obesity levels in children as well as (in)appropriate physical ability is recognised as an important issue. Despite all the efforts, 2 to 3 classes of physical education cannot fully satisfy the need for physical activity, a fact which has led a large number of experts to join the fight against obesity (Ivanović and Gajević, 2013). A group of Greek authors (Christodoulos et al., 2006) concluded that an additional 30 minutes of physical activity every day would be an excellent way to prevent obesity. These conclusions were based on research conducted on a sample of 178 children of school age. Morphological characteristics, with special attention to obese children, as well as physical ability, were monitored during the school year and after children returned from their summer holidays. Ahmedov and his associates (Ahmedov et al., 2006) attempted to explain the issue of obesity, and the causes behind its origins in relation to physical fitness. In the course of their research they monitored children aged 9 to 11 from different regions in Cyprus. The study comprised 7425 children and the obtained results showed that children from rural areas possess a higher level of physical fitness compared to their peers from urban parts of the state. They also demonstrated a smaller share of fat mass within overall body mass.

In order to differentiate between physical abilities and activities among children with obesity issues and those who have no such problems, Deforche and his associates (Deforche et al., 2003) tested 3214 Flemish children. It was found that those who were overweight achieved lower scores in all the tests that involved manipulating their own body weight, but generally did not fall behind other children with regard to the values of the fitness index. One possible conclusion based on these results, was that there was a need to adapt physical activity programmes to the abilities of obese children. In many countries around the world, as well as here at home, schools attach enormous importance to their physical education programmes, as these are seen to involve not just physical fitness, but overall development among young people. Physical education programmes are seen to involve mental development in children, i.e., health in the general sense, proper physical growth, optimal physical abilities, physical education social values such as self-discipline, responsibility, fair play and a high level of tolerance for diversity. Basically, physical education can be said to be one of the most important tools for social integration (Hardman, 2009).

However, physical education objectives and programmes are often a source of conflict, owing to the situation faced by many schools, whereby a lack of funds is often an obstacle to the provision of organised training courses; facilities in schools and at the local level are often inadequate and insufficiently equipped, and programme content is often maladjusted. Research from Ivanović (Ivanović et al., 2009) indicated that awareness among physical education teachers regarding this topic is poor. Most certainly, the appropriate and permanent training of personnel, professional-advisory assistance and greater supervision in the implementation of programmes could contribute more to the planned physical training exercise programmes. For this reason, several papers have been aimed at examining, among others issues, the effectiveness of physical education. Koutedakis and Bouziotas (2003) divided a sample of 84 boys of secondary school age into two groups: one experimental (this group was involved in extra-curricular physical activities 3 times per week) and one control. As expected, the control group, which did not engage in additional activities, demonstrated poorer health. The authors concluded that the National Plan does not meet the needs of health status improvement in children, and that it must be reviewed and appropriately modified.

With respect to the observed characteristics of physical ability at the level of the total sample in the function of age testing and trend changes, the results showed:

Generally, a tendency of change was observed and recognised for the characteristics of physical fitness in relation to the initial stratum sample of boys measured in 2009. At this point the given tendency can be quantified using the following values of directions and intensity changes:

- Trend change for the ability to establish body balance is *0,93 attempts* to establish balance in 60 seconds, a *reduction* in comparison to the observed stratum in 2009, which represents *an improvement in results*,
- Trend change in speed of movement is *0,25* seconds less for performing 25 regular cycles in comparison to the observed stratum in 2009, which represents *an improvement in results*,
- Trend change of mobility in the hip joint showed an 0.12 cm increase in comparison to the observed stratum in 2009, which represents *an improvement in results*,
- The trend of leg extensors explosive force changed by 0.44 cm, a deterioration in comparison to the observed stratum in 2009, which represents *a deterioration in results*,
- The trend of flexor isometric force for the dominant hand changed by 0.35 kg, a decrease in comparison to the observed stratum in 2009, which represents *a deterioration in results*,
- The trend for repetitive muscle force for abdominal and flexor muscles in the hip joint changed by 0.12 for lifting the upper body into the sitting position from the prone position, which is achieved in 30 seconds in comparison to the observed stratum in 2009, which represents *a deterioration in results*,
- The trend for the static force of the arm and shoulder muscles changed by 0.56 seconds, an improvement in comparison to the observed stratum in 2009, which represents *an improvement in results*,
- The trend for speed changed by 0.20 seconds, an improvement in comparison to the observed stratum in 2009, which represents *an improvement in results*.

Generally, a tendency of change was observed and recognised for the characteristics of physical fitness in relation to the initial stratum sample of girls measured in 2009. At this point the given tendency can be quantified using the following values of directions and intensity changes:

- Trend change for the ability to establish body balance is *0,93 attempts* to establish balance in 60 seconds, a *reduction* in comparison to the observed stratum in 2009, which represents *an improvement in results*,
- Trend change for speed of movement is *0.11* seconds less for performing 25 regular cycles in comparison to the observed stratum in 2009, which represents *an improvement in results*,

- Trend change of mobility in the hip joint is an 0.11 cm decrease in comparison to the observed stratum in 2009, which represents *a deterioration in results,*
- The positive trend of leg extensors explosive force changed by 0.50 cm in comparison to the observed stratum in 2009, which represents *an improvement in results,*
- The trend of flexor isometric force for the dominant hand changed by 0.17 kg, a decrease in comparison to the observed stratum in 2009, which represents *a deterioration in results,*
- The trend for repetitive muscle force for the abdominal and flexor muscles in the hip joint changed by 0.06 for lifting the upper body into the sitting position from the prone position, which is achieved in 30 seconds in comparison to the observed stratum in 2009, which represents *an improvement in results,*
- The trend for the static force of arm and shoulder muscles changed by 0.13 seconds, an improvement in comparison to the observed stratum in 2009, which represents *an improvement in results,*
- The trend for speed changed by 0.08 seconds, a decrease in comparison to the observed stratum in 2009, which represents *a deterioration in results.*

CONCLUSION

At this point, based on current research and a comparative analysis of the test results obtained in 2009 and 2014, the precise reason for the determined differences and trend changes for the characteristics of physical fitness in children of primary school age cannot be assessed. This is not possible owing to a combination of numerous factors that were not covered in the course of this research, for example:

- Number of physical education classes,
- The structure and efficiency of the physical education programme,
- Extra-curricular physical activities,
- Other social or personal factors.

For the purpose of general application of the obtained results, it is necessary to conduct extensive research that will include an examination of the aforementioned factors.

Regarding the results obtained using a comparative analysis of current testing and previous research, at a general level it can be concluded that children from our primary schools are still recording results which indicate that physical fitness fails to follow physical development adequately. The measures to be taken in order to improve the physical fitness of children should on one hand focus on increasing the efficiency of physical education in schools (the number of hours, improved conditions, availability of school facilities for use, a precise programme and its implementation from the 1st grade of elementary school, increasing the number of extra-curricular physical activities, and so on), and on the other hand improving measures relating to the community and providing better conditions for sport.

Understanding and becoming acquainted with physical abilities is only one part of physical education, which is in turn one part of general education. Physical ability among children is a reflection of their lifestyles. If the inactive lifestyle and inadequate nutrition are to be ignored by the family, the community and the media, attempts to solve the problem of rising obesity in children and the issue of (in)appropriate physical abilities will fail. Thus, physical ability is a concern that is equally important for children, parents, physical education teachers and, ultimately, society in general. Society should generally become more involved and interested in the physical status and abilities of children. This would facilitate and contribute to developing a positive attitude towards the body, leading individuals to become more involved in physical activities and thus to be additionally motivated to maintain or improve the status of their physical fitness. This is especially important in the context of modern life trends.

REFERENCES

Ahmedov, S., Emiroglu, O., Atamtürk, H., Burgul, C., Tinazci, C. (2006). Level of physical fitness among young Turkish Cypriot population. *The 11th Annual Congress of the European College of Sport Science International Congress Proceedings*, July 5-8, Lausanne, Swutzerland: ECSS, (pp.135).

Booth, M. (2000). Assessment of physical activity: An international perspective. *Research Quarterly for Exercise and Sport, 71(2),* 114-120.

Christodoulos, A., Flouris, A., Tokmakidis, S. (2006). Obesity and physical fitness of pre-adolescent children during the academic year and the summer period: effects of organized physical activity. *Journal of Child Health Care, 10,* 199-212.

Council of Europe, Committee of Experts on Sports Research. (1993). *EUROFIT: Handbook for the EUROFIT tests of physical fitness (2nd ed.).* Strasbourg: Council of Europe.

Deforche, B., Lefevre, J., De Bourdeaudhuij, I., et al. (2003). Physical fitness and physical activity in obese and nonobese flemish youth. The North American Association for the Study of Obesity. *Obesity Research, 11,* 434-441.

Ekblom, O., Oddsson, K., Ekblom, B. (2005). Physical performance and body mass index in Swedish children and adolescents. *Scandinavia Journal of Nutrition, 49(4),* 172-179.

Eminović, F., Gajević, A. (2011). Differences in physical development and physical fitness in children of school age. *I International scientific conference of Special education and rehabilitation.* Belgrade: Faculty for Special education and rehabilitation.

Gajević, A. (2009). *Physical development and physical fitness in children of school age.* Belgrade: Serbian Institute for sport (in Serbian).

Gajević, A. (2010). *Monitoring the physical fitness in children of school age in the Republic of Serbia.* Project, Serbian Institute for sport, Belgrade (in Serbian).

Hair, J., Anderson, R., Tatham, R., Black, W. *Multivariate Data Analysis (Fifth Ed.).* (1998). New Jersey, USA: Prentice - Hall, Inc.

Hardman, K. (2009). Elected issues, challenges and resolutions in physical education. *International scientific conference "Theoretical methodology and methodical aspects of physical education."* Faculty of sport and physical education, University of Belgrade. (pp. 11-20).

Ivanović, J., Dragojević, M., Karalić, B., Milenković, T. (2009). The information habits in pedagogues of physical culture. *International scientific conference "Theoretical methodology and methodical aspects of physical education.*" Faculty of sport and physical education, University of Belgrade. (pp.120).

Ivanović, J., Gajević, A. (2013). Monitoring the physical fitness in children of school age. *First national fitness conference.* Belgrade: Serbian institute for sport and sports medicine.

Ivanović, J., Gajević, A., Badnjarević, N. (2013). Changes in speed, agility and endurance in football players regarding different age categories – transversal model. *8th FIEP European Congress "Physical Education and Sports Perspective of Children and Youth in Europe"* from August 29th to September 1st 2013, Bratislava, Slovakia.

Kallings, L.V., Leijon, M., Hellénius, M.L., Ståhle, A. (2008). Physical activity on prescription in primary health care: a follow-up of physical activity level and quality of life. *Scandinavian Journal of Medicine and Science in Sports, 18,* 154-161.

Keane, A., Scott, M.A., Dugdill, L., Reilly, T. (2010). Fitness test profiles as determined by the Eurofit Test Battery in elite female Gaelic football players. *Journal of Strength and Conditioning Research, 24(6),* 1502-6.

Koutedakis, Y., Bouziotas, C. (2003). National physical education curriculum: motor and cardiovascular health related fitness in Greek adolescents. *British Journal of Sports Medicine, 37,* 311- 4.

Michaud, P., Narring, F., Cauderay, M., et al. (1999). Sports activity, physical activity and fitness of 9- to 19-year-old teenagers in the canton of Vaud (Switzerland). *Schweizerische medizinische Wochenschrift, 129,* 691-99.

Sauka, M., Priedite, I.S., Artjuhova, L., Larins, V., Selga, G., Dahlström, O., Timpka T. (2011). Physical fitness in northern European youth: reference values from the Latvian Physical Health in Youth Study. *Scandinavian Journal of Public Health, 39(1),* 35-43.

Serbescu, C., Flora, D., Hantiu, I., et al. (2006). Effect of a six month training programme on the physical capacities of Romanian schoolchildren. *Acta Paediatrica, 95,* 1258–65.

Strel, J., Bizjak, K., Starc, G., Kovač, M. (2009). Longitudinal comparison of development of certain physical characteristics and motor abilities of two generations of children and youth, aged 7 to 18, in Slovenian primary and secondary schools in the period 1990-2001 and 1997-2008. *International scientific conference "Theoretical methodology and methodical aspects of physical education."* Faculty of sport and physical education, University of Belgrade. (pp.26).

Tomkinson, G. R. (2007). Global changes in anaerobic fitness test performance of children and adolescents (1958-2003). *Scandinavian Journal of Medicine and Science in Sports, 17,* 497-507.

Vuori, I. (2004). Physical inactivity is a cause and physical activity is a remedy for major public health problems. *Kinesiology, 36(2),* 123-153.

Westerstahl, M., Barnekow-Bergkvist, M., Hedberg, G., Jansson, E. (2003). Secular trends in body dimensions and physical fitness among adolescents in Sweden from 1974 to 1995. *Scandinavian Journal of Medicine and Science in sports, 13,* 128-137.

Wilsgaard, T., Jacobsen, B.K., Arnesen, E. (2005). Determining lifestyle correlates of body mass index using multilevel analyses: The Tromsø study, 1979-2001. *American Journal of Epidemiology, 162(12),* 1-10.

www.who.int/gho/ncd/risk_factors/overweight/en/index.html.

Chapter 5

THE EFFECTS OF LINEAR AND CHANGE-OF-DIRECTION SPEED TRAINING ON THE SPRINT PERFORMANCE OF YOUNG ADULTS

Robert Lockie[*]

California State University, Department of Kinesiology, Northridge, CA, US

ABSTRACT

Individuals from a range of different sports require linear and change-of-direction (COD) speed. Linear speed incorporates the ability to maximally run in a straight line. COD speed involves the ability to decelerate, stop and cut, and reaccelerate in a new direction. These capacities are specific, in that the ability to run fast in a straight line does not always translate to faster COD speed. There are a number of important technique characteristics specific to linear and COD speed that must be understood by strength and conditioning coaches and sport and exercise practitioners prior to training program implementation. Following this, there are a range of training protocols that can be used to enhance linear and COD speed in young adults. There are some similarities in the modalities utilized for both linear and COD speed, as most training modalities target some type of technique, force, or power adaptation. Coaches should be aware of how force and power are expressed within these training modalities, and how this could then be transferred to linear and COD speed. Free sprinting typically forms the basis for linear speed training. When training for linear speed, it is important that the distances used (acceleration is approximately the first 15 meters of a maximal sprint; maximum velocity is typically attained within 30-60 meters) during training are specific to the individual's requirements. Additional protocols such as resistance or strength training, plyometrics, resisted sprinting, and assisted sprinting have also been utilized to enhance linear speed. COD speed requires different technical movements to linear sprinting, such as the ability to cut from each leg. Strength training and plyometrics can also be used to develop strength and power specific to COD speed. A variety of COD drills have been used in training to develop COD speed, with deceleration training being one novel training variation. If a coach or practitioner has knowledge of the individual's training

---

[*] Corresponding Author, Email: robert.lockie@csun.edu.

background, their sport, and can appropriately implement different training modalities, they will be able to enhance the linear and COD speed for their athletes.

Keywords: sprinting, planned agility, resistance training, power, strength and conditioning

INTRODUCTION

Speed is an essential quality for many individuals. This includes not only track athletes competing in the sprint events (e.g., 100 meters [m] and 200 m), but also athletes from a range of field and court sports. Field sports include soccer, American and Australian football, rugby union and league, and field hockey. Basketball, netball, European handball, and racket sports (e.g., tennis, squash, and badminton) are all court sports. Although all of these athletes have a reliance on speed, the sprint distances covered during match-play are sport-specific. Furthermore, athletes from field and court sports will be required to change direction while sprinting. As a result, change-of-direction (COD) speed becomes another important physical capacity for these athletes. Strength and conditioning coaches must be aware that linear and COD speed are different physical capacities, and must be trained specifically.

This chapter will define both linear and COD speed. The technique characteristics of linear and COD speed will be described, as it is these factors that will be manipulated during training. A review of the different training practices used to enhance linear and COD speed will be presented. How these training protocols influence the technical characteristics of linear and COD speed will be investigated, and practical information will be documented for the strength and conditioning coach and exercise practitioner.

LINEAR SPEED DEFINED

Linear speed is as the name suggests; the ability to generate a high velocity in a straight line without changes of direction. There are several components to a maximal sprint. A velocity curve produced from a 100 m sprint provides a good example of this (Figure 1). A sprint velocity curve is a fundamental signature of human motion. The shape of this curve will essentially be the same for any individual starting from a stationary position – only the magnitudes of the values will change. A maximal 100 m sprint is characterized by an initial period of acceleration which involves a great increase in velocity from the initiation of movement, with the most pronounced period of acceleration occurring over the first 15 m (Delecluse, 1997; Majumdar and Robergs, 2011). Following this period of acceleration, the sprinter will attain their maximum velocity. Once maximal velocity is reached, the sprinter will attempt to maintain this speed for as long as possible; this is referred to as speed endurance (Delecluse, 1997; van Ingen Schenau et al., 1994).

In many sports, the ability to reach a high sprinting velocity is very important, as high velocities contribute to faster sprint performances. Evidence of this is provided by elite male sprinters, who can attain peak velocities in excess of 11-12 meters per second (m·s^{-1}) (Majumdar and Robergs, 2011; Slawinski et al., 2010). While most field or court sport athletes may not attain as great a sprinting velocity as this, many can still reach a high speed appropriate for their sport. For example, elite rugby union players (Duthie et al., 2006), and Australian rules footballers (Benton, 2001) can achieve peak velocities of 8-9 m·s⁻¹ in a linear maximal sprint.

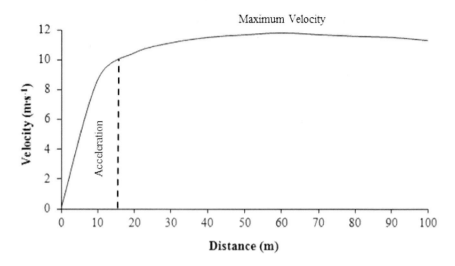

Figure 1. Sprint velocity curve of an elite sprinter, highlighting the phases of acceleration and maximum velocity. Velocity is measured in meters per second (m·s⁻¹); distance is measured in meters (m). Adapted from Müller and Hommel (1997).

Track sprinters will tend to reach peak velocity in the 40-60 m range of a 100 m sprint (Müller and Hommel, 1997; Slawinski et al., 2010; Majumdar and Robergs, 2011). However, acceleration distances as long as this are often not practical for field or court sport athletes. These athletes do not attain maximum velocity very frequently during a match, as the nature of these sports generally does not allow participants to cover the distance required to attain peak speed (Young et al., 1995). For example, in Australian football (Dawson et al., 2004), rugby union (Deutsch et al., 2007; Docherty et al., 1988), and soccer (Bangsbo et al., 1991; Krustrup et al., 2005; Reilly and Vaughan, 1976), the mean duration of a linear sprint during a match is approximately two seconds. Sprints of this short a duration will not allow for the attainment of peak velocity, particularly if starting from a stationary position. Benton (2001) suggests that to make full use of their speed, field sport athletes should try and reach their maximum velocity as soon as possible. As a result, athletes from team sports, such as male rugby union players (Duthie et al., 2006) and female soccer players (Vescovi, 2012), attain their peak velocity after approximately 30 m of a maximal sprint. Nevertheless, attaining a high sprint velocity, especially over a short distance, can be an important contributor to successful team sport performance.

TECHNICAL FACTORS IMPORTANT TO LINEAR SPEED

The Sprinting Gait

The sprinting gait cycle has been divided into two phases; the stance and swing phases (Gittoes and Wilson, 2010). The stance phase is the period in which the contact or drive leg is in contact with the ground. This phase can be further sub-divided into foot-strike and toe-off (Hinrichs, 1992). The swing or recovery phase occurs when the leg is airborne just prior to the contralateral limb contacting the ground (Gittoes and Wilson, 2010). As the running action is cyclic, when one leg is in the stance phase, the other leg is completing the swing phase. Due to variations between individuals, there may be no single, ideal sprinting technique (Unitas and Dintiman, 1979). Nonetheless, the investigation of sprint technique can still demonstrate changes over time as a result of training. It is important for the strength and conditioning practitioner to understand the technical components of sprinting, as it is these factors that can be manipulated to enhance linear speed.

Step Kinematics

Sprinting velocity is the product of step length and step frequency (Donati, 1995; Hunter et al., 2004). In order to improve sprint performance, there must be an increase in one or both of these factors. Step length is the distance between alternating contacts of the left and right feet, and is reliant on the force produced by the leg in contact with the ground (Hunter et al., 2004; Lockie et al., 2013c). Stride length is the distance between successive contacts of the same foot (i.e., left foot to left foot contact, and right foot to right foot contact), and is typically twice the distance of step length (Webster and Roberts, 2011). Step frequency is the rate that each step can be reproduced, and this is dependent on the neural firing rate within the muscles of the lower limbs (Donati, 1995; Gottschall and Palmer, 2002). Both of these variables will increase with a rise in sprint velocity (Mann and Hagy, 1980). During acceleration, there has been research that has demonstrated the value of having both a longer step length (Callaghan et al., 2014; Callaghan et al., 2015; Lockie et al., 2014b; Lockie et al., 2013b; Lockie et al., 2013c) and higher step frequency (Hewit et al., 2013; Lockie et al., 2011; Murphy et al., 2003). As running speed surpasses 7 m·s^{-1}, however, step length will plateau (Luhtanen and Komi, 1978; Kuitunen et al., 2002). This means any further increases in sprint velocity are dependent on step frequency (Young et al., 2001a), and a high step frequency is a technical characteristic of elite sprinters at maximum velocity (Čoh et al., 2001).

The temporal characteristics of gait are also an important consideration. Contact time is the period between touchdown and toe-off of one foot during ground support. During acceleration, an individual needs a longer period of time to generate the force needed to overcome their body's inertia (Brughelli et al., 2011; Mero et al., 1986). Nonetheless, relatively shorter contact times have been related to faster speed during acceleration in field sport athletes (Lockie et al., 2011; Murphy et al., 2003). Murphy et al. (2003) posited that quicker athletes had a superior capability to generate velocity through decreasing the time in contact with the ground, which also contributed to a higher step frequency. The efficiency of ground contact has also been suggested as being the key contributor to maximal velocity in elite sprinters (Čoh et al., 2001).

Flight time is the duration between toe-off and touchdown of the opposing feet, and is a function of step length. If the length of the step is longer, then the time of flight should also increase (Lockie et al., 2013c; Mero et al., 1986). Conceptually, it would seem if an athlete increases their flight time during gait, this would indicate an increase in step length. However, athletes from certain sports should avoid excessive flight during their gait (Benton, 2001; Sayers, 2000). Players involved in contact sports (e.g., American and Australian football, rugby union and league) cannot change direction if they are airborne, and this can affect their body positioning prior to a collision. Hunter et al. (2005) affirmed flight time should only be long enough to allow the limbs to reposition.

Upper-Body Kinematics

During the gait cycle the arms act in opposition to the legs. This means that when the arm is in a position of maximum shoulder flexion (i.e., the arm is in its foremost position), the opposing leg is extending. Maximum shoulder extension occurs when the arm is in its rearmost position. These arm movements are pivotal to the transfer of angular momentum between the upper- and lower-body about the vertical axis (Bhowmick and Bhattacharyya, 1988; Hinrichs, 1992). Although this needs to substantiated in the literature, Bhowmick and Bhattacharyya (1988) suggested that the horizontal component of the arm swing during acceleration assists in increasing step length and regulating leg movement, while the vertical component creates a condition that enhances leg drive during ground contact. When comparing elite to well-trained male track sprinters, Slawinski et al. (2010) did find that elite sprinters displayed a greater arm range of motion during block clearance. Slawinski et al. (2010) further stated that these arm actions aided in shifting the sprinter's center of mass further forwards during the initial stages of acceleration.

During acceleration, all individuals will experience a degree of forward lean. An appropriate trunk lean and angle of trajectory (or total body take-off angle) can aid in the production of the horizontal forces (Lockie et al., 2003), and trajectory angles closer to the horizontal contribute to faster sprint times (Čoh et al., 1998; Lockie and Vickery, 2013). What will influence trunk lean and trajectory during acceleration is how the individual begins the sprint. For example, a sprinter leaving the starting blocks is best positioned to achieve optimal trunk lean and trajectory angles, as opposed to field and court sport athletes, who generally begin sprints from an upright position. A further consideration for field and court sport athletes is that a greater trunk lean when sprinting will lower the individual's center of mass, which is advantageous for dynamic balance (Sayers, 2000), and producing the force needed for lateral movements (Young et al., 2002). Regardless of the starting position, as an individual progresses from acceleration to maximum velocity trunk lean should gradually diminish (Atwater, 1982; Korneljuk, 1982; Woicik, 1983). During the period of maximum velocity, correct sprint technique involves a relatively upright body position (Mann, 1986; Young et al., 2001a).

Lower-Body Kinematics

The actions of the lower limbs will ultimately determine sprint performance. Hip range of motion will rise with sprint velocity (Mann and Hagy, 1980), and the muscles about the hip are the prime movers for increasing linear speed (Belli et al., 2002; Bezodis et al., 2008; Mann et al., 1986). Several authors have indicated that maximum hip extension occurs just prior to or at toe-off (Dillman, 1975; Novacheck, 1998); however, the thigh may extend further after toe-off in some individuals (Mann, 1986; Webster and Roberts, 2011). Following maximum extension the hip will flex during recovery, which reduces the rotational inertia and aids clearance of the swing leg (Ambrose, 1978; Mero et al., 1992; Lockie et al., 2014b). Maximum hip flexion during sprinting is associated with the end of forward swing, which occurs just prior to foot-strike (Mann and Herman, 1985). Impact with the ground will result in hip flexion (Mann and Hagy, 1980). This action will assist with the initial absorption of GRF, prior to force generation through stance and into take-off for the next step.

There are existing recommendations that the knee be greatly extended at toe-off during acceleration (Korchemny, 1992; van Ingen Schenau et al., 1994). In contrast to acceleration, during maximal velocity the angle of the knee tends to be abbreviated at toe-off, which is indicative of reduced extension (Mann, 1986; Mann and Herman, 1985; Mann and Sprague, 1980). Interestingly, Murphy et al. (2003) also found this phenomenon in field sport athletes during the first two steps of a 10 m sprint. This led Murphy et al. (2003) to suggest that the reduction in knee range of motion allowed for a more rapid turnover of the limbs, shortening contact time and increasing step frequency. Knee flexion during the recovery period of the step increases as sprinting speed increases (Dillman, 1975). This reduces the rotational inertia of the leg about the hip joint, which allows the leg to be recovered faster (Ambrose, 1978). Upon impact with the ground and through the initial stages of stance, there will be a degree of knee flexion (Mann and Hagy, 1980; Novacheck, 1998). This action will facilitate power transfer from the hip to the ankle during stance (Bezodis et al., 2008).

The ankle joint is a vital lever during sprinting (McFarlane, 1987; Baxter et al., 2012), and is important for force attenuation during stance (Hunter et al., 2005). The ankle is dorsi flexed at foot-strike to facilitate GRF absorption, prior to rapid plantar flexion (Mann and Hagy, 1980). The muscles that plantar flex the ankle contribute to power generation during this period of the step (Bezodis et al., 2008). For correct sprinting technique, the individual should remain on the ball of the foot throughout stance, without the heel contacting the ground (Mann and Sprague, 1980; Novacheck, 1998). Novacheck (1998) indicated that during the swing phase in sprinting, ankle dorsi flexion is less than that for both walking and running. This is because dorsi flexing the ankle to a neutral position is not required for leg clearance in the sprint step, due to the increase in hip and knee flexion of the swing leg.

Stance Kinetics

Stance kinetics refers to the force produced by an individual during ground support. Ground reaction force (GRF) can be divided into its three orthogonal components; vertical, horizontal (anterior-posterior, or braking and propulsive), and medial-lateral. For linear sprinting, the force produced in the vertical and horizontal (braking and propulsive) planes are of the greatest consequence to performance (Hunter et al., 2005). GRF in both of these planes will increase as running speed increases (Mann and Hagy, 1980). General recommendations for sprinting are that individuals should attempt to minimize braking forces (Mero et al., 1992), while maximizing propulsive forces (Hunter et al., 2005; Mero et al., 1992). This is true for both acceleration and maximum velocity sprinting. During acceleration, Harland and Steele (1997) and Kraan et al. (2001) have both suggested that to optimize performance, the foot contact should be behind the individual's center of mass. The block start used for track events puts the sprinter in the best position to do this. Indeed, Mero (1988) established a positive correlations between maximal force (correlation coefficient [r] = 0.63), average force (r = 0.66), and impulse (force x time; r = 0.79) out of a block start with 3 m sprint velocity in experienced track sprinters.

This underlies the importance of the force produced during ground contact in the initial movements of acceleration, as well as the time over which it is produced.

Further to this, Lockie et al. (2011) has stated that reducing the time to peak force in both the vertical and horizontal plane is beneficial for acceleration in field sport athletes. Hunter et al. (2005) affirmed that relative propulsive impulse was an important contributor to higher velocities when measured at the 16 m point of a 25 m sprint in athletes. Although acceleration will feature relatively longer contact times than maximum velocity sprinting (Brughelli et al., 2011; Mero et al., 1986), individuals still should attempt to generate force as quickly as possible (Lockie et al., 2011; Murphy et al., 2003).

Force production is also important during the period of maximum velocity. Previous research has suggested that faster sprint speeds are achieved by applying greater vertical force to the ground during contact (Weyand et al., 2000). During treadmill sprinting at maximum velocity, Weyand et al. (2000) found that when comparing faster and slower sprinters, there was no variation in the time needed to reposition the legs during each step. Rather, it was the force generated during each contact in relation to the time taken for force generation that proved to be the differentiating factor.

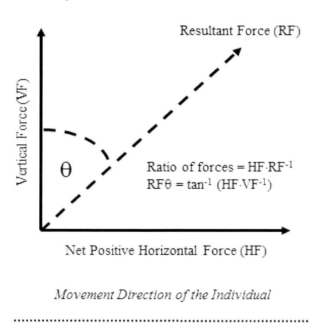

Figure 2. Schematic representation of the ratio of forces, resultant ground reaction, and resultant ground reaction force angle (RFθ), as a function of vertical and net positive horizontal force. Adapted from Kugler and Jansen (2010) and Lockie et al. (2014c).

More recently, however, Kugler and Jansen (2010) stated that rather than maximal force production, there should be a focus on 'optimal' force production during sprinting. This relates to the resultant magnitude and direction of the forces generated in the vertical and horizontal planes (Figure 2). Morin et al. (2011) described this as technical ability, in that it is the way in which individuals apply force to the ground. The importance of horizontal force production in particular has been related to acceleration (Hunter et al., 2005; Kawamori et al., 2013; Kugler and Janshen, 2010; Morin et al., 2011), where the individual must overcome their inertia to initiate a maximal sprint. Moreover, a greater ratio of horizontal to resultant ground reaction force in physical education students (Morin et al., 2011), and greater horizontal force production in Australian football players (Brughelli et al., 2011) and rugby league players (de Lacey et al., 2014), has been linked to higher maximal sprint velocities.

Interestingly, Lockie et al. (2013c) found that vertical force correlated with higher 10 m sprint velocities, and vertical impulse was associated with longer step lengths and shorter contact times within this interval in male field sport athletes. These results tended to suggest a greater importance on vertical GRF, similar to Weyand et al. (2000). However, Lockie et al. (2013c) discussed that due to the nature of their sports, field sport athletes may be better conditioned to produce horizontal GRF during acceleration. Indeed, when compared to the physical education student sample from Kugler and Janshen (2010), the participants from Lockie et al. (2013c) produced superior resultant horizontal GRF within the first two steps of a sprint. Nonetheless, for faster linear speed during both acceleration and maximum velocity sprinting, the correct balance between vertical and horizontal GRF production must be found, and this force must be generated efficiently.

CHANGE-OF-DIRECTION SPEED DEFINED

There has historically been conjecture as to the definition of agility. Sheppard et al. (2014) detailed the ambiguity with which agility has been described in the past, and how any movement that incorporated a direction change could be classed as 'agility.' This led to much clearer definitions of agility and COD speed being presented in the literature (Sheppard and Young, 2006; Young et al., 2002). Agility has now been defined as the initiation of body movement, change of direction, or rapid acceleration or deceleration, often in response to some form of stimulus (Sheppard and Young, 2006). Therefore, for a movement to be described as agility, there must be a cognitive component, which will incorporate perception, decision-making, visual scanning, and knowledge of situations (Sheppard and Young, 2006). There are several reviews that have investigated agility (Sheppard et al., 2014; Sheppard and Young, 2006; Young and Farrow, 2006, 2013; Young et al., 2015). For this chapter, however, the focus will be on COD speed.

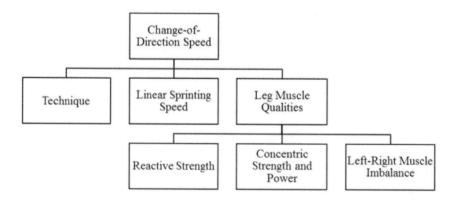

Figure 3. The physical factors of change-of-direction speed than can be targeted by strength and conditioning practitioners to enhance performance. Adapted from Sheppard and Young (2006).

COD speed is the physical component of agility, and incorporates factors such as the individual's anthropometry, COD and sprint technique, and leg muscle qualities (Sheppard and Young, 2006). Adapted from the model presented by Sheppard and Young (2006), Figure 3 displays the qualities that can be targeted by strength and conditioning coaches and exercise practitioners to enhance COD speed. There is a degree of crossover in the conditioning modalities that can be used to improve linear and COD speed. Nonetheless, there are specific technical aspects to COD speed that must be considered by coaches before training program implementation.

TECHNICAL FACTORS IMPORTANT TO COD SPEED

COD Gait Kinematics

The actual foot placement and direction change during a COD movement has been labelled a 'cut' (Sacco et al., 2006), although these terms have been used interchangeably (Green et al., 2011; Lockie et al., 2014c; Lockie et al., 2013a). Nonetheless, Sacco et al. (2006) categorized cuts as sharp changes in direction, which consist of a linear deceleration and angular acceleration about the stance leg, as the individual decelerates before moving towards the new direction. In a planned COD, an individual knows which direction they are going to cut. In unplanned circumstances, the individual must be prepared to move in different directions depending on the task demands. Due to the nature of the tasks, the mechanics of a planned and unplanned cut are different (Brown et al., 2014; McLean et al., 2004; Wheeler and Sayers, 2010). While the kinematics required for a reactive cut are important for athletes involved in sports where there is temporal and spatial uncertainty, the focus of this section will be on the mechanics of planned COD speed.

The orientation of the body during a COD will indicate the direction an individual will ultimately move. A forward lean is required to accelerate, a backward lean to decelerate, and a sideward lean for lateral movement (Young and Farrow, 2006). These body positions are required so that the individual can produce the necessary GRF to change direction. What complicates the analysis of COD gait kinematics is it can be specific to the type of cut performed. The mechanics to best complete a 45° cut would likely be different to that for a 90° or 180° cut. Nonetheless, Hewit et al. (2013) detailed some of the general kinematic requirements of an effective COD. These included making appropriate step adjustments, suitably positioning the plant or stance leg, and ensuring the correct sequencing of joint and body movements both prior to and after the cut.

The first component of a COD is the entry into the cut. This is the deceleration phase, as the individual is decreasing their velocity prior to the COD. The entry into a COD particularly differentiates between planned and reactive cuts. During reactive conditions, an individual is more likely to perform an open maneuver (i.e., a side-step cut) where the cut is initiated by the opposite leg to that of the target direction (Rand and Ohtsuki, 2000). As the name suggests, the stance will be more open, such that individual's resulting center of pressure between the feet does not favor movement to one side, and the cut can be initiated in any direction (Lockie et al., 2013a; Tateuchi et al., 2006). In planned conditions, the width of stance will not be as pronounced. A cross maneuver (i.e., a crossover cut) may be performed, where the leg on the same side as the target direction initiates the COD (Rand and Ohtsuki, 2000).

Prior to a direction change, there is an increase in lateral speed in the direction of the intended movement (Wheeler and Sayers, 2010). Depending on the angle of the cut, the COD can resemble linear speed kinematics, such as during a 45° cut (Spiteri et al., 2013). A more severe COD (i.e., a 180° cut) will alter the gait kinematics produced by the individual. Nevertheless, a faster COD should feature a lowered center of mass, shorter steps leading into the foot plant, with the feet positioned closer to the individual's center of mass (Wheeler and Sayers, 2010). In team sports where the demands of match-play involve a high volume of direction changes, especially invasion sports with tackles and collisions, one adaptation to running technique an individual makes is to sprint with a greater forward lean (Sayers, 2000; Young et al., 2002). This body position should not only better prepare an individual for a collision, but should also assist with a quick COD as match-play demands.

The next component of a COD is the stance phase. The stance leg needs to be positioned appropriately to halt movement in one direction, before initiating movement in the new direction (Hewit et al., 2013). During a COD, initial contact with the ground results in hip flexion, due to the forward and downward momentum of the trunk (McLean et al., 2004). Greater knee flexion and hip abduction can also facilitate horizontal braking during the initial stages of stance (Spiteri et al., 2013). Following impact, the stance leg needs to be extended into toe-off, as extension of this leg will initiate reacceleration. Green et al. (2011) found higher-level rugby union players begin knee extension earlier, which results in a faster COD. While extension occurs in the stance leg, the free or swing leg must rotate around into the new direction before driving upward (Hewit et al., 2013). The knee must be rapidly flexed so that the hip can more easily rotate this leg (Hase and Stein, 1999). Much like linear sprinting, shorter contact times have been associated a more efficient COD (Green et al., 2011).

The actions of the upper-body will also facilitate the COD. Brown and Vescovi (2003) state that following positioning of the stance leg, the head will turn and face the intended direction. The inside arm will pull in a posterior direction, while the outside arm drives forward to generate angular momentum and facilitate rotation of the body about the longitudinal axis. Brown and Vescovi (2003) further assert that any action that results in the arms being too far away from the body will create more resistive forces for the body to overcome, resulting in a slower COD. The torso should also be orientated towards the intended direction (Young and Farrow, 2006). In addition to this, if the trunk is leaning or rotated towards the opposite direction of the cut, this increases the load experienced and risk of injury at the knee of the stance leg (Dempsey et al., 2007).

The final phase involves the acceleration out of the cut. The kinematics through this component of the COD will draw from technical information for the acceleration phase of linear sprinting. This includes appropriate extension of the drive leg (Korchemny, 1992; Murphy et al., 2003; van Ingen Schenau et al., 1994), and fast repositioning of the swing leg (Ambrose, 1978; Lockie et al., 2014b; Mero et al., 1992). Furthermore, coaching information for team sport athletes recommends taking shorter steps within a COD (Benton, 2001; Sayers, 2000). Hewit et al. (2013) found that faster female netball players had a greater step frequency over 2.5 m following a 180° cut, when compared to their slower counterparts (5.55 ± 0.21 Hertz vs. 5.31 ± 0.22 Hertz). To optimize acceleration following a cut, individuals should transition to their typical sprint kinematics as quickly as possible.

COD Stance Kinetics

The correct application of force during stance is required for an effective COD. While linear speed places an emphasis the vertical and horizontal GRF, COD speed will also rely on medial-lateral force production (Glaister et al., 2008; Houck, 2003; McClay et al., 1994). A schematic representation of GRF in each of these planes is shown in Figure 4. There are several factors that will influence the magnitude and timing of GRF during a cut, including the mass of the individual, the approach velocity, the body position adopted during stance, and the intended direction of the cut. The resultant force vector following stance will dictate the final movement direction after the cut (Dayakidis and Boudolos, 2006; Glaister et al., 2008).

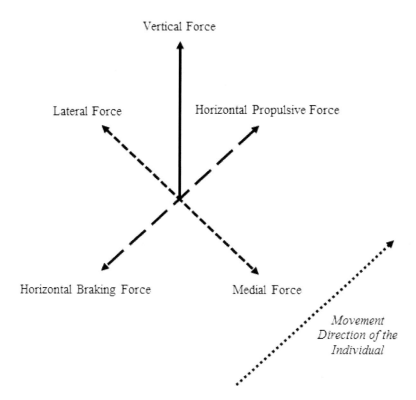

Figure 4. Schematic representation of the ground reaction forces present during a change-of-direction movement.

With regards to the vertical GRF pattern, there is an initial impact peak early in stance, followed by a propulsive peak when the individual reaccelerates (Dayakidis and Boudolos, 2006; Sacco et al., 2006). During a V-cut, Dayakidis and Boudolos (2006) observed that in male basketball players the initial impact peak was approximately 3 x body weight, while the propulsive peak was 2½ x body weight. The higher initial impact peak would be associated with the need to stop the momentum of the body prior to the COD. Spiteri et al. (2013) illustrated the value of vertical GRF during a cut. Stronger male and female recreational athletes (as measured by the isometric mid-thigh pull), who were faster in a 45° cut, produced greater vertical braking and propulsive impulse, and relative vertical propulsive force, when compared to weaker athletes. The importance of vertical propulsive force is notable, as this mirrors research into linear sprint acceleration (Lockie et al., 2013c). Thus, for an effective COD, an individual must generate an appropriate magnitude of vertical GRF.

Any movement involving a cut will result in an increase in braking GRF in the horizontal plane (Houck, 2003). The ability to produce greater braking force is important, as this will arrest movement in one plane (Glaister et al., 2008; Jindrich et al., 2006; Spiteri et al., 2013). McClay et al. (1994) documented that during a basketball cut, a braking force equivalent to approximately 1.1 x body weight was exerted against the ground. To stop movement in the original direction, a force greater than body weight would need to be exerted. Once this is done, the individual can accelerate in the new direction during propulsion. The magnitude of the propulsive force component will influence the resulting direction of the cut (Dayakidis and Boudolos, 2006; Glaister et al., 2008; McClay et al., 1994). McClay et al. (1994) found that propulsive force was much lower during a basketball cut, with a mean GRF of approximately to 0.3 x body weight. Interestingly, although the stronger participants from Spiteri et al. (2013) tended to exert greater propulsive force, there was not a significant difference when compared to the weaker participants. This would be reflective of the fact that the V-cut measured by McClay et al. (1994), and the 45° cut from Spiteri et al. (2013), involved only a component of horizontal force. Force in the medial-lateral plane is also a contributor to the resultant GRF vector.

The intended direction of the cut will affect the magnitude of force produced medially or laterally. A planned cut will often place greater prominence on medial-lateral force production, as the individual knows the intended direction (Wheeler and Sayers, 2010). McClay et al. (1994) also investigated medial-lateral forces during several basketball-specific movements. In each of the movements (running at 3.8 m·s^{-1}, lay-up and jump shot take-off and landings, vertical jumping), medial forces were higher, which indicated the resultant GRF was directed towards the midline of the players. In most cases, the movements resulted in a medial GRF that was low (0.2-0.7 x body weight). However, during a cut, the medial force was equal to 1 x body weight, and during a shuffle, the medial GRF was approximately 1.5 x body weight. Shuffling in basketball is a side-to-side movement commonly used on defense where movement speed is critical (Whitting et al., 2013). This provides an indication why medial force would be in excess of body weight, as the individual pushes off from the outside leg to drive themselves laterally as quickly as possible. The importance of GRF in each of the planes during a cut is clear. Strength and conditioning coaches must therefore select training protocols that can enhance the magnitude and efficiency of force production during stance for COD speed.

INTRODUCTION TO SPEED TRAINING

Although sprinting does incorporate a large degree of natural ability, it is generally accepted that appropriate training can lead to the improvement of an individual's speed (Delecluse, 1997; Ross and Leveritt, 2001). The specificity of the training must be taken into account and should be such that it stresses the individual in conditions similar to those that they will experience in competition. Research has shown the existence of movement-specific, in addition to velocity-specific, effects on the neuromuscular system, whereby the greatest gains are made at or near the training velocity (Behm, 1995; Behm and Sale, 1993). Therefore, when prescribing speed training programs, consideration must be made of the factors affecting performance, including the speed of the movement patterns used, required force output, distances covered, and optimal technique for the individual's sport.

Another important consideration is that the ability to sprint linearly and change direction rapidly are recognized as separate skill components (Little and Williams, 2005; Salaj and Markovic, 2011; Vescovi and McGuigan, 2008; Young et al., 2001b). What this means is that athletes who can run fast in a straight line may not necessarily be able to change direction at speed. Coaches must carefully consider what modalities they will prescribe to improve linear and COD speed, with the knowledge that each must be trained specifically.

There are a number of different modalities that can be implemented to enhance speed in young adults. This includes free sprinting and technique drills, resistance or strength training, plyometrics, and resisted and assisted sprinting (Cronin et al., 2008; Lockie et al., 2012a; Rumpf et al., in press). Most of these will be used in combination within an athlete's program. The concentration of this chapter, however, will be on how each modality could individually influence sprinting speed, more so than combined methods of training. In addition to this, the focus of the discussion will not be to say that one modality is better than another. Rather, the discussion will highlight how each individual modality can impact speed, and this information can then drive how a coach would construct a training program for their athletes.

MODALITIES USED FOR LINEAR SPEED TRAINING

Free Sprint Training

Free sprinting forms the basis for any linear speed training program (Lockie et al., 2012a), and commonly features a series of sprints over a variety of distances (Dintiman and Ward, 2003; Korchemny, 1992; Martinopoulou et al., 2011). As a general rule, these sprint exercises remain central to any program designed for improving speed. Interval training is the most common method used in the development of speed, and will generally involve a defined number of repetitions, with sufficient recovery periods between each repetition. The distances covered for each sprint will depend on the individual's sport, as well as their training cycle. If acceleration is a focus, then shorter sprints (20 m or less) should be incorporated into training. When training for maximum velocity, longer sprints (30 m and above) must be used.

Research has established that free sprint training can effectively enhance linear sprinting speed, although adaptations tend to be distance-specific (Rumpf et al., in press). For example, in a program that specifically used sprint acceleration intervals (5 m, 10 m, 15 m, and 20 m), Spinks et al. (2007) found sprint velocity over 15 m significantly increased following eight weeks of training. Kristensen et al. (2006) found six weeks of training with sprint intervals of 22 m led to an increase in 20 m sprint velocity in trained recreational athletes. Markovic et al. (2007) used interval distances of 10-50 m to decrease 20 m sprint time in male physical education students. A speed training program administered by Young et al. (2001b), which led a decrease in 30 m sprint time in male team sport athletes, featured sprint intervals of 20-40 m. These studies illustrate that improvements in linear speed can be achieved over the distances specifically used in training.

Free sprint training can also cause favorable adaptations to technique. Contact time for the first two contacts in a 15 m sprint has been found to decrease following eight weeks of free sprint training (Spinks et al., 2007). Kristensen et al. (2006) observed that the increases in 20 m sprint velocity were primarily a function of an increase in step length. The findings of Kristensen et al. (2006) were supported by two studies featuring six weeks of sprint training, and both used 5-20 m distances which led to a faster 10 m sprint courtesy of step length increases (Lockie et al., 2014d; Lockie et al., 2012a). However, concurrent with increases in step length over 0-5 m, 5-10 m, and 0-10 m, Lockie et al. (2012a) documented decreases in step frequency over each of these intervals. This would relate to the phenomenon proposed by Hunter et al. (2004), in that should one of these variables increase, the other would likely decrease. Lockie et al. (2012a) also found contact time increased in the 0-5 m and 0-10 m intervals, and suggested that this was due to participants requiring more time to produce the force necessary to lengthen the step. Coaches should be cognizant as to what technical adaptations result from free sprint training, and whether other speed training modalities should be used to target other technical developments.

The value of using other modalities is reflected by research indicating free sprint training alone was not sufficient to elicit significant improvement in linear speed. Rimmer and Sleivert (2000) found that eight weeks of speed training using 10 m and 40 m intervals led to non-significant changes in 0-10 m and 0-40 times in male rugby union players, and no changes in technical variables such as step length. A free sprint program featuring repetition distances of 20 m and 50 m led to no significant changes in velocity over the 0-10 m, 10-20 m, and 0-20 m intervals in a 50 m sprint in male university students (Zafeiridis et al., 2005). Upton (2011) documented that four weeks of free sprint training was not sufficient to improve speed over 36.58 m in Division I collegiate female soccer players. Especially in trained athletes, free sprint training by itself may not always significantly enhance linear speed (Rimmer and Sleivert, 2000; Upton, 2011). This has been referred to as the 'speed barrier,' where new stimuli are required to enhance sprint performance (Martinopoulou et al., 2011; Tabachnik, 1992). Therefore, strength and conditioning coaches should be mindful of other linear speed training modalities.

Resistance Training

Resistance training consists of weights training, as well as any other modality that is designed to make an athlete overcome a resistance greater than what they will encounter under competitive conditions (Young, 1991). The focus of this section will be on strength training. Traditional strength training generally involves heavy weights (80-90% of maximum) being lifted for relatively few repetitions (5-6 repetitions or less) (Wilson et al., 1993). Strength development aids in forming the foundation to support further sport-specific training, such as speed development, as a high degree of power is dependent on high maximum strength (Tan, 1999; Young, 1991).

When an individual accelerates, strength is needed to overcome the inertia of their body mass. As evidence of this, average and peak concentric power, as measured by a back squat and split squat, was significantly related to 5 m sprint time in male athletes ($r = -0.64$ to -0.68) (Sleivert and Taingahue, 2004). Absolute one-repetition maximum (1RM) squat correlated with 10 m ($r = -0.94$) and 30 m ($r = -0.71$) sprint times in male soccer players (Wisloff et al.,

2004). Relative 1RM squat strength has been significantly related to 9.14 m (r = -0.54) and 36.58 m (r = -0.60) sprint times in collegiate football players (McBride et al., 2009), 10 m (r = -0.87), 17.9 m (r = -0.84), and 35.8 m (r = -0.84) sprint times in female softball players (Nimphius et al., 2010), and 10 m (r = -0.62) and 20 m (r = -0.60) sprint times in recreationally trained men (Comfort et al., 2012a). Strength has also been shown to differentiate between faster and slower individuals, such as female track sprinters and recreationally-trained individuals (Meckel et al., 1995), and collegiate American football players from Division I competition when compared to Division II (Garstecki et al., 2004).

There have been some conflicting findings as to the benefits of strength training for linear speed within the literature. Moir et al. (2007) detailed that an eight-week strength training program failed to improve 0-10 m sprint times in physically active males, despite increases in strength measured by a 1RM squat. Hoffman et al. (2004) composed a 15-week, periodized full-body strength program for collegiate American footballers. While lower-body strength measured by a 1RM squat increased by 13%, the time for a 36.58 m sprint did not significantly decrease. However, two systematic reviews of the literature, conducted by Seitz et al. (2014) and Bolger et al. (2015), documented that there was general consensus that strength training would positively influence linear speed. Exercises such as the back squat, loaded jump squat, deadlift, and clean typically form the foundation for strength training programs that enhance linear speed (Bolger et al., 2015; Delecluse, 1997; Seitz et al., 2014). Interestingly, Seitz et al. (2014) found that any improvements in speed occurred independent of the average load intensity. Although it is commonly thought that strength will have a greater influence on sprint acceleration (Sleivert and Taingahue, 2004; Young et al., 2001a; Young et al., 1995), Seitz et al. (2014) also detailed that there were no significant differences in improvements made in sprints less than 20 m, or between 20-40 m. As a result, Seitz et al. (2014) proposed that strength training could provide benefits for both short (acceleration) and longer distance (maximal velocity) sprinting.

To provide some specific examples, Delecluse et al. (1995) found acceleration over the first 10 m in a 100 m sprint improved by 7% in physical education students following nine weeks of full-body resistance training. Lower-body strength, trained by the leg press, half-squat, and calf raise, was targeted from weeks 4-9, when ranges of 3-6 repetitions were employed. Lockie et al. (2012a) investigated the effects of a six-week strength training program on 10 m sprint performance in field sport athletes. The program included back squats, step-ups, cable hip flexion, and calf raises, and the repetition ranges decreased from 10-12 repetitions in week 1, to 4 repetitions in week 6, with concomitant increases in load. Following the intervention, the participants increased their three-repetition maximum (3RM) squat from 114.40 ± 26.80 kilograms (kg) to 131.73 ± 23.54 kg. Concurrent with this 15% increase in 3RM squat, the participants significantly increased 0-5 m velocity by 10%, 5-10 m velocity by 3%, and 0-10 m velocity by 7%. The primary kinematic adaptations were increases in step length. Lockie et al. (2012a) stated that the external loading provided with strength training aided in the development of force production, which participants were able to express during stance to lengthen the step. As asserted by Seitz et al. (2014), strength improvements can also influence maximum velocity sprinting. Cormie et al. (2010) detailed that 10 weeks of strength training utilizing the back squat, where intensity varied between 75-90% of the individual's 1RM, caused a significant 2.2% decrease in 40 m sprint time in relatively untrained men.

Improvements in strength for highly-trained athletes can also contribute to improved linear speed. Following an eight-week pre-season program (back squats, mid-thigh clean pull, Romanian deadlift, Nordic curls), that featured four-week strength (85-90% 1RM) and power (85% 1RM) mesocycles, professional rugby league players improved their 1RM back squat from 170.6 ± 21.4 kg to 200.8 ± 19.0 kg (Comfort et al., 2012b). Parallel with the improved strength, Comfort et al. (2012b) also observed decreases in 0-5 m, 0-10 m, and 0-20 m sprint times from a 20-m sprint, by 8%, 7%, and 6%, respectively. Ronnestad et al. (2008) investigated the effects of a seven-week strength program incoporating a half squat and hip flexion exercise in elite soccer players. 1RM half squat improved by approximately 25% following the intervention (pre-test = 179 ± 6 kg; post-test = 220 ± 3 kg). There were also significant, albeit slight (1-2%), improvements in the 0-10 m (acceleration) and 30-40 m (maximum velocity) intervals in a 40 m sprint. Interestingly, Ronnestad et al. (2008) found a significant correlation (r = 0.40) between the change in relative 1RM half squat and the 40 m sprint time. This provided an indication of the transfer of training effect from strength to linear speed.

The long-term effects of strength training on linear speed has also been investigated in elite softball (Nimphius et al., 2012) and rugby union (Barr et al., 2014) players. Nimphius et al. (2012) tracked female softball players over the course of a 20-week season, which included a 14-week strength training program. The exercises in the strength program included the power and hang clean, squat, split squat, and deadlift. The effect of training was investigated through a number of variables, including muscle architecture and linear speed measured by a 17.9 m (the distance from home plate to first base in softball), and 35.8 m sprint (the distance from home plate to second base). The data was analyzed by calculating correlations between the percent change in these variables following the intervention. Nimphius et al. (2012) found very large (r = -0.80) and large (r = -0.55) correlations between the changes in vastus lateralis (VL) muscle thickness and 17.9 m and 35.8 m sprint times, respectively. Increases in VL thickness have been noted as an adaptation to strength training that can increase the force output necessary to improve maximal speed (Cormie et al., 2010). Nimphius et al. (2012) also found a very large correlation (r = -0.84) for the percent change in VL fiber length and 35.8 m sprint time, and inferred that the changes in muscle physiology that resulted from strength training had a positive influence on linear speed.

Barr et al. (2014) charted a group of elite male rugby union players over the course of a year to determine changes in several physical characteristics courtesy of strength training, including linear speed measured by a 40 m sprint. Technique characteristics, such as contact and flight time, and stride length and frequency, were also investigated. The strength training program incorporated upper- (e.g., presses, pulls) and lower-body (e.g., squats, cleans, snatches, jerks) exercises specific to rugby union. Barr et al. (2014) also calculated correlations between the percent change in strength and speed variables following the intervention. With regards to strength changes, there was a significant, moderate change in 1RM power clean relative to body mass (effect size [d] = 0.60), and trivial changes in relative 1RM front squat (d = 0.07). Barr et al. (2014) acknowledged that when working with highly-trained, elite athletes, the principle of diminishing returns applies, where a high training load may not be reflected with significant changes to physical performance. This was also seen with linear speed, where there was no change in acceleration (0-10 m interval) or maximal velocity (30-40 m interval) times in a 40 m sprint. However, Barr et al. (2014) did find there was a large change in stride length during acceleration over the course of the year, and the changes in maximal velocity stride length had a very large relationship (r = 0.70) with the change in relative 1RM power clean. Given the importance of step and stride length to higher sprint velocities (Callaghan et al., 2014; Callaghan et al., 2015; Lockie et al., 2014b; Lockie et al., 2014d; Lockie et al., 2013b; Lockie et al., 2013c; Lockie et al., 2012a), this is a notable effect for the long-term benefits of strength training.

This section has discussed strength training that has used fixed plane resistance, which means the exercises are performed in the one location (Bolger et al., 2015). Linear speed clearly involves locomotion. Furthermore, sprinting incorporates a large eccentric element in the action (Belli et al., 2002; Bezodis et al., 2008; Mann and Sprague, 1980). As resistance training with weights primarily develops the concentric portions of a movement (Wilson et al., 1996), high levels of strength will not always directly correlate with linear speed (Baker and Nance, 1999; Cronin and Hansen, 2005). Consequently, strength and conditioning coaches will also program exercises that incorporate a more explosive element to transition from high force to high power output in athletic movements. One such example is plyometrics.

Plyometrics Training

Plyometrics are a group of exercises where the movement is performed more rapidly than typical resistance exercises, and can be modelled to closely match those actions performed in sports. Jump training is the most common form of plyometrics, although this modality can also include pushing, pulling, or throwing movements. All of these actions will incorporate the stretch-shortening cycle (SSC) capacities of the musculature. The SSC is made up of three components; the eccentric contraction, amortization phase, and concentric contraction (Potach and Chu, 2008). The eccentric contraction loads the muscle with elastic energy. The amortization phase is the period of time prior to the initiation of the concentric contraction. The subsequent concentric contraction is where this energy is utilized, with the muscle shortening taking advantage of the additional elastic energy to augment the power and speed of the movement. Plyometrics training can enhance the rate of eccentric lower body force production (Wilson et al., 1996). Additionally, these exercises allow the individual to accelerate all the way through the movement to the point of projection of the resistance, such as during the take-off in a jump (Newton and Kraemer, 1994).

Numerous studies have indicated relationships between jump performance and linear speed over a variety of distances. For example, 30 m sprint times in elite sprinters have been significantly correlated with vertical ($r = 0.91$) and standing broad ($r = 0.87$) jumps (Baker and Bell, 1994). Cronin and Hansen (2005) illustrated that squat and countermovement jump height were the best correlates with 5 m, 10 m, and 30 m sprint times ($r = -0.56$ to -0.66) in elite male rugby league players. In female collegiate soccer and lacrosse players, Vescovi and McGuigan (2008) found that the countermovement jump correlated ($r = -0.66$ to -0.79) with sprint times over 9.1 m, 18.3 m, 27.4 m, and 36.58 m. Unilateral jump performance in male recreational field sport athletes has also been related to sprinting speed, with moderate-to-very large correlations ($r = -0.40$ to -0.73) found between single-leg vertical, standing broad, and lateral jumps, and 0-5 m, 0-10 m, and 0-20 sprint times (Lockie et al., 2014a). Mero and Komi (1994) affirmed that plyometric movements, such as hopping and bounding, are comparable to sprint movements, due to the relative similarity of the ground contact times produced during both types of activities. This should make plyometrics very applicable for the development of linear speed.

However, it must be acknowledged that there is research documenting that plyometrics training can have limited effects on linear speed. While a training program for male physical education students involving hurdle and drop jumps led to increases in vertical, reactive and horizontal power, there were no significant improvements in 20 m sprint performance (Markovic et al., 2007). A periodized drop jump training program led to no changes in the 30 m sprint time of experienced weight trainers (Wilson et al., 1993). Additionally, nine weeks of unilateral lower-limb plyometrics training did not significantly decrease 12 m sprint time in novice tennis players (Salonikidis and Zafeiridis, 2008). It is possible that the exercises used and program design from these studies may not have been specific enough to linear speed, which would influence any changes to performance. This is especially pertinent when considering the work of Saez de Villarreal et al. (2012). In a meta-analysis of the effects of plyometrics training on sprint performance, Saez de Villarreal et al. (2012) noted that there is general agreement in the literature that plyometrics training can enhance linear speed. The importance of using specific exercises that have a horizontal force component, such as skipping and travelling jumps, were highlighted, as well as the use of high-intensity plyometrics. This supports the findings of Mero and Komi (1994), and Dawes and Lentz (2012) have also recommended utilizing vertical and horizontal jump exercises for the development of linear speed. Saez de Villarreal et al. (2012) further stated that the most improvements in speed following plyometrics training were made in sprints over 10-40 m distances.

To illustrate some specific examples, although 12 m sprint time did not change, Salonikidis and Zafeiridis (2008) observed an 8% decrease in 4 m time for their participants. Plyometrics training improved speed over 10 m in male physical education students (1995), rugby union players (2000), and field sport athletes (Lockie et al., 2014d; Lockie et al., 2012a). Not only did Lockie et al. (2012a) find that 0-10 m velocity was improved by a six-week plyometrics program incorporating box jumps, bounding, forward hops, hurdle jumps, and drop jumps, but so was 0-5 m and 5-10 m velocity. Ozbar et al. (2014) used an eight-week plyometrics program for experienced female soccer players. There was a significant, 8.1% decrease in 20 m sprint time following the intervention that utilized unilateral vertical, horizontal, and lateral jumps, and jumps and hops over cones. An eight-week, in-season program (hurdles and drop jumps) was adopted by Chelly et al. (2010) for implementation with experienced male soccer players. Chelly et al. (2010) discerned that within a 40 m sprint, velocity during the first step, acceleration (0-5 m) and maximum speed (35-40 m) all improved, by 18%, 10%, and 10%, respectively.

Extra load can also be added to plyometric exercises in an attempt to increase power output. The jump squat is the most commonly used exercise for this, and training with loaded jump squats can enhance SSC function and rate of force development during dynamic activities (Cormie et al., 2010). Wilson et al. (1993) originally documented that peak power for a loaded jump squat occurred with 30% of 1RM back squat in trained males. However, Baker et al. (2001) observed that for stronger athletes, peak power can be achieved with a heavier load (55-59% of 1RM). Although there are some studies that have suggested loaded jump squat training does not enhance linear speed (Hoffman et al., 2005; Wilson et al., 1993), and Saez de Villarreal et al. (2012) suggested it was not necessary, there is research that has documented benefits. McBride et al. (2002) found that eight weeks of jump squat training with 30% of 1RM back squat showed a trend towards improved 20 m sprint performance in club-level male athletes. Using the same load, Cormie et al. (2010) observed that in relatively untrained men, 10 weeks of jump squat training significantly improved 0-20 m, 0-30 m, and

0-40 m time in a 40 m sprint. As an example of how stronger athletes can generate peak power at heavier loads, Harris et al. (2008) noted that seven weeks of jump squat training with either a maximal power load (20-44% of 1RM back squat) or a heavy load (80% of 1RM back squat) improved 10 m and 30 m sprint performance in elite rugby league players.

Plyometrics training can also cause technical changes in an individual. Lockie et al. (2014d) noted that the primary technique adaptations following plyometrics training were increased step length within a 10 m sprint, and increased vertical force production in the first, second, and last step over this distance. As field sport athletes are conditioned to produce horizontal force in their sports, Lockie et al. (2014d) suggested that in order to make the kinetic adaptations required to improve step length there was a change in vertical GRF. In addition to this, Maćkala and Fostiak (2015) documented that a two-week, high-intensity (squat, tuck, hurdle, and depth jumps; hopping; bilateral and unilateral bounding) plyometrics program could increase step frequency and reduce contact time in a flying 20 m sprint in experienced male sprinters. Taken together, these findings indicate that an appropriately designed plyometrics training program can lead to favorable changes to sprint technique, and thus enhanced linear speed.

Resisted Sprint Training

Resistance exercises that involve movement away from one location are can be termed as locomotor exercises (Bolger et al., 2015). Resisted sprinting is an example of this, and is an extension to strength training. This modality involves adding resistance to the athlete while they are running, which can come in the form of uphill sprinting, weighted vests, small weights attached to individual segments, parachutes, or weighted sleds (Costello, 1985; Faccioni, 1994b). Depending on the applied load, this modality has the potential to be specific to any individual that needs to sprint, as the gait pattern can be maintained while they are under resistance. As a result of the need for high force development to overcome additional inertia, resisted sprinting has primarily been thought of as a modality for improving speed during acceleration (Bachero-Mena and Gonzalez-Badillo, 2014; Cronin et al., 2008; Lockie et al., 2003; Spinks et al., 2007).

When using resisted sprint training modalities, an approximate 10% decrease in maximum velocity for a given distance has been recommended (Jakalski, 1998; Lockie et al., 2003; Spinks et al., 2007). Through a regression analysis of load versus sprint velocity over 15 m in field sport athletes, Lockie et al. (2003) derived a formula that could calculate the mass (%body mass) required to cause a specific decrease in speed. This formula, which had a correlation coefficient of 0.99, was:

%body mass = (-1.96 x %velocity) + 188.99

where %velocity = the required training velocity as a percentage of maximum velocity over a given distance (e.g., 90% of maximum velocity).

Lockie et al. (2003) found the load that caused a 10% decrease in velocity equated to approximately 12.59% of body mass. As will be discussed, there were several studies that utilized this load during training programs that led to improvements in linear speed (Harrison and Bourke, 2009; Lockie et al., 2012a; Spinks et al., 2007; Upton, 2011; Wagganer et al., 2015; West et al., 2013).

Alcaraz et al. (2009) extended this research by examining loads for maximum velocity sprint training in track and field athletes. Six national level sprinters completed flying 30 m sprints towing sleds with different loads so that Alcaraz et al. (2009) could calculate a regression formula for longer distance sprints. The formula had a correlation coefficient of 0.82, and was:

$$\%body\ mass = (-0.8674 \times \%velocity) + 87.89$$

Therefore, the load that caused a 10% decrease in velocity equated to approximately 9.82% of body mass, which was less than that derived by Lockie et al. (2003). Whether the use of this load during training can enhance maximum velocity needs to be confirmed by research.

Although this modality does not require the addition of weight to the individual, uphill sprinting is a form of resisted sprinting. The influence of gravity while sprinting uphill provides the overload, and a 3° incline has been previously used (Barr et al., 2014; Paradisis and Cooke, 2001, 2006). An acute technical adaptation to uphill sprinting is a decrease in step length and flight time, which contributes to reduced sprint velocity (Paradisis and Cooke, 2001). However, when using a 3° incline on a custom-built platform for sprint training over six weeks, Paradisis and Cooke (2006) found no significant changes to 35 m sprint performance or the associated step kinematics in physical education students. A limitation for using uphill sprinting is controlling the incline of the slope, as well as access to a slope that allows for the use of a range of sprint distances. Thus, other forms of resisted sprinting may be more practical for linear speed training.

One method for resisted sprinting is to add load directly to the individual, either via weights attached to body segments (Ropret et al., 1998; Bennett et al., 2009), or a weighted vest (Cronin et al., 2008; Clark et al., 2010; Zafeiropoulos et al., 2014). Ropret et al. (1998) examined the effects of arm or leg loading on 30 m sprint performance in male physical education students. While arm loading (0.22-0.66 kg lead rods held in each hand) had no effect on 30 m sprint performance, adding 0.6-1.8 kg load belts around each ankle led to significant 7.8-12.8% decreases in velocity, which was due to reductions in stride frequency. Bennett et al. (2009) added the equivalent of 10% of segment mass to the thighs and shanks of male competitive beach sprinters, and assessed 40 m sprint performance. Except for the 0-10 m interval, there were significant increases in sprint time in all other 10 m intervals of the 40 m sprint, although the changes were relatively small (between 3-7%). Bennett et al. (2009) also found almost no changes to step kinematics, with only a slight decrease in hip flexion between the 25 m and 30 m mark of the sprint.

Weighted vests tend to have a more pronounced acute influence on linear speed. Zafeiropoulos et al. (2014) investigated the use of vests equivalent to 8%, 15%, and 20% of body mass in male university students, and found they caused a 4-10% increase in 0-10 m, 0-20 m, 0-40 m, and 0-50 m times within a 50 m sprint. In trained male and female athletes, wearing a vest equal to 15% and 20% of body mass led to a 7.5-10% increase in 0-10 m time, and 9.3-11.7% increase in 0-30 m time (Cronin et al., 2008). In contrast to Bennett et al. (2009), Cronin et al. (2008) noted numerous technical changes to gait, including increased contact time, and decreased swing phase time, step length and trunk lean, at the 5 m, 15 m, and 25 m points within a 30 m sprint. As a more upright body position resulted from sprinting with a weighted vest, Cronin et al. (2008) suggested that this modality would be best suited for developing maximum velocity, and that the greater eccentric load that resulted from weighted vest sprinting could be an appropriate form of overload for free sprinting. Despite this, Clark et al. (2010) found that sprint training with weighted vest equivalent to 18.5% of body mass over seven weeks with male collegiate lacrosse players led to only trivial improvements 18.3 and 54.9 sprint velocity. Nevertheless, further research should be conducted into the effects of sprint training with a weighted vest.

Sprinting with parachutes is another form of resisted sprinting. An argument for the use of parachutes is that they should cause minimal disruptions to sprint technique (Pauletto, 1993; Tabachnik, 1992; Martinopoulou et al., 2011). This idea is supported by analysis into the acute effects of parachute sprinting (Alcaraz et al., 2008; Paulson and Braun, 2011). Even though Paulson and Braun (2011) found a 4.4% decrease in speed over 36.58 m, and Alcaraz et al. (2008) a 6.6% decrease in a flying 30 m sprint, both studies documented minimal to no changes in sprint technique in male and female track sprinters. Paulson and Braun (2011) did find there was an increase in shoulder flexion at take-off within the step at the 18.3 m mark of the sprint, but this was the only difference when compared to free sprinting. With regards to longitudinal effects, Martinopoulou et al. (2011) found that four weeks of sprint training with a parachute, using 30 m and 50 m intervals, improved 0-20 m and 40-50 m velocity by 3% in male track sprinters. The improvements in the acceleration phase were due to an increase in step length, while the maximal velocity improvements were supported by step frequency increases.

There are, however, some limitations associated with parachute sprint training. The size of available parachutes are often limited by the manufacturer (Paulson and Braun, 2011). Furthermore, a parachute may not stay directly behind an athlete while they are sprinting, as they tend to move from side to side. This can lead to the individual attempting to maintain balance during each repetition, which could limit the attainment of maximum speed (Faccioni, 1994b; Jakalski, 1998). Jakalski (1998) suggested that these sudden shifts due to crosswinds may lead to injuries for the athlete, although this claim has not been substantiated by any research. Nonetheless, coaches should be cognizant of other resisted sprinting modalities that could allow for a greater degree of control on the external load.

Weighted sled towing is one of the more popular forms of resisted sprinting. This protocol allows the coach to exercise some measure of control on the load experienced by the athlete (Alcaraz et al., 2009; Lockie et al., 2003). Descriptive studies of resisted sled towing have shown some common results. For example, the acute effects of load increases on female sprinters at maximum velocity were decreases in stride length and frequency, and increased contact time, upper body lean, and hip joint angle at the beginning of stance (Letzelter et al., 1995). More recent investigations of the acute changes in acceleration kinematics in field sport athletes using sled towing found greater decreases in stride length than stride frequency, in addition to increases in contact time, trunk lean, hip flexion, and shoulder range of motion (Cronin et al., 2008; Lockie et al., 2003; Murray et al., 2005). The body position attained from sled towing typically realigns an individual such that their trunk lean and angle of trajectory are closer to the horizontal, which would also place a greater emphasis on horizontal force production during stance (Lockie et al., 2003). This further illustrates why sled towing is often used in an attempt to improve acceleration, due to the increased emphasis on horizontal GRF.

An argument against sled towing is that because it can significantly slow down the athlete, it could contravene sprinting technique (Lavrienko et al., 1990; Martinopoulou et al., 2011; Mouchbahani et al., 2004; Pauletto, 1993; Saraslanidis, 2000). Further, there is research that has illustrated resisted sprint training provides no benefit to linear speed. Saraslanidis (2000) found no improvements in the 20-50 m interval of a 50 m sprint performance for male physical education student who sprint trained for eight weeks towing a 5 kg sled. However, Saraslanidis (2000) did not provide justification for the use of this load. Kristensen et al. (2006) observed that 20 m sprint performance did not change in university students following six weeks of a sprint training program while being resisted by a load that decreased maximum velocity by 8.5%. Given the Lockie et al. (2003) recommendations, this load may not have been sufficient to provide the necessary overload for speed improvements. Indeed, there has been more research demonstrating that resisted sprinting can be effective in improving linear speed.

Zafeiridis et al. (2005) conducted an eight-week program using a 5 kg load which led to increases in 0-10 m and 0-20 m velocity in male university students. Even though the load was relatively light, linear speed still improved. Bachero-Mena and Gonzalez-Badillo (2014) investigated the use of loads equivalent to 5%, 12.5%, and 20% of body mass in male college students. Six weeks of training with each load improved 40 m sprint performance, and the 20% load induced significant changes in 0-20 m and 0-30 m time. Interestingly, the 12.5% load was very similar to that of Lockie et al. (2003). Six separate studies have used or adapted the load recommended by Lockie et al. (2003), and found that resisted sled training can improve speed (Harrison and Bourke, 2009; Lockie et al., 2012a; Spinks et al., 2007; Upton, 2011; Wagganer et al., 2015; West et al., 2013).

Spinks et al. (2007) demonstrated that resisted sprint towing can enhance speed over 15 m in male field sport athletes. Furthermore, Spinks et al. (2007) observed a reduction in second stride contact time, and an increase in trunk lean at take-off into the second stride. The increase in trunk lean could place an individual in a more advantageous position to produce horizontal force during stance. As a reflection of this, Lockie et al. (2012a) found sprint training with sleds, also in male field sport athletes, improved 0-5 m and 0-10 m sprint performance. These improvements were due to increases in step length over these intervals. Longer steps result from greater impulse generated during ground support (Lockie et al., 2013c), so these results suggest sled towing can improve force relative to the sprint step. In addition to this, sprint training while towing sleds has also been shown to improve 0-5 m, 0-10 m, and 0-30 m sprint performance in elite male rugby union players (Harrison and Bourke, 2009; West et al., 2013).

Resisted sprint training using sleds can also improve linear speed in females. While also incorporating free sprint drills and assisted sprinting, Wagganer et al. (2015) investigated the effects of sled towing in collegiate female soccer players. This combined, four-week training program led to a reduction in 36.58 m sprint time. Upton (2011) found that while using a device that allowed for resistance to be scaled and set at 12.6% of the participant's body mass, improvements were made in the 22.86-36.58 m interval of a 36.58 m sprint in collegiate female soccer players. This led Upton (2011) to suggest that resisted sprint training could improve maximum velocity in female soccer players. Lastly, Makaruk et al. (2013) used loads between 7.5%-10% of body mass when investigating sled towing in female physical education students. Following a nine-week program, the participants improved 20 m sprint velocity, which was primarily due to increases in step length. This was in line with the results from Lockie et al. (2012a), and the step length changes found by Makaruk et al. (2013)

were facilitated by increased knee extension at take-off into each step within the 20 m sprint. These studies collectively illustrate that resisted sled towing can be used in training to improve linear speed in both males and females, and cause favorable changes in the biomechanics of the sprint step.

Coaching literature has also suggested using a resisted sprinting system that can release the individual (Mouchbahani et al., 2004; Sebestyen, 1996), or completing unloaded sprint repetitions following the resisted repetitions (Verkhoshansky, 1996). Mouchbahani et al. (2004) implied that this practice will enhance the transferability of resisted sprinting to normal sprinting. Completing a free sprint after a resisted sprint also attempts to use the phenomenon of post-activation potentiation (Whelan et al., 2014). Whelan et al. (2014) stated that post-activation potentiation presents as an acute enhancement of performance or an enhancement of factors affecting performance after a preload stimulus. However, using a range of recovery times between 1-10 minutes, Whelan et al. (2014) found no clear evidence of any benefits for completing a free sprint after a resisted sprint with 25-30% of body mass in physically active men. This included sprint velocity, and technical factors such as step length, step frequency, and contact time.

What should be investigated further are the training effects of using a heavy load (i.e., 30% of body mass or greater) for resisted sled towing. As stated, a common critique of using heavy sled loads is that sprint technique will deteriorate too much, and this will negatively affect linear speed (Lavrienko et al., 1990; Martinopoulou et al., 2011; Mouchbahani et al., 2004; Pauletto, 1993; Saraslanidis, 2000). However, Lockie et al. (2003) found few significant changes in joint angular velocities, even with a load above 30% of body mass. Furthermore, Kawamori et al. (2014) observed that towing a sled load equating to 30% of body mass induced significant increases in second contact net horizontal and propulsive impulses when compared to a free sprint, but a 10% load did not. There may be further benefits for athletes to use a heavier sled load, especially trained athletes. Indeed, given elite strength-trained athletes can develop peak power at greater loads during a jump squat (Baker et al., 2001), this could also apply to an action such as resisted sprinting. This needs to be confirmed in future research.

Assisted Sprint Training

Assisted sprint training modalities allow an athlete to increase their speed or frequency of movement by receiving assistance from an external person or device (Faccioni, 1994a). Also referred to as overspeed sprinting, this modality involves an individual completing sprints that attain speeds above the velocity that they could otherwise achieve unaided (i.e., supramaximal velocities). Due to the importance of step frequency to increasing maximum velocity (Kuitunen et al., 2002; Luhtanen and Komi, 1978), assisted sprinting has typically been used with a view to enhancing this kinematic parameter. Sprinting using a towing device has indeed been shown to lead to acute increases in step frequency during sprinting (Mero and Komi, 1985). However, research has tended to show greater acute changes in step length with assisted sprint modalities (Mero and Komi, 1985; Paradisis and Cooke, 2001; Corn and Knudson, 2003).

As for resisted sprinting, there are suggested guidelines for how much assistance should be provided while sprinting. Clark et al. (2009) recommended that individuals should not exceed 106-110% of their unassisted maximal sprint velocity. Bartolini et al. (2011) proposed that 30% of body mass assistance should be used when training with elastic cords for sprints over distances of up to 13.72 m (i.e., 15 yards). The issue for coaches is using assisted modalities where there is explicit control over the sprint velocities that result. There are a number of different modalities that can be used to provide assisted conditions. Some examples include: towing via an or elastic cord and harness connected to another sprinter and then stretched; towing via an elastic cord and harness that is connected to an immovable object and then stretched; a towing machine that 'reels in' the sprinter; high-speed treadmill sprinting; and downhill sprinting (Costello, 1985; Faccioni, 1994a).

Sprinting with assistance provided by a towing mechanism will lead to acute changes in technique. For example, 5 kg of assistance via a towing machine led to a reduction in mean contact time (0.795 seconds [s]) when compared to free sprinting (0.899 s) over 20 m in track sprinters (Mouchbahani et al., 2004). Elastic cord assistance that provided a towing force of 10-30% body weight led to progressive decreases in sprint times over 18.29 m (Bartolini et al., 2011). A partner-assisted towing system that provided 30-45 Newtons (N) of force in male and female sprinters caused an 8.5% increase in sprint velocity after a 35 m flying start (Mero and Komi, 1985, 1987). Other technical changes to performance in track sprinters include a 1.7% increase in stride frequency and 6.8% increase in stride length (Mero and Komi, 1985), as well as increases in flight time and braking force (Mero and Komi, 1987). The increase in braking force could be an issue with sprint towing. If the towing force is too great, the individual will lose some control of their sprint step and over-stride. This may actually cause the individual to slow down (Bartolini et al., 2011), which could then adversely affect any adaptations that result with training. Lastly, Corn and Knudson (2003) used a partner-assisted towing that provided 40-50 N of horizontal force in male and female collegiate sprinters over a 20 m sprint. Sprint velocity increased by 7.1%, and there was also an increase in stride length, although stride frequency did not change.

Partner-assisted towing from another sprinter via an elasticized cord is arguably the most practical field modality for assisted sprint training. A limitation of this method is that the amount of assistance provided during a sprint is often dictated by the equipment design from the manufacturer (Corn and Knudson, 2003). Nonetheless, some of the acute changes that result following assisted towing are also reflected in training adaptations. As previously acknowledged, Wagganer et al. (2015) utilized a combined sprint training protocol in collegiate female soccer players. The assistive force provided by the elastic towing device equated to approximately 6-10% of body weight. The sprint repetitions were over 18.3 m, and the program by Wagganer et al. (2015) improved 36.58 m sprint performance. The four-week speed training program utilized by Upton (2011) also included an exclusive assisted sprint training group. The assisted towing device provided a mean towing force of 14.7 ± 0.8% of body weight. Although assisted sprint training modalities were traditionally thought to be most valuable for improving maximum velocity sprinting, Upton (2011) found more benefit to acceleration in female soccer players. Indeed, the players who completed assisted sprint training improved performance in the 0-4.6 m, 0-13.7 m, and 4.6-13.7 m intervals in a 36.58 m sprint. Upton (2011) inferred that the improvements in speed were due to neurological adaptations, and recommended using assisted sprint training for acceleration development.

A treadmill can also be used to provide overspeed conditions, as the moving belt assists with repositioning the legs underneath the body during the sprint step (Frishberg, 1983). If the individual's maximum velocity is known, then the treadmill can be programmed above this value, and the action of the treadmill belt can force the individual to sprint at a higher speed than they otherwise could. Ross et al. (2009) investigated treadmill sprint training in trained men, using maximal treadmill sprints that equated to 40-560 m over an eight-week period. Following the intervention, 30 m sprint performance improved by 0.08 s, although this was a non-significant change. There may be merit in using high-speed treadmill sprinting to enhance linear speed, although further research is needed to confirm this.

Downhill sprinting is another form of assisted sprinting. As for uphill sprinting, a limitation is the ability to control the slope used in training, as well as the availability of slopes. Anecdotal information suggested that a decline of 3° was appropriate for assisted sprint training (Costello, 1985; Paradisis and Cooke, 2006; Pauletto, 1993), although this initially was not based upon scientific research. Subsequently, there was analysis conducted as to the benefits of using a 3° slope for assisted sprint training, using a custom-built running platform (Paradisis et al., 2009; Paradisis and Cooke, 2006). Paradisis and Cooke (2006) found that six weeks of completing 3° downhill sprints led to a 1.1% increase in 35 m sprint velocity, and 2.4% increase in step frequency, in physical education students. However, a group that completed combined 3° uphill and 3° downhill sprints experienced a 3.5% increase in 35 m sprint velocity, and 3.4% increase in step frequency. This led Paradisis et al. (2009) to compare combined uphill-downhill sprint training to free sprint training over an eight-week program. Physical education students were again the sample population. The results indicated that although both groups improved linear speed, the combined uphill-downhill group experienced relatively greater gains in 35 m sprint velocity (4.3% increase), step frequency (4.3% increase), and contact time (5.1% decrease). Taken together, the results from Paradisis and Cooke (2006) and Paradisis et al. (2009) imply some benefit to using a 3° downhill speed training modality.

Nonetheless, there was contention as to whether 3° is the most appropriate decline angle to use for downhill sprinting. Ebben (2008) and Ebben et al. (2008) measured the 36.58 m sprint performance of Division III collegiate male athletes over a range of different decline slopes (0°, 2.1°, 3.3°, 4.7°, 5.8°, and 6.9°). The combined results indicated that the fastest performance for both the 0-9.14 m (Ebben et al., 2008) and 0-36.58 m (Ebben, 2008; Ebben et al., 2008) interval resulted from the 5.8° slope. Much like increasing pulling force in a towing system, a greater downhill slope will provide more assistance when sprinting, and could potentially provide more benefit to an individual who wishes to enhance acceleration and maximal velocity sprinting. However, the training effects of using a more pronounced slope, both from a speed and technique perspective, requires further investigation.

MODALITIES USED FOR COD SPEED TRAINING

Resistance Training for COD Speed

A strong base of strength should not just benefit linear speed; it should also positively influence COD speed. Indeed, strength forms part of the model for COD speed illustrated by Sheppard and Young (2006). There is also research that has established relationships between strength and COD speed (Delaney et al., 2015; Lockie et al., 2012b; Spiteri et al., 2013; Spiteri et al., 2014). However, there has been debate suggesting significant (Sheppard et al., 2014) or relatively minor (Brughelli et al., 2008) influences of strength training on COD speed. The reason for this is that there is research showing improvement (Barr et al., 2014;

Keiner et al., 2014; Nimphius et al., 2012) or no significant change (Fry et al., 1991; Hoffman et al., 2004; Tricoli et al., 2005) in COD speed following strength training.

For example, Tricoli et al. (2005) observed that eight weeks of strength training using Olympic lifts did not significantly improve COD speed measured by a custom test (three circuits of three 45° cuts completed within a 4 m square) in male physical education students. In an investigation of a 12-week off-season strength training program in collegiate female volleyball players, Fry et al. (1991) found a significant 3% increase in T-test time, which indicated a decline in COD speed. The strength training program used many traditional exercises, such as back and split squats, hang power cleans, calf raises, and a range of upper-body exercises. Hoffman et al. (2004) investigated the effects of an Olympic lifting versus a powerlifting program in Division III collegiate male American football players. After 15 weeks, neither group improved COD speed measured by the T-test. The T-test is a very dynamic assessment, which incorporates a linear acceleration, side-shuffling, and backwards running (Semenick, 1990). Potentially, the exercises used in the strength programs by Fry et al. (1991) and Hoffman et al. (2004) were not specific enough to improve the movement patterns in a COD speed assessment such as the T-test. In addition to this, the afore-mentioned studies all used exercises (e.g., squats, deadlifts, and Olympic-style lifts) that predominantly generate vertical force. Brughelli et al. (2008) stated that one of the limitations of traditional strength exercises eliciting improvements in COD speed is that most focus on vertical force production. This could restrict the direct transfer of strength improvements to COD speed.

A counterpoint to Brughelli et al. (2008) was provided by Sheppard et al. (2014). Sheppard et al. (2014) asserted that the transfer of training effect should be measured, as this takes into consideration the change in strength as it relates to the change in another variable, such as COD speed (Nimphius et al., 2012; Barr et al., 2014; Sheppard et al., 2014). Sheppard et al. (2014) also advised that there were limitations in interpreting the findings of Fry et al. (1991) and Hoffman et al. (2004), as they did not present relative strength results. Given that a COD requires the effective control of body mass (Sheppard et al., 2014; Spiteri et al., 2013), relative strength should contribute greatly to these actions. In corroboration of this, Delaney et al. (2015) discovered that the strongest predictor (67% of the common variance) of performance of the 505 COD speed test by elite rugby league players was relative strength as measured by a 3RM squat. If changes in relative strength are not considered in relation to COD speed, this may not be the best interpretation as to the effects of strength training.

The value of strength for COD speed was illustrated by Spiteri et al. (2013) and Spiteri et al. (2014). As previously stated, Spiteri et al. (2013) found that stronger recreational male and female team sport athletes produced greater levels of braking, vertical, and propulsive force during a 45° cut when compared to weaker athletes. The ability to generate great vertical (Lockie et al., 2013c; Weyand et al., 2000) and propulsive (Brughelli et al., 2011; de Lacey et al., 2014; Hunter et al., 2005; Kawamori et al., 2013; Kugler and Janshen, 2010; Morin et al., 2011) forces are essential for linear speed, which would have contributed to the faster post-stride velocity in the COD for the stronger (2.50 ± 0.37 m·s^{-1}) when compared to the weaker (2.28 ± 0.27 m·s^{-1}) participants. In a separate study, Spiteri et al. (2014) discovered that eccentric strength as measured by the isometric mid-thigh pull predicted both T-test (77% of the common variance) and 505 COD speed test (75% of the common variance) time in elite female basketball players. Spiteri et al. (2014) concluded that the number of directional changes required in the T-test, and the severity of the 180° cut in the 505, placed a greater emphasis on the eccentric strength that needed to be expressed when braking. As further support, Lockie et al. (2012b) observed that recreational male team sport athletes who had a smaller between-leg difference in knee flexor eccentric work (measured by isokinetic dynamometry at an angular velocity of 30° per second [$°·s^{-1}$]) were faster in the T-test when compared to those participants with a larger difference. Indeed, strength imbalances between the legs have been recognized as a limiting factor in COD speed (Sheppard and Young, 2006). Collectively, these studies provide support to Sheppard et al. (2014), and thus there should be further discussion as to the transfer of training from strength to COD speed.

Within the longer-term analysis of strength training and female softball players, Nimphius et al. (2012) found a very large correlation (r = -0.70) between the change in 1RM squat relative to body mass (12.22% increase) and 505 COD test time from the dominant leg (1.09% decrease), and a large correlation (r = -0.51) with 505 COD test time from the non-dominant leg (5.48% decrease), following the intervention. Additionally, the decrease in non-dominant leg 505 COD test time was a significant change. Although the non-dominant leg would have a greater capacity for improvement when compared to the dominant leg (Newton et al., 2006; Nimphius et al., 2012), this is still a noteworthy result, given that elite, highly-trained athletes will experience diminishing returns with training (Barr et al., 2014). Nimphius et al. (2012) concluded that the correct implementation of a periodized strength program over the course of a season can improve measures of strength and sport performance, in this instance COD speed in elite female athletes.

Keiner et al. (2014) investigated the long-term effects of strength training on young male soccer players across a range of different ages. However, only those participants 18 years of age or older will be considered for this chapter. The players were tracked over the course of two years, and the training program included front and back squats, deadlifts, bench presses, rows, and trunk muscle exercises. Maximum strength was measured by 1RM front and back squats; COD speed was measured by a custom-designed test that involved a total distance of 10 m, with 2.5 m and 5 m sprints interspersed with two direction changes. The results indicated that those players who resistance trained significantly improved relative strength measured by both front and back squats when compared to a control group that did not. More importantly, the effect size for the between-group differences in the time changes for the custom COD speed test were large (*d* > 1), with strength-trained participants completing the test faster. Lastly, a correlation analysis showed relative 1RM front and back squat significantly related to the agility test times (r = -0.45 to 0.64). Keiner et al. (2014) linked the higher maximum strength levels with faster COD times and improvements in deceleration, which the authors suggested was due to enhanced eccentric strength. This coalesces with previous research that established relationships between eccentric strength and COD speed in males (Lockie et al., 2012b) and females (Spiteri et al., 2014).

Sheppard et al. (2014) asserted that the results of Nimphius et al. (2012) and Keiner et al. (2014) was evidence that longitudinal changes in strength led to a moderate to very large transfer of training effects to COD speed. This occurred even with the use of traditional exercises that emphasized vertical force production. In addition to this, strength and conditioning coaches should also be aware of other resistance exercises that can more closely match the movement patterns of COD speed. For example, lateral walking lunges and lateral-step-ups are examples of strength exercises adapted for COD movements (Dawes and Lentz, 2012; Twist and Benicky, 1996; Yap et al., 2000). Intuitively, it would seem that strength exercises incorporating lateral movements should engender some crossover into COD speed performance. However, there is no research that categorically documents this, and this should be confirmed in future investigations.

Plyometrics Training for COD Speed

Leg power also forms part of the model for COD speed (Sheppard and Young, 2006). Multiple plyometrics exercises have been used in an attempt to improve COD speed, and examples of these exercises are available in numerous sources (Brown and Ferrigno, 2015; Dawes and Roozen, 2012; Radcliffe and Farentinos, 2015). However, similar to resistance training, Brughelli et al. (2008) acknowledged that many standard plyometrics exercises, such as the countermovement or squat jump, place a greater emphasis of vertical force production. This is also reflected in studies that show limited relationships between COD speed performance and an assessment such as the vertical countermovement jump (Alemdaroglu, 2012; Vescovi and McGuigan, 2008), even though both stress the stretch-shortening capacities of the muscles in the lower-body. However, several different studies have indicated relationships between leg power measured by jumps in multiple directions (vertical, horizontal, and lateral) and COD speed.

Chaouachi et al. (2012) observed that peak power measured during a countermovement jump contributed to the predictive model for the 5 m shuttle run-sprint test in elite male soccer players. In a similar analysis of elite rugby league players, two variables that contributed to a predictive model for the 505 COD speed test performed off the non-dominant leg was dominant leg lateral jump distance, and peak power from a 40 kg loaded jump squat (Delaney et al., 2015). The squat jump, which emphasizes concentric power, significantly correlated with an up-and-back COD speed test ($r = -0.44$), and the T-test ($r = -0.41$), in female collegiate athletes (Sekulic et al., 2013). The 5-jump (or 5-bound) test, which places a great emphasis on horizontal power generation, was significantly correlated ($r = -0.61$) with T-test time in elite professional basketball players (Chaouachi et al., 2009). Lockie et al. (2014a) examined relationships between unilateral (vertical, standing broad, and lateral) jumps with COD speed measured by a modified, smaller version of the T-test and the 505 COD speed test. A range of significant correlations were found between jump performance and the COD speed test times ($r = -0.38$ to -0.72). The results from these studies suggest that improving lower-body power should contribute to positive changes in COD speed.

Previous research has indeed shown that specific plyometrics training can improve COD speed (McBride et al., 2002; Miller et al., 2006; Salonikidis and Zafeiridis, 2008; Váczi et al., 2013). In a six-week program that incorporated jumps emphasizing vertical (standing jump and reach), horizontal (standing long jump and travelling hops), and lateral (multidirectional jumps and hops) projection, Miller et al. (2006) found significant 5% and 3% decreases in T-test and Illinois Agility Test time, respectively, in college-aged males. Váczi et al. (2013) also documented that six weeks of plyometrics training can improve T-test (2.5% decrease) and Illinois Agility Test (1.7% decrease) times in experienced male soccer players. Although the percent changes were smaller than those of Miller et al. (2006), the significant improvements found by Váczi et al. (2013) occurred with the use of a program that had a short duration (10-20 minutes) within the context of the team training sessions. Váczi et al. (2013) inferred that even relatively brief plyometrics training sessions can positively influence aspects of athletic performance, such as COD speed. Salonikidis and Zafeiridis (2008) examined the effects of a plyometrics program incorporating unilateral jumps, hops-in-place, stair hops, and single-leg tuck, drop and lateral jumps, on novice tennis players. The nine-week program led to an improvement in a 4 m lateral sprint, as well as a reaction time test involving side-stepping.

Plyometrics exercises can also be completed with extra load, such as with weighted jump squats. Although a jump squat almost purely emphasizes vertical force production, this exercise incorporates high velocities with large eccentric forces (Cormie et al., 2008; McBride et al., 2002). Brughelli et al. (2008) stated that this could provide similar conditions to a COD action, which could then engender crossover into performance. As evidence of this, McBride et al. (2002) found that an eight-week training program utilizing jump squats with either 30% or 80% of 1RM squat both resulted in significant 2% decreases in T-test time in club-level male athletes. The collective results from these studies designate the value of using plyometrics training, whether purely incorporating body weight exercises or jumps with additional load, for improving COD speed in young adults.

Much like linear speed training programs, however, coaches will rarely use plyometrics in isolation. Rather, they will often be incorporated into COD speed training programs with COD drills. Several research studies have combined plyometrics with specific drills in training programs to investigate the overall effects on COD speed (Bloomfield et al., 2007; Jovanovic et al., 2011; Lockie et al., 2014e; Milanovic et al., 2013; Polman et al., 2004). This will be discussed in the following section.

Specific COD Drills

COD speed requires the effective use of an individual's neuromuscular characteristics (Neptune et al., 1999). As a result, training for COD speed will generally involve the completion of drills that target specific movement patterns and cutting actions. Many COD drills focus on developing footwork, correct body position, and acceleration capacity. There are a multitude of COD drills that can and have been used in training, and there is available literature that contains examples and explanations of different drills (Brown and Ferrigno, 2015; Dawes and Roozen, 2012). A coach may use their own discretion to design a particular drill, but they must ensure that the prescribed exercises are specific to the movement patterns of the individual's sport. Within the scientific literature, COD speed training research has incorporated a range of activities, including specific COD and technique drills, maximal sprint running, and plyometrics (Bloomfield et al., 2007; Jovanovic et al., 2011; Lockie et al., 2014e; Milanovic et al., 2013; Polman et al., 2004). The results have generally shown that the correct implementation of COD drills within training can improve COD speed.

Jovanovic et al. (2011) investigated the effects of an eight-week COD speed training program on young, high-level soccer players. Although the study methodology did not include a COD speed test, the program, which involved linear and COD speed drills, resisted lateral runs, and multidirectional plyometrics, improved 10 m sprint and vertical jump performance. As noted in Figure 3, linear speed and leg power both contribute to COD speed (Sheppard and Young, 2006). Milanovic et al. (2013) examined the effects of a 12-week COD speed program in a similar population, with similar training exercises to those of Jovanovic et al. (2011). However, Milanovic et al. (2013) did assess COD speed, and found multiple tests of this capacity (sprint with 180° turns, 4 x 5 m shuttle sprints, slalom test, sprint with a 90° turn) all improved after the training intervention.

A range of different equipment can be used when training COD speed. However, the use of expensive equipment is not imperative to improving COD speed. As evidence of this, Polman et al. (2004) investigated the use of specialized COD training equipment (e.g., speed ladders, resistance cords, breakaway cords, and hurdles) in elite female soccer players. Exercises were grouped under general headings of sprint mechanics, speed, agility, power, and speed endurance, and the program ran for 10 weeks. One training group used specialized equipment, while the other did not. COD speed was measured by a custom soccer test that incorporated 90° and 180° turns, covering a total distance of approximately 18 m, and an up-and-back test featuring a 180° turn within an approximate 9 m sprint. Both training groups improved COD speed measured by the two tests, with no real between-group differences, irrespective of equipment use. Bloomfield et al. (2007) substantiated these findings in an analysis of COD speed training in untrained males and females. A six-week program featuring drills that targeted sprint technique, footwork development, lateral shuffling, back pedaling, and linear acceleration, either with or without equipment, was implemented. The results indicated that the improvements in a 15 m linear sprint, T-test, and standing broad jump all occurred regardless of whether COD training equipment was used or not. Coaches who do not have access to specialized COD speed training equipment can still elicit improvements in the indivdiuals whom they are training, as long as their program design is appropriate.

All of this research jointly indicates that the correct use of specific training drills can enhance COD speed. These improvements can occur irrespective of whether specialized equipment is used or not, as long as the training program is appropriately designed and specific to the desired outcomes. What is worthy of further investigation is a method that can be used to manipulate COD drills by enforcing a stop at the end of an exercise (Dawes and Roozen, 2012; Lockie et al., 2014e). This has been referred to as deceleration training.

Deceleration Training

As previously discussed, a component of COD speed is deceleration. Deceleration has not been widely analyzed in the current scientific literature, although there is available coaching theory (Dawes and Roozen, 2012; Hewit et al., 2011; Kovacs et al., 2008). Kovacs et al. (2008) stated that deceleration features four major components: power, reactive strength, eccentric strength, and dynamic balance or stability. The relationship between strength, power, and COD speed has been discussed in this chapter. What has yet to be explored is dynamic stability, which is the ability to maintain balance while transitioning from a dynamic to static state (Wikstrom et al., 2005). During a COD movement, individuals must maintain stability when shifting from a dynamic (deceleration) to a static (stopping to cut), before returning to a dynamic (acceleration) state.

To this end, Sekulic et al. (2013) demonstrated that two basic tests of dynamic stability (overall stability index and limit of stability score) correlated (r = 0.40 to 0.58) with several different COD speed tests involving lateral cutting, side-shuffling, and up-and-back sprinting in male collegiate athletes. However, both of these dynamic stability tests were performed from a bilateral stance, as opposed to a unilateral stance which is typical for cutting. Thus, Lockie et al. (in press) investigated the relationship between dynamic stability, measured by a modified version of the Star Excursion Balance Test (mSEBT), and COD speed, measured by the T-test and change-of-direction and acceleration test (CODAT). The mSEBT, shown in Figure 5, involves an individual adopting a unilateral stance and performing a series of single-leg squats while maximally reaching with the other leg (Gribble, 2003; Hertel et al., 2000; Lockie et al., in press). A further reach indicates better dynamic stability. The CODAT features four 45° cuts within a sprint distance of approximately 24 m (Lockie et al., 2013d). Thus, both the T-test and CODAT contain pronounced cuts (i.e., 45°, 90°, or 180°) which should stress an individual's ability to maintain stability while changing direction. In support of this, Lockie et al. (in press) noted a range of significant relationships (r = -0.51 to -0.64) between mSEBT excursion distances for both legs, and T-test and CODAT times. Thus, dynamic stability is a capacity that could influence COD speed (Lockie et al., in press; Sekulic et al., 2013).

Lockie et al. (2014e) then investigated whether specifically training the aspect of cutting where dynamic stability would be important (i.e., the deceleration phase) would enhance COD speed in male and female recreational team sport athletes. One training group completed COD drills in the traditional manner; the other completed the same drills except they had an enforced stop at the end of each repetition. Novel assessments were included in the study methodology, such as isokinetic strength of the knee extensors and flexors, and dynamic stability measured by the mSEBT. The six-week program included linear speed and speed ladder drills, COD speed drills (Y-cuts, T-drill, W-drill, Z-drill), and medicine ball throws. For the enforced stopping group, participants stopped: at a marker at the end of a COD drill; after 3 m following a 10-20 m sprint; or after 6 m following a 30-40 m sprint. The stop position used by Lockie et al. (2014e) is shown in Figure 6. Position A was used at the end of drills which had a side-shuffle or back pedal to finish. Position B was used for drills that finished with a linear sprint.

For the group that completed traditional COD speed training, Lockie et al. (2014e) found 0-10 m, 0-20 m, and 0-40 m sprint times, as well as T-test and CODAT times, decreased following the intervention. This supported other research documenting the benefits of training with specific drills to enhance COD speed (Bloomfield et al., 2007; Jovanovic et al., 2011; Milanovic et al., 2013; Polman et al., 2004). There were no significant changes in isokinetic strength, but mSEBT performance did improve. For those in the enforced stopping group, there were improvements in 0-40 m sprint, T-test, CODAT, and mSEBT performance. However, even though time in the 0-10 m and 0-20 m intervals in the 40 m sprint decreased by 4% and 2%, respectively, these changes were not significant. Lockie et al. (2014e) suggested that participants may have started slowing down prior to the end of the shorter sprints if they felt they could not decelerate quickly enough within the stopping distance. The practical implication of this is that coaches should use stopping distances that allow their athletes to maximally complete the sprint distances required within the drill. Furthermore, shortening stopping distances could be used as a progressive overload within COD speed training.

The enforced stopping training group also increased relative left-leg concentric knee extensor torque measured at an angular velocity of $240°·s^{-1}$ by 8%, and eccentric knee flexor torque at $30°·s^{-1}$ by 19%. More notably, there was a significant increase in the between-leg difference in concentric knee flexor torque at $240°·s^{-1}$ (7.00 ± 6.65% to 11.61 ± 6.15%). Although a clinical significance level for a strength asymmetry has been stated as being 15% (Bennell et al., 1998; Dauty et al., 2007; Knapik et al., 1991), and these values were below this, Lockie et al. (2014e) still made an important point. As individuals generally have a preferred starting leg for sprinting (Lockie et al., 2012c; Vagenas and Hoshizaki, 1986), they would also likely have a preferred braking leg to stop. Coaches who use enforced stopping or deceleration drills must ensure there is an equal balance between the legs used to stop. Otherwise, over the long term they may unwittingly cause a lower-body strength imbalance in their athletes, which would negatively influence COD speed (Lockie et al., 2012b; Sheppard and Young, 2006). Lockie et al. (2014e) concluded that there was merit in using enforced stopping COD drills, but an entire program built around these drills was likely not required. The collective findings from the discussed research clearly indicate that the correct implementation of COD speed training drills, of which specific deceleration drills can be included, will enhance this capacity in individuals from a range of athletic backgrounds.

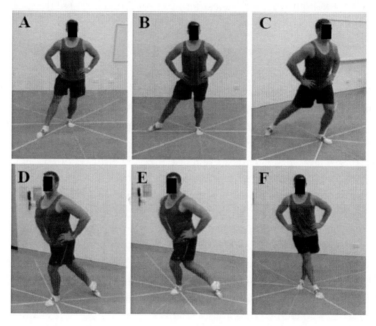

Figure 5. The modified Star Excursion Balance Test (mSEBT) used by Lockie et al. [105]. The figure depicts mSEBT performance with a left stance leg and right reach leg for the (A) anterolateral; (B) lateral; (C) posterolateral; (D) posteromedial; (E) medial; and (F) anteromedial excursions.

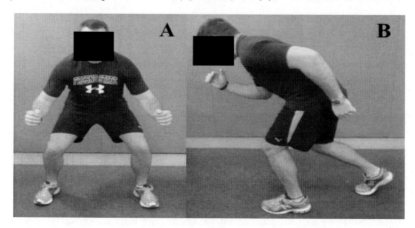

Figure 6. Stopping positions used for deceleration training during change-of-direction speed training. Lockie et al. (2013a) utilized Position A following a lateral shuffle or back pedal, and Position B following a linear sprint.

CONCLUSION

Linear and COD speed are essential requirements within many different sports. There are number of different modalities that can be used to train speed, although coaches must be cognizant of the fact that linear and COD speed are different qualities and must be developed specifically. Most training protocols target some type of technique, force, or power adaptation. Coaches should be aware of how force and power are expressed within specific training modalities, how this could be transferred to the sprinting gait, and ultimately how this could influence technique adaptations for linear and COD speed. The correct use of specific sprint intervals, resistance training for strength, plyometrics, and resisted and assisted sprint training modalities should improve linear speed in young adults. Strength training and plyometrics can also positively influence COD speed. Specific COD speed drills should also be used to improve this capacity, and deceleration training could also be incorporated in some manner. With appropriate knowledge of the individual's training background, their sport, and the appropriate implementation of training, coaches should be able to enhance the linear and COD speed of their athletes.

REFERENCES

Alcaraz, P.E., Palao, J.M. and Elvira, J.L. (2009). Determining the optimal load for resisted sprint training with sled towing. *Journal of Strength and Conditioning Research, 23,* 480-485.

Alcaraz, P.E., Palao, J.M., Elvira, J.L., Linthorne, N.P. (2008). Effects of three types of resisted sprint training devices on the kinematics of sprinting at maximum velocity. *Journal of Strength and Conditioning Research, 22,* 890-897.

Alemdaroglu, U. (2012). The relationship between muscle strength, anaerobic performance, agility, sprint ability and vertical jump performance in professional basketball players. *Journal of Human Kinetics, 31,* 149-158.

Ambrose, W.T. (1978). The dynamics of sprinting. *Track and Field Quarterly Review, 78,* 11-14.

Atwater, A. E. (1982). Kinematic analyses of sprinting. *Track and Field Quarterly Review, 82,* 12-16.

Bachero-Mena, B., Gonzalez-Badillo, J.J. (2014). Effects of resisted sprint training on acceleration with three different loads accounting for 5, 12.5, and 20% of body mass. *Journal of Strength and Conditioning Research, 28,* 2954-2960.

Baker, D., Nance, S. (1999). The relation between running speed and measures of strength and power in professional rugby league players. *Journal of Strength and Conditioning Research, 13,* 230-235.

Baker, D., Nance, S., Moore, M. (2001). The load that maximizes the average mechanical power output during jump squats in power-trained athletes. *Journal of Strength and Conditioning Research, 15,* 92-97.

Baker, J.S., Bell, W. (1994). Anaerobic performance and sprinting ability in elite male and female sprinters. *Journal of Human Movement Studies, 27,* 235-244.

Bangsbo, J., Nørregaard, L., Thorsø, F. (1991). Activity profile of competition soccer. *Canadian Journal of Sport Sciences, 16,* 110-116.

Barr, M.J., Sheppard, J.M., Agar-Newman, D. J., Newton, R.U. (2014). Transfer effect of strength and power training to the sprinting kinematics of international rugby players. *Journal of Strength and Conditioning Research, 28,* 2585-2596.

Bartolini, J.A., Brown, L.E., Coburn, J.W., Judelson, D.A., Spiering, B.A., Aguirre, N.W., Carney, K.R., Harris, K.B. (2011). Optimal elastic cord assistance for sprinting in collegiate women soccer players. *Journal of Strength and Conditioning Research, 25,* 1263-1270.

Baxter, J.R., Novack, T.A., Van Werkhoven, H., Pennell, D.R. and Piazza, S.J. (2012). Ankle joint mechanics and foot proportions differ between human sprinters and non-sprinters. *Proceedings of Biological Science, 279,* 2018-2024.

Behm, D.G. (1995). Neuromuscular implications and applications of resistance training. *Journal of Strength and Conditioning Research, 9,* 264-274.

Behm, D. G., Sale, D. G. (1993). Velocity specificity of resistance training. *Sports Medicine, 15,* 374-388.

Belli, A., Kyröläinen, H. and Komi, P.V. (2002). Movement and power of lower limb joints in running. *International Journal of Sport Medicine, 23,* 136-141.

Bennell, K., Wajswelner, H., Lew, P., Schall-Riaucour, A., Leslie, S., Plant, D., Cirone, J. (1998). Isokinetic strength testing does not predict hamstring injury in Australian Rules footballers. *British Journal of Sports Medicine, 32,* 309-314.

Bennett, J.P., Sayers, M.G. and Burkett, B.J. (2009). The impact of lower extremity mass and inertia manipulation on sprint kinematics. *Journal of Strength and Conditioning Research, 23,* 2542-2547.

Benton, D. (2001). Sprint running needs of field sport athletes: a new perspective. *Sports Coaching, 24,* 12-14.

Bezodis, I.N., Kerwin, D.G., Salo, A.I. (2008). Lower-limb mechanics during the support phase of maximum-velocity sprint running. *Medicine and Science in Sports and Exercise, 40,* 707-715.

Bhowmick, S., Bhattacharyya, A.K. (1988). Kinematic analysis of arm movements in sprint start. *Journal of Sports Medicine and Physical Fitness, 28,* 315-323.

Bloomfield, J., Polman, R., O'Donoghue, P., McNaughton, L. (2007). Effective speed and agility conditioning methodology for random intermittent dynamic type sports. *Journal of Strength and Conditioning Research, 21,* 1093-1100.

Bolger, R., Lyons, M., Harrison, A.J., Kenny, I.C. (2015). Sprinting performance and resistance-based training interventions: a systematic review. *Journal of Strength and Conditioning Research, 29,* 1146-1156.

Brown, L.E., Ferrigno, V.A. (2015). *Training for Speed, Agility, and Quickness* (3rd ed.). Champaign: Human Kinetics.

Brown, S.R., Brughelli, M., Hume, P.A. (2014). Knee mechanics during planned and unplanned sidestepping: a systematic review and meta-analysis. *Sports Medicine, 44,* 1573-1588.

Brown, T.D., Vescovi, J.D. (2003). Efficient arms for efficient agility. *Strength and Conditioning Journal, 25,* 7-11.

Brughelli, M., Cronin, J., Chaouachi, A. (2011). Effects of running velocity on running kinetics and kinematics. *Journal of Strength and Conditioning* Research, *25,* 933-939.

Brughelli, M., Cronin, J., Levin, G., Chaouachi, A. (2008). Understanding change of direction ability in sport. *Sports Medicine*, *38*, 1045-1063.

Callaghan, S.J., Lockie, R.G., Jeffriess, M.D. (2014). The acceleration kinematics of cricket-specific starts when completing a quick single. *Sports Technique, 7*, 39-51.

Callaghan, S.J., Lockie, R.G., Jeffriess, M.D., Nimphius, S. (2015). The kinematics of faster acceleration performance of the quick single in experienced cricketers. *Journal of Strength and Conditioning Research, 29*, 2623-2634.

Chaouachi, A., Brughelli, M., Chamari, K., Levin, G.T., Ben Abdelkrim, N., Laurencelle, L., Castagna, C. (2009). Lower limb maximal dynamic strength and agility determinants in elite basketball players. *Journal of Strength and Conditioning Research*, *23*, 1570-1577.

Chaouachi, A., Manzi, V., Chaalali, A., Wong del, P., Chamari, K., Castagna, C. (2012). Determinants analysis of change-of-direction ability in elite soccer players. *Journal of Strength and Conditioning* Research, *26*, 2667-2676.

Chelly, M.S., Ghenem, M.A., Abid, K., Hermassi, S., Tabka, Z., Shephard, R.J. (2010). Effects of in-season short-term plyometric training program on leg power, jump- and sprint performance of soccer players. *Journal of Strength and Conditioning Research*, *24*, 2670-2676.

Clark, D.A., Sabick, M.B., Pfeiffer, R.P., Kuhlman, S.M., Knigge, N.A., Shea, K.G. (2009). Influence of towing force magnitude on the kinematics of supramaximal sprinting. *Journal of Strength and Conditioning Research*, *23*, 1162-1168.

Clark, K.P., Stearne, D.J., Walts, C.T., Miller, A.D. (2010). The longitudinal effects of resisted sprint training using weighted sleds vs. weighted vests. *Journal of Strength and Conditioning Research*, *24*, 3287-3295.

Čoh, M., Jošt, B., Škof, B., Tomažin, K., Dolenec, A. (1998). Kinematic and kinetic parameters of the sprint start and start acceleration model of top sprinters. *Gymnica, 28,* 33-42.

Čoh, M., Mihajloviè, S. and Praprotnik, U. (2001). Morphologic and kinematic characteristics of elite sprinters. *Collegium Antropologicum*, *25*, 605-610.

Comfort, P., Bullock, N. and Pearson, S.J. (2012a). A comparison of maximal squat strength and 5-, 10-, and 20-meter sprint times, in athletes and recreationally trained men. *Journal of Strength and Conditioning Research*, *26*, 937-940.

Comfort, P., Haigh, A. and Matthews, M.J. (2012b). Are changes in maximal squat strength during preseason training reflected in changes in sprint performance in rugby league players? *Journal of Strength and Conditioning Research*, *26*, 772-776.

Cormie, P., McBride, J.M., McCaulley, G.O. (2008). Power-time, force-time, and velocity-time curve analysis during the jump squat: impact of load. *Journal of Applied Biomechanics*, *24*, 112-120.

Cormie, P., McGuigan, M.R., Newton, R.U. (2010). Adaptations in athletic performance after ballistic power versus strength training. *Medicine and Science in Sports and Exercise*, *42*, 1582-1598.

Corn, R.J., Knudson, D. (2003). Effect of elastic-cord towing on the kinematics of the acceleration phase of sprinting. *Journal of Strength and Conditioning Research*, *17*, 72-75.

Costello, F. (1985). Training for speed using resisted and assisted methods. *National Strength and Conditioning Association Journal*, *7*, 74-75.

Cronin, J., Hansen, K., Kawamori, N., McNair, P. (2008). Effects of weighted vests and sled towing on sprint kinematics. *Sports Biomechanics, 7,* 160-172.

Cronin, J. B., Hansen, K. T. (2005). Strength and power predictors of sports speed. *Journal of Strength and Conditioning Research, 19*, 349-357.

Dauty, M., Dupré, M., Potiron-Josse, M. and Dubois, C. (2007). Identification of mechanical consequences of jumper's knee by isokinetic concentric torque measurement in elite basketball players. *Isokinetics and Exercise Science, 15,* 37-41.

Dawes, J., Lentz, D. (2012). Methods of developing power to improve acceleration for the non-track athlete. *Strength Conditioning Journal, 34,* 44-51.

Dawes, J., Roozen, M. (Eds.). (2012). *Developing Agility and Quickness.* Champaign: Human Kinetics.

Dawson, B., Hopkinson, R., Appleby, B., Stewart, G., Roberts, C. (2004). Player movement patterns and game activities in the Australian Football League. *Journal of Science and Medicine in Sport, 7,* 278-291.

Dayakidis, M.K., Boudolos, K. (2006). Ground reaction force data in functional ankle instability during two cutting movements. *Clinical Biomechanics, 21,* 405-411.

de Lacey, J., Brughelli, M. E., McGuigan, M. R. and Hansen, K.T. (2014). Strength, speed and power characteristics of elite rugby league players. *Journal of Strength and Conditioning Research, 28,* 2372-2375.

Delaney, J.A., Scott, T.J., Ballard, D.A., Duthie, G.M., Hickmans, J.A., Lockie, R.G. and Dascombe, B.J. (2015). Contributing factors to change-of-direction ability in professional rugby league players. *Journal of Strength and Conditioning Research, 29,* 2688-2696.

Delecluse, C. (1997). Influence of strength training on sprint running performance: current findings and implications for training. *Sports Medicine, 24,* 147-156.

Delecluse, C., Van Coppenolle, H., Willems, E., Van Leemputte, M., Diels, R., Goris, M. (1995). Influence of high-resistance and high-velocity training on sprint performance. *Medicine and Science in Sports and Exercise, 27,* 1203-1209.

Dempsey, A.R., Lloyd, D.G., Elliott, B.C., Steele, J. R., Munro, B. J. and Russo, K. A. (2007). The effect of technique change on knee loads during sidestep cutting. *Medicine and Science in Sports and* Exercise, *39,* 1765-1773.

Deutsch, M.U., Kearney, G.A. and Rehrer, N.J. (2007). Time-motion analysis of professional rugby union players during match-play. *Journal of Sports Sciences, 25,* 461-472.

Dillman, C.J. (1975). Kinematic analyses of running. *Exercise and Sport Sciences Reviews, 3,* 193-218.

Dintiman, G.B., Ward, R.D. (2003). *Sports Speed* (3rd ed.). Champaign: Human Kinetics.

Docherty, D., Wenger, H.A., Neary, P. (1988). Time-motion analysis related to the physiological demands of rugby. *Journal of Human Movement Studies, 14,* 269-277.

Donati, A. (1995). The development of stride length and stride frequency in sprinting. *New Studies in Athletics, 10,* 51-66.

Duthie, G.M., Pyne, D. B., Marsh, D. J., Hooper, S. L. (2006). Sprint patterns in rugby union players during competition. *Journal of Strength and Conditioning Research, 20,* 208-214.

Ebben, W.P. (2008). The optimal downhill slope for acute overspeed running. *International Journal of Sports Physiology and Performance, 3,* 88-93.

Ebben, W.P., Davies, J. A., Clewien, R. W. (2008). Effect of the degree of hill slope on acute downhill running velocity and acceleration. *Journal of Strength and Conditioning Research, 22,* 898-902.

Faccioni, A. (1994a). Assisted and resisted methods for speed development: Part 1. *Modern Athlete and Coach, 32,* 3-6.

Faccioni, A. (1994b). Assisted and resisted methods for speed development: Part 2. *Modern Athlete and Coach, 32*, 8-12.

Frishberg, B.A. (1983). An analysis of overground and treadmill sprinting. *Medicine and Science in Sports and Exercise, 15*, 478-485.

Fry, A. C., Kraemer, W.J., Weseman, C.A., Conroy, B.P., Gordon, S.E., Hoffman, J.R., Maresh, C.M. (1991). The effects of an off-season strength and conditioning program on starters and non-starters in women's intercollegiate volleyball. *Journal of Strength and Conditioning Research, 5*, 174-181.

Garstecki, M.A., Latin, R.W., Cuppett, M.M. (2004). Comparison of selected physical fitness and performance variables between NCAA Division I and II football players. *Journal of Strength and Conditioning Research, 18*, 292-297.

Gittoes, M.J., Wilson, C. (2010). Intralimb joint coordination patterns of the lower extremity in maximal velocity phase sprint running. *Journal of Applied Biomechanics, 26*, 188-195.

Glaister, B. C., Orendurff, M. S., Schoen, J. A., Bernatz, G. C., Klute, G. K. (2008). Ground reaction forces and impulses during a transient turning maneuver. *Journal of Biomechanics, 41*, 3090-3093.

Gottschall, J.S., Palmer, B.M. (2002). The acute effects of prior cycling cadence on running performance and kinematics. *Medicine and Science in Sports and Exercise, 34*, 1518-1522.

Green, B.S., Blake, C., Caulfield, B.M. (2011). A comparison of cutting technique performance in rugby union players. *Journal of Strength and Conditioning Research, 25*, 2668-2680.

Gribble, P. (2003). The star excursion balance test as a measurement tool. *Athletic Therapy Today, 8*, 46-47.

Harland, M. J., Steele, J. R. (1997). Biomechanics of the sprint start. *Sports* Medicine, *23*, 11-20.

Harris, N.K., Cronin, J. B., Hopkins, W. G., Hansen, K. T. (2008). Squat jump training at maximal power loads vs. heavy loads: effect on sprint ability. *Journal of Strength and Conditioning Research, 22*, 1742-1749.

Harrison, A.J., Bourke, G. (2009). The effect of resisted sprint training on speed and strength performance in male rugby players. *Journal of Strength and Conditioning Research, 23*, 275-283.

Hase, K., Stein, R. B. (1999). Turning strategies during human walking. *Journal of Neurophysiology, 81*, 2914-2922.

Hertel, J., Miller, S. J., Denegar, C. R. (2000). Intratester and intertester during the Star Excursion Balance Tests. *Journal of Sport Rehabilitation, 9*, 104-116.

Hewit, J., Cronin, J., Button, C., Hume, P. (2011). Understanding deceleration in sport. *Strength and Conditioning Journal, 33*, 47-52.

Hewit, J.K., Cronin, J. B., Hume, P. A. (2013). Kinematic factors affecting fast and slow straight and change-of-direction acceleration times. *Journal of Strength and Conditioning Research, 27*, 69-75.

Hinrichs, R.N. (1992). Case studies of asymmetrical arm action in running. *International Journal of Sport Biomechanics, 8*, 111-128.

Hoffman, J.R., Cooper, J., Wendell, M., Kang, J. (2004). Comparison of Olympic vs. traditional power lifting training programs in football players. *Journal of Strength and Conditioning Research, 18*, 129-135.

Hoffman, J.R., Ratamess, N. A., Cooper, J. J., Kang, J., Chilakos, A., Faigenbaum, A. D. (2005). Comparison of loaded and unloaded jump squat training on strength/power performance in college football players. *Journal of Strength and Conditioning Research, 19*, 810-815.

Houck, J. (2003). Muscle activation patterns of selected lower extremity muscles during stepping and cutting tasks. *Journal of Electromyography and Kinesiology, 13*, 545-554.

Hunter, J.P., Marshall, R. N., McNair, P. J. (2004). Interaction of step length and step rate during sprint running. *Medicine and Science in Sports and Exercise, 36*, 261-271.

Hunter, J.P., Marshall, R. N., McNair, P. J. (2005). Relationships between ground reaction force impulse and kinematics of sprint-running acceleration. *Journal of Applied Biomechanics, 21*, 31-43.

Jakalski, K. (1998). Parachutes, tubing, and towing: the pros and cons of using resisted and assisted training methods with high school sprinters. *Track Coach, 144*, 4585-4589; 4612.

Jindrich, D.L., Besier, T. F., Lloyd, D. G. (2006). A hypothesis for the function of braking forces during running turns. *Journal of Biomechanics, 39*, 1611-1620.

Jovanovic, M., Sporis, G., Omrcen, D., Fiorentini, F. (2011). Effects of speed, agility, quickness training method on power performance in elite soccer players. *Journal of Strength and Conditioning Research, 25*, 1285-1292.

Kawamori, N., Newton, R., Nosaka, K. (2014). Effects of weighted sled towing on ground reaction force during the acceleration phase of sprint running. *Journal of Sports Sciences, 32*, 1139-1145.

Kawamori, N., Nosaka, K., Newton, R. U. (2013). Relationships between ground reaction impulse and sprint acceleration performance in team sport athletes. *Journal of Strength and Conditioning Research, 27*, 568-573.

Keiner, M., Sander, A., Wirth, K., Schmidtbleicher, D. (2014). Long-term strength training effects on change-of-direction sprint performance. *Journal of Strength and Conditioning Research, 28*, 223-231.

Knapik, J.J., Bauman, C.L., Jones, B.H., Harris, J.M., Vaughan, L. (1991). Preseason strength and flexibility imbalances associated with athletic injuries in female collegiate athletes. *American Journal of Sports Medicine, 19*, 76-81.

Korchemny, R. (1992). A new concept for sprint start and acceleration training. *New Studies in Athletics, 7*, 65-72.

Korneljuk, A. O. (1982). Scientific basis of sprinting speed development. *Track and Field Quarterly Review, 82*, 6-9.

Kovacs, M.S., Roetert, E. P., Ellenbecker, T. S. (2008). Efficient deceleration: the forgotten factor in tennis-specific training. *Strength and Conditioning Journal, 30*, 58-69.

Kraan, G.A., van Veen, J., Snijders, C. J., Storm, J. (2001). Starting from standing; why step backwards? *Journal of Biomechanincs, 34*, 211-215.

Kristensen, G.O., van den Tillar, R., Ettema, G. J. C. (2006). Velocity specificity in early-phase sprint training. *Journal of Strength and Conditioning Research, 20*, 833-837.

Krustrup, P., Mohr, M., Ellingsgaard, H., Bangsbo, J. (2005). Physical demands during an elite female soccer game: importance of training status. *Medicine and Science in Sports and Exercise, 37*, 1242-1248.

Kugler, F., Janshen, L. (2010). Body position determines propulsive forces in accelerated running. *Journal of Biomechanincs, 43*, 343-348.

Kuitunen, S., Komi, P. V., Kyröläinen, H. (2002). Knee and ankle joint stiffness in sprint running. *Medicine and Science in Sports and Exercise, 34*, 166-173.

Lavrienko, A., Kravtsev, J., Petrova, Z. (1990). Non-traditional training. *Modern Athlete and Coach, 28*, 3-5.

Letzelter, M., Sauerwein, G., Burger, R. (1995). Resistance runs in speed development. *Modern Athlete and Coach, 33*, 7-12.

Little, T., Williams, A. G. (2005). Specificity of acceleration, maximum speed, and agility in professional soccer players. *Journal of Strength and Conditioning Research, 19*, 76-78.

Lockie, R. G., Callaghan, S. J., Berry, S. P., Cooke, E. R., Jordan, C. A., Luczo, T. M., Jeffriess, M. D. (2014a). Relationship between unilateral jumping ability and asymmetry on multidirectional speed in team-sport athletes. *Journal of Strength and Conditioning Research, 28*, 3557-3566.

Lockie, R.G., Callaghan, S. J. and Jeffriess, M.D. (2014b). Acceleration kinematics in cricketers: Implications for performance in the field. *Journal of Sports Sciences and Medicine, 13*, 128-136.

Lockie, R.G., Callaghan, S.J., McGann, T.S. and Jeffriess, M.D. (2014c). Ankle muscle function during preferred and non-preferred 45° directional cutting in semi-professional basketball players. *International Journal of Performance Analyses in Sport, 14*, 574-593.

Lockie, R.G., Jeffriess, M.D., McGann, T.S., Callaghan, S.J., Schultz, A.B. (2013a). Planned and reactive agility performance in semi-professional and amateur basketball players. *International Journal of Sports Physiology and Performance, 9*, 766-771.

Lockie, R.G., Murphy, A.J., Callaghan, S.J., Jeffriess, M.D. (2014d). Effects of sprint and plyometrics training on field sport acceleration technique. *Journal of Strength and Conditioning Research, 28*, 1790-1801.

Lockie, R.G., Murphy, A.J., Jeffriess, M.D., Callaghan, S.J. (2013b). Step kinematic predictors of short sprint performance in field sport athletes. *Serbian Journal of Sports Sciences, 7*, 71-77.

Lockie, R.G., Murphy, A.J., Knight, T.J., Janse de Jonge, X.A.K. (2011). Factors that differentiate acceleration ability in field sport athletes. *Journal of Strength and Conditioning Research, 25*, 2704-2714.

Lockie, R.G., Murphy, A.J., Schultz, A.B., Jeffriess, M.D., Callaghan, S.J. (2013c). Influence of sprint acceleration stance kinetics on velocity and step kinematics in field sport athletes. *Journal of Strength and Conditioning Research, 27*, 2494-2503.

Lockie, R.G., Murphy, A.J., Schultz, A.B., Knight, T.J., Janse de Jonge, X.A.K. (2012a). The effects of different speed training protocols on sprint acceleration kinematics and muscle strength and power in field sport athletes. *Journal of Strength and Conditioning Research, 26*, 1539-1500.

Lockie, R.G., Murphy, A.J., Spinks, C.D. (2003). Effects of resisted sled towing on sprint kinematics in field-sport athletes. *Journal of Strength and Conditioning Research, 17*, 760-767.

Lockie, R.G., Schultz, A.B., Callaghan, S.J., Jeffriess, M.D. (2014e). The effects of traditional and enforced stopping speed and agility training on multidirectional speed and athletic performance. *Journal of Strength and Conditioning Research, 28*, 1538-1551.

Lockie, R.G., Schultz, A.B., Callaghan, S.J., Jeffriess, M.D. (in press). The relationship between dynamic stability and multidirectional speed. *Journal of Strength and*

Conditioning Research, Publish Ahead of Print: doi: 10.1519/JSC.1510b 1013e3182a1744b1516.

Lockie, R.G., Schultz, A.B., Callaghan, S.J., Jeffriess, M.D., Berry, S. P. (2013d). Reliability and validity of a new test of change-of-direction speed for field-based sports: the Change-of-Direction and Acceleration Test (CODAT). *Journal of Sports Science and Medicine, 12,* 88-96.

Lockie, R.G., Schultz, A.B., Jeffriess, M.D., Callaghan, S.J. (2012b). The relationship between bilateral differences of knee flexor and extensor isokinetic strength and multi-directional speed. *Isokinetic and Exercise Science, 20,* 211-219.

Lockie, R.G., Vickery, W.M. (2013). Kinematics that differentiate the beach flags start between elite and non-elite sprinters. *Biology of Sport, 30,* 255-261.

Lockie, R.G., Vickery, W.M., de Jonge, X. A. K. J. (2012c). Kinematics of the typical beach flags start for young adult sprinters. *Journal of Sports Science and Medicine, 11,* 444-451.

Luhtanen, P., Komi, P. V. (1978). Mechanical factors influencing running speed. In E. Asmussen and K. Jorgensen (Eds.), *Biomechanics V1-B* (pp. 23-29). Baltimore: University Park Press.

Maćkala, K., Fostiak, M. (2015). Acute effects of plyometric intervention - performance improvement and related changes in sprinting gait variability. *Journal of Strength and Conditioning Research, 29,* 1956-1965.

Majumdar, A.S., Robergs, R. A. (2011). The science of speed: determinants of performance in the 100 m sprint. *International Journal of Sports Science and Coaching, 6,* 479-494.

Makaruk, B., Sozański, H., Makaruk, H. and Sacewicz, T. (2013). The effects of resisted sprint training on speed performance in women. *Human Movement, 14,* 116-122.

Mann, R. (1986). The biomechanical analysis of sprinters. *Track Technique, 94,* 3000-3003.

Mann, R., Herman, J. (1985). Kinematic analysis of Olympic sprint performance: men's 200 meters. *International Journal of Sport Biomechanics, 1,* 151-162.

Mann, R., Sprague, P. (1980). A kinetic analysis of the ground leg during sprint running. *Research Quarterly in Exercise and Sport, 51,* 334-348.

Mann, R. A., Hagy, J. (1980). Biomechanics of walking, running, and sprinting. *American Journal of Sports Medicine, 8,* 345-350.

Mann, R. A., Moran, G. T., Dougherty, S. E. (1986). Comparative electromyography of the lower extremity in jogging, running, and sprinting. *American Journal of Sports Medicine, 14,* 501-510.

Markovic, G., Jukic, I., Milanovic, D., Metikos, D. (2007). Effects of sprint and plyometric training on muscle function and athletic performance. *Journal of Strength and Conditioning Research, 21,* 543-549.

Martinopoulou, K., Argeitaki, P., Paradisis, G., Katsikas, C., Smirniotou, A. (2011). The effects of resisted training using parachute on sprint performance. *Journal of Biology of Exercise, 7,* 7-23.

McBride, J.M., Blow, D., Kirby, T.J., Haines, T.L., Dayne, A.M., Triplett, N.T. (2009). Relationship between maximal squat strength and five, ten, and forty yard sprint times. *Journal of Strength and Conditioning Research, 23,* 1633-1636.

McBride, J.M., Triplett-McBride, T., Davie, A., Newton, R.U. (2002). The effect of heavy- vs. light-load jump squats on the development of strength, power, and speed. *Journal of Strength and Conditioning Research, 16,* 75-82.

McClay, I.S., Robinson, J.R., Andriacchi, T.P., Frederick, E.C., Gross, T., Martin, P., Valiant, G., Williams, K. R., Cavanagh, P. C. (1994). A profile of ground reaction forces in professional basketball. *Journal of Applied Biomechanics, 10,* 222-236.

McFarlane, B. (1987). A look inside the biomechanics and dynamics of speed. *National and Strength and Conditioning Association Journal, 9,* 35-41.

McLean, S.G., Lipfert, S.W., van den Bogert, A.J. (2004). Effect of gender and defensive opponent on the biomechanics of sidestep cutting. *Medicine and Science in Sports and Exercise, 36,* 1008-1016.

Meckel, Y., Atterbom, H., Grodjinovsky, A., Ben-Sira, D., Rotstein, A. (1995). Physiological characteristics of female 100 metre sprinters of different performance levels. *Journal of Sports Medicine and Physical Fitness, 35,* 169-175.

Mero, A. (1988). Force-time characteristics and running velocity of male sprinters during the acceleration phase of sprinting. *Research Quarterly in Exercise and Sport, 59,* 94-98.

Mero, A., Komi, P.V. (1985). Effects of supramaximal velocity on biomechanical variables in sprinting. *International Journal of Sport Biomechanics, 1,* 240-252.

Mero, A., Komi, P.V. (1987). Electromyographic activity in sprinting at speeds ranging from sub-maximal to supra-maximal. *Medicine and Science in Sports and Exercise, 19,* 266-274.

Mero, A., Komi, P. V. (1994). EMG, force, and power analysis of sprint-specific strength exercises. *Journal of Applied Biomechanics, 10,* 1-13.

Mero, A., Komi, P. V., Gregor, R. J. (1992). Biomechanics of sprint running: a review. *Sports Medicine, 13,* 376-392.

Mero, A., Luhtanen, P., Komi, P. (1986). Segmental contribution to velocity of center of gravity during contact at different speeds in male and female sprinters. *Journal of Human Movement Studies, 12,* 215-235.

Milanovic, Z., Sporis, G., Trajkovic, N., James, N., Samija, K. (2013). Effects of a 12 Week SAQ training programme on agility with and without the ball among young soccer players. *Journal of Sports Sciences and Medicine, 12,* 97-103.

Miller, M. G., Herniman, J. J., Ricard, M. D., Cheatham, C. C., Michael, T. J. (2006). The effects of a 6-week plyometric training program on agility. *Journal of Sports Sciences and Medicine, 5,* 459-465.

Moir, G., Sanders, R., Button, C., Glaister, M. (2007). The effect of periodized resistance training on accelerative sprint performance. *Sports Biomechanics, 6,* 285-300.

Morin, J.-B., Edouard, P., Samozino, P. (2011). Technical ability of force application as a determinant factor of sprint performance. *Medicine and Science in Sports and Exercise, 43,* 1680-1688.

Mouchbahani, R., Gollhofer, A., Dickhuth, H. (2004). Pulley systems in sprint training. *Modern Athlete and Coach, 42,* 14-17.

Müller, H., Hommel, H. (1997). Biomechanical research project at the VIth world championships in athletics, Athens 1997: preliminary report. *New Studies in Athletics, 12,* 43-73.

Murphy, A. J., Lockie, R. G., Coutts, A. J. (2003). Kinematic determinants of early acceleration in field sport athletes. *Journal of Sports Sciences and Medicine, 2,* 144-150.

Murray, A., Aitchison, T. C., Ross, G., Sutherland, K., Watt, I., McLean, D., Grant, S. (2005). The effect of towing a range of relative resistances on sprint performance. *Journal of Sport Sciences, 23,* 927-935.

Neptune, R. R., Wright, I. C., van den Bogert, A. J. (1999). Muscle coordination and function during cutting movements. *Medicine and Science in Sports and Exercise, 31,* 294-302.

Newton, R.U., Gerber, A., Nimphius, S., Shim, J.K., Doan, B.K., Robertson, M., Pearson, D. R., Craig, B.W., Hakkinen, K., Kraemer, W.J. (2006). Determination of functional strength imbalance of the lower extremities. *Journal of Strength and Conditioning Research, 20,* 971-977.

Newton, R.U., Kraemer, W.J. (1994). Developing explosive muscular power: implications for a mixed methods training strategy. *Strength and Conditioning Journal, 16,* 20-31.

Nimphius, S., McGuigan, M.R., Newton, R.U. (2010). Relationship between strength, power, speed, and change of direction performance of female softball players. *Journal of Strength and Conditioning Research, 24,* 885-895.

Nimphius, S., McGuigan, M.R., Newton, R.U. (2012). Changes in muscle architecture and performance during a competitive season in female softball players. *Journal of Strength and Conditioning Research, 26,* 2655-2666.

Novacheck, T.F. (1998). The biomechanics of running. *Gait and Posture, 7,* 77-95.

Ozbar, N., Ates, S., Agopyan, A. (2014). The effect of 8-week plyometric training on leg power, jump and sprint performance in female soccer players. *Journal of Strength and Conditioning Research, 28,* 2888-2894.

Paradisis, G.P., Bissas, A., Cooke, C.B. (2009). Combined uphill and downhill sprint running training is more efficacious than horizontal. *International Journal of Sports Physiology and Performance, 4,* 229-243.

Paradisis, G.P., Cooke, C.B. (2001). Kinematic and postural characteristics of sprint running on sloping surfaces. *Journal of Sport Sciences, 19,* 149-159.

Paradisis, G.P., Cooke, C.B. (2006). The effects of sprint running training on sloping surfaces. *Journal of Strength and Conditioning Research, 20,* 767-777.

Pauletto, B. (1993). Speed-power training: how to get that last 10% effort to assure a good speed workout. Part III: special apparatus. *Scholastic Coach, 63,* 54-55.

Paulson, S., Braun, W. A. (2011). The influence of parachute-resisted sprinting on running mechanics in collegiate track athletes. *Journal of Strength and Conditioning Research, 25,* 1680-1685.

Polman, R., Walsh, D., Bloomfield, J., Nesti, M. (2004). Effective conditioning of female soccer players. *Journal of Sports Sciences, 22,* 191-203.

Potach, D.H., Chu, D.A. (2008). Plyometric training. In T. R. Baechle and R. W. Earle (Eds.), *Essentials of Strength Training and Conditioning* (3rd ed., pp. 413-456). Champaign: Human Kinetics.

Radcliffe, J.C., Farentinos, R.C. (2015). *High-Powered Plyometrics* (2nd ed.). Champaign: Human Kinetics.

Rand, M.K., Ohtsuki, T. (2000). EMG analysis of lower limb muscles in humans during quick change in running directions. *Gait and Posture, 12,* 169-183.

Reilly, T., Vaughan, T. (1976). A motion analysis of work-rate in different positional roles in professional football match-play. *Journal of Human Movement Studies, 2,* 87-97.

Rimmer, E., Sleivert, G. (2000). Effects of a plyometrics intervention program on sprint performance. *Journal of Strength and Conditioning Research, 14,* 295-301.

Ronnestad, B.R., Kvamme, N.H., Sunde, A., Raastad, T. (2008). Short-term effects of strength and plyometric training on sprint and jump performance in professional soccer players. *Journal of Strength and Conditioning Research, 22,* 773-780.

Ropret, R., Kukolj, M., Ugarkovic, D., Matavulj, D., Jaric, S. (1998). Effects of arm and leg loading on sprint performance. *European Journal of Applied Physiology and Occupational Physiology, 77,* 547-550.

Ross, A., Leveritt, M. (2001). Long-term metabolic and skeletal muscle adaptations to short-sprint training: implications for sprint training and tapering. *Sports Medicine, 31,* 1063-1082.

Ross, R.E., Ratamess, N.A., Hoffman, J.R., Faigenbaum, A.D., Kang, J., Chilakos, A. (2009). The effects of treadmill sprint training and resistance training on maximal running velocity and power. *Journal of Strength and Conditioning Research, 23,* 385-394.

Rumpf, M. C., Lockie, R. G., Cronin, J. B., Jalilvand, F. (in press). The effect of different sprint training methods on sprint performance over various distances: a brief review. *Journal of Strength and Conditioning Research,* Publish Ahead of Print, doi:10.1519/jsc.0000000000001245.

Sacco, I. d. C.N., Takahasi, H.Y., Suda, E.Y., Battistella, L.R., Kavamoto, C.A., Lopes, J.A. F., Vasconcelos, J.C.P. (2006). Ground reaction force in basketball cutting maneuvers with and without ankle bracing and taping. *Sao Paulo Medical Journal, 124,* 245-252.

Saez de Villarreal, E., Requena, B., Cronin, J.B. (2012). The effects of plyometric training on sprint performance: a meta-analysis. *Journal of Strength and Conditioning Research, 26,* 575-584.

Salaj, S., Markovic, G. (2011). Specificity of jumping, sprinting, and quick change-of-direction motor abilities. *Journal of Strength and Conditioning Research, 25,* 1249-1255.

Salonikidis, K., Zafeiridis, A. (2008). The effects of plyometric, tennis-drills, and combined training on reaction, lateral and linear speed, power, and strength in novice tennis players. *Journal of Strength and Conditioning Research, 22,* 182-191.

Saraslanidis, P. (2000). Training for the improvement of maximum speed: flat running or resistance training? *New Studies in Athletics, 15,* 45-51.

Sayers, M. (2000). Running techniques for field sport players. *Sports Coach, 23,* 26-27.

Sebestyen, E. (1996). Speed improvement with the Speedy-System. *New Studies in Athletics, 11,* 149-154.

Seitz, L. B., Reyes, A., Tran, T. T., Saez de Villarreal, E., Haff, G. G. (2014). Increases in lower-body strength transfer positively to sprint performance: a systematic review with meta-analysis. *Sports Medicine, 44,* 1693-1702.

Sekulic, D., Spasic, M., Mirkov, D., Cavar, M., Sattler, T. (2013). Gender-specific influences of balance, speed, and power on agility performance. *Journal of Strength and Conditioning Research, 27,* 802-811.

Semenick, D. (1990). Tests and measurements: the t-test. *National Strength and Conditioning Association Journal, 12,* 36-37.

Sheppard, J.M., Dawes, J.J., Jeffreys, I., Spiteri, T., Nimphius, S. (2014). Broadening the view of agility: a scientific review of the literature. *Journal of Australian Strength and Conditioning, 22,* 6-25.

Sheppard, J.M., Young, W.B. (2006). Agility literature review: classifications, training and testing. *Journal of Sports Sciences, 24,* 919-932.

Slawinski, J., Bonnefoy, A., Leveque, J. M., Ontanon, G., Riquet, A., Dumas, R., Cheze, L. (2010). Kinematic and kinetic comparisons of elite and well-trained sprinters during sprint start. *Journal of Strength and Conditioning Research, 24,* 896-905.

Sleivert, G., Taingahue, M. (2004). The relationship between maximal jump-squat power and sprint acceleration in athletes. *European Journal of Applied Physiology and Occupational Physiology, 91,* 46-52.

Spinks, C.D., Murphy, A.J., Spinks, W.L., Lockie, R.G. (2007). Effects of resisted sprint training on acceleration performance and kinematics in soccer, rugby union and Australian football players. *Journal of Strength and Conditioning Research, 21,* 77-85.

Spiteri, T., Cochrane, J. L., Hart, N. H., Haff, G. G., Nimphius, S. (2013). Effect of strength on plant foot kinetics and kinematics during a change of direction task. *European Journal of Sport Sciences, 13,* 646-652.

Spiteri, T., Nimphius, S., Hart, N.H., Specos, C., Sheppard, J.M., Newton, R.U. (2014). Contribution of strength characteristics to change of direction and agility performance in female basketball athletes. *Journal of Strength and Conditioning Research, 28,* 2415-2423.

Tabachnik, B. (1992). The speed chute. *National Strength and Conditioning Association Journal, 14,* 75-80.

Tan, B. (1999). Manipulating resistance training program variables to optimize strength in men: a review. *Journal of Strength and Conditioning Research, 13,* 289-304.

Tateuchi, H., Yoneda, T., Tanaka, T., Kumada, H., Kadota, M., Ohno, H., Tanaka, K., Yamaguchi, J. (2006). Postural control for initiation of lateral step and step-up motions in young adults. *Journal of Physical Therapy Science, 18,* 49-55.

Tricoli, V., Lamas, L., Carnevale, R., Ugrinowitsch, C. (2005). Short-term effects on lower-body functional power development: weightlifting vs. vertical jump training programs. *Journal of Strength and Conditioning Research, 19,* 433-437.

Twist, P.W., Benicky, D. (1996). Conditioning lateral movement for multi-sport athletes: practical strength and quickness drills. *Strength and Conditioning Journal, 18,* 10-19.

Unitas, J., Dintiman, G. (1979). Sprinting speed improvement: how to run faster. In J. Unitas and G. Dintiman (Eds.), *Improving Health and Performance in the Athlete* (pp. 236-271). Englewood Cliffs: Prentice-Hall.

Upton, D.E. (2011). The effect of assisted and resisted sprint training on acceleration and velocity in Division IA female soccer athletes. *Journal of Strength and Conditioning Research, 25,* 2645-2652.

Váczi, M., Tollár, J., Meszler, B., Juhász, I., Karsai, I. (2013). Short-term high intensity plyometric training program improves strength, power and agility in male soccer players. *Journal of Human Kinetics, 36,* 17-26.

Vagenas, G., Hoshizaki, T. B. (1986). Optimization of an asymmetrical motor skill: sprint start. *International Journal of Sport Biomechanics, 2,* 29-40.

van Ingen Schenau, G. J., de Koning, J. J., de Groot, G. (1994). Optimisation of sprinting performance in running, cycling and speed skating. *Sports Medicine, 17,* 259-275.

Verkhoshansky, Y.V. (1996). Speed training for high level athletes. *New Studies in Athletics, 11,* 39-49.

Vescovi, J.D. (2012). Sprint speed characteristics of high-level American female soccer players: Female Athletes in Motion (FAiM) study. *Journal of Science and Medicine in Sport, 15,* 474-478.

Vescovi, J.D., McGuigan, M.R. (2008). Relationships between sprinting, agility, and jump ability in female athletes. *Journal of Sports Sciences, 26,* 97-107.

Wagganer, J.D., Williams, J., Ronald, D., Barnes, J.T. (2015). The effects of a four week primary and secondary speed training protocol on 40 yard sprint times in female college soccer players. *Journal of Human Sport and Exercise, 9,* 713-725.

Webster, J., Roberts, J. (2011). Determining the effect of cricket leg guards on running performance. *Journal of Sports Sciences, 29,* 749-760.

West, D.J., Cunningham, D.J., Bracken, R.M., Bevan, H.R., Crewther, B.T., Cook, C.J., Kilduff, L.P. (2013). Effects of resisted sprint training on acceleration in professional rugby union players. *Journal of Strength and Conditioning Research, 27,* 1014-1018.

Weyand, P.G., Sternlight, D.B., Bellizzi, M.J., Wright, S. (2000). Faster top running speeds are achieved with greater ground forces not more rapid leg movements. *Journal of Applied Physiology, 89,* 1991-1999.

Wheeler, K.W., Sayers, M.G.L. (2010). Modification of agility running technique in reaction to a defender in rugby union. *Journal of Sports Science and Medicine, 9,* 445-451.

Whelan, N., O'Regan, C., Harrison, A.J. (2014). Resisted sprints do not acutely enhance sprinting performance. *Journal of Strength and Conditioning Research, 28,* 1858-1866.

Whitting, J.W., de Melker Worms, J.L., Maurer, C., Nigg, S.R., Nigg, B.M. (2013). Measuring lateral shuffle and side cut performance. *Journal of Strength and Conditioning Research, 27,* 3197-3203.

Wikstrom, E.A., Tillman, M.D., Smith, A.N., Borsa, P.A. (2005). A new force-plate technology measure of dynamic postural stability: the dynamic postural stability index. *Journal of Athletic Training, 40,* 305-309.

Wilson, G.J., Murphy, A.J., Giorgi, A. (1996). Weight and plyometric training: effects on eccentric and concentric force production. *Canadian Journal of Applied Physiology, 21,* 301-315.

Wilson, G.J., Newton, R.U., Murphy, A.J., Humphries, B.J. (1993). The optimal training load for the development of dynamic athletic performance. *Medicine and Science in Sports and Exercise, 25,* 1279-1286.

Wisloff, U., Castagna, C., Helgerud, J., Jones, R., Hoff, J. (2004). Strong correlation of maximal squat strength with sprint performance and vertical jump height in elite soccer players. *British Journal of Sports Medicine, 38,* 285-288.

Woicik, M. (1983). Sprinting. *Track and Field Quarterly Review, 83,* 16-17.

Yap, C.W., Brown, L.E., Woodman, G. (2000). Development of speed, agility, and quickness for the female soccer athlete. *Strength and Conditioning Journal, 22,* 9-12.

Young, W. (1991). The planning of resistance training for power sports. *National Strength and Conditioning Association Journal, 13,* 26-29.

Young, W., Benton, D., Duthie, G., Pryor, J. (2001a). Resistance training for short sprints and maximum-speed sprints. *Strength and Conditioning Journal, 23,* 7-13.

Young, W., Farrow, D. (2006). A review of agility: practical applications for strength and conditioning. *Strength and Conditioning Journal, 28,* 24-29.

Young, W., Farrow, D. (2013). The importance of a sport-specific stimulus for training agility. *Strength and Conditioning Journal, 35,* 39-43.

Young, W., McLean, B., Ardagna, J. (1995). Relationship between strength qualities and sprinting performance. *Journal of Sports Medicine and Physical Fitness, 35,* 13-19.

Young, W.B., Dawson, B., Henry, G.J. (2015). Agility and change-of-direction speed are independent skills: Implications for training for agility in invasion sports. *International Journal of Sports Science and Coaching, 10,* 159-169.

Young, W.B., James, R., Montgomery, I. (2002). Is muscle power related to running speed with changes of direction? *Journal of Sports Medicine and Physical Fitness, 42,* 282-288.

Young, W.B., McDowell, M.H., Scarlett, B.J. (2001b). Specificity of sprint and agility training methods. *Journal of Strength and Conditioning Research, 15,* 315-319.

Zafeiridis, A., Saraslandis, P., Manou, V., Ioakimidis, P., Dipla, K., Kellis, S. (2005). The effects of resisted sled-pulling sprint training on acceleration and maximum speed performance. *Journal of Sports Medicine and Physical Fitness, 45,* 284-290.

Zafeiropoulos, K., Smirniotou, A., Argeitaki, P., Paradisis, G., Zacharogiannis, E., Tsolakis, C. (2014). Acute effects of different loading conditions using weighted vest on running performance. *Journal of Biology of Exercise, 10,* 52-65.

In: Physical Activity Effects on the Anthropological Status …   ISBN: 978-1-63484-782-7
Editors: Fadilj Eminović and Milivoj Dopsaj   © 2016 Nova Science Publishers, Inc.

Chapter 6

RELATIONSHIP BETWEEN PHYSICAL FITNESS CHARACTERISTICS AND SPORTS EXPERIENCE IN CHILDHOOD AND ADOLESCENCE AMONG JAPANESE FEMALE UNIVERSITY STUDENTS

*Itaru Enomoto**

Kamakura Women's University, Kanagawa, Japan

ABSTRACT

The relationship between lifestyle-related illnesses and health-related physical fitness has recently become an increasingly prevalent public health concern. University students, who typically range between 18 and 22 years of age, should have long-term plans in order to maintain their good health. However, researchers have reported that the fitness levels of young university students have been decreasing in recent decades. The influence of long-term sports experience in childhood and adolescence on the physical fitness of university students remains unknown. The purpose of this chapter is to clarify the relationship between sports experience and performance scores on a health-related physical fitness test among female university freshmen in Japan. A total of 149 female university freshmen participated in the Japanese physical fitness test (Ministry of Education, Culture, Sports, Science and Technology-Japan test; MEXT test), which consists of eight assessments, including of upper and lower body strength, flexibility, and aerobic capacity. Participants were divided into five groups by self-reported length of sports experience from childhood to adolescence. Most of the correlation coefficients among test scores were low to moderate. The results indicated no significant relationships between sports experience and handgrip strength, 50-m sprint running, and standing long jump scores among female university students. On the other hand, the group of students with longer sports experience showed statistically higher scores in sit ups, side stepping, 20-m shuttle running, and handball throwing scores compared to those in students with less sports experience.

Keywords: University student, fitness test, sports career

---

* Corresponding Author, Email: ienomoto@kamakura-u.ac.jp.

INTRODUCTION

The physical fitness levels of athletes are evaluated with motor-related physical fitness tests, while the physical fitness levels of individuals from the general public are evaluated with health-related physical fitness tests. Mountjoy et al. (2011) indicated in an International Olympic Committee consensus statement that the health consequences of a lack of physical fitness, physical activity, and/or sports participation were summarized as follows: obesity, injury, and decreased cardiovascular and metabolic health, bone health, and mental health. The relationship between lifestyle-related illnesses and health-related physical fitness has become a more significant public health concern in recent decades. Health-related fitness ability has a very close relationship with daily human lifestyle. Franks et al. (2004) observed a strong and significant inverse association between physical activity energy expenditure and metabolic syndrome. Katzmarzyk et al. (2005) suggested that cardiorespiratory fitness, which is observed as the VO2 max in the treadmill test, is an important effect modifier in the relationships among obesity, metabolic status, and mortality from cardiovascular disease. Decreased fitness levels may form the basis of future lifestyle-related illness. Steele et al. (2008) reviewed recent studies and suggested that physical activity is associated with metabolic risk factors in children.

University students, typically ranging in age from 18 to 22 years, should have long-term plans in order to maintain good health throughout their lives. However, research has suggested that the fitness levels of young university students has been decreasing in recent decades (Suzuki et al., 1999). Kuribayashi et al. (2007) suggested that university students with low physical fitness test scores also have low functional fitness test scores. The Ministry of Education, Culture, Sports, Science and Technology (MEXT) in Japan had reported that, in spite of increasing height and weight, the fitness levels of young adolescents (a 16-year-old group and a 13-year-old group) have decreased dramatically over the past 25 years (MEXT 2012).

It is well known that fitness levels decrease after adolescence. Nishijima et al. (2003) clarified that the overall physical fitness test scores of 17-year-olds have been decreasing since 1980 in Japan. On the other hand, for people who engaged in regular sports and exercise as adolescents, fitness levels may decrease at a slower rate because of their histories of regular exercise. Itaki et al. (2001) reported that 21-year-old university students with long-term, regular exercise habits (twice per week for more than 6 months) had lower total cholesterol, lower LDL cholesterol, and higher HDL cholesterol compared to those in same-aged university students who were not engaged in regular, long-term exercise. Cavill et al. (2001) recommended an average of 1 hour of physical activity per day, and although the majority of young people currently engage in 30 min of moderate physical activity per day on most days of the week, childhood overweight and obesity rates are increasing in the UK.

Many countries have some kind of health-related physical fitness test. The EUROFIT Fitness Testing Battery was established for use in 1993 in Europe (Council of Europe, 1993). The Canadian Standard Fitness Test was established in 1987 (Government of Canada, Fitness and Amateur Sport, 1987). In Japan, a survey of physical and motor abilities has been conducted nationwide since 1964 by the MEXT (Suzuki and Nishijima, 2005). The MEXT later established a modified fitness test to address health-related physical fitness rather than motor-related physical fitness (MEXT-test; MEXT 2000).

There has been no research regarding the relationship between health-related fitness levels and length of sports experience in childhood and adolescence among Japanese university students. The purpose of this chapter is to clarify the relationship between sports experience and performance scores on health-related physical fitness tests for female university freshmen in Japan.

METHODS

Participants

A total of 149 female university freshmen (18–19 years old) participated in this research. The Means ± Standard Deviation (SD) for the height, weight, and body mass index (BMI) of the participants were 159.6 ± 7.4 cm, 51.5 ± 6.8 kg, and 20.2 ± 2.5 kg/m2, respectively. The purpose of the research and risks associated with each testing protocol were explained to all participants before their participation.

Testing Procedure

The MEXT test, which requires participants to perform a handgrip strength test, sit-ups, the sit and reach test, side stepping, a 20-m shuttle run, a 50-m sprint run, overhand handball throwing, and a standing long jump, was performed to evaluate participants' fitness levels. Except for overhand handball throwing, measurements were carried out under stable conditions in an indoor gymnasium. Overhand handball throwing was completed outside to ensure sufficient height for the throwing capacity of each participant. A regular 15-min warm-up was implemented before beginning of all the test.

Handgrip Strength

The purpose of testing handgrip strength is to measure the maximal handgrip muscle strength of the forearm. Forearm muscles are small and easily fatigued, so the best scores are generally achieved during 3–5 seconds of effort. A hand dynamometer with an adjustable grip was used (TKK5101 Grip D; Takei, Tokyo, Japan). Participants squeezed the dynamometer gradually and continuously, performing the test with both the right and left hands two times each, using the optimal grip span. The average of the scores achieved during both handgrip trials was used in analysis.

Sit-Ups

For the sit-up test, the legs of the participant were bent to a 90° angle. A helper held the participant's feet to avoid having participants raise their legs during testing. Participants were instructed to raise their upper body until their knees touched their elbows and then to return to the prone position. They performed as many sit-ups as possible within 30 s. Only accurately performed cumulative sit-ups were recorded.

The timed sit-up test has been widely described not only as a test of abdominal muscle strength but also of the possible relationship between poor abdominal strength and the incidence of low back pain (Hall et al., 1992). An important difference in positioning between the famous Kraus–Weber test and the MEXT test is related to the posture of the arms during the test. In the Kraus–Weber test manuals, fingers are to be interlocked behind the head. However, in the MEXT test, both arms are folded in front of the chest to avoid neck pain that can occur when the palms push too strongly against the head while the upper body is moving into a vertical position.

Sit and Reach

The purpose of the sit and reach test is to measure flexibility. The most logical way to measure it is to set the level of the feet as the 0 measurement, so that any measure that does not reach the toes has a negative value and any reach past the toes has a positive value. However, using negative values is difficult for statistical analyses and for comparing results. Therefore, as in the EUROFIT manual, Minkler and Petterson (1994) suggested setting the level of the feet as 15 cm. In both methods, the feet remain fixed, and the angle of the ankles is fixed as well. This fixed position can be painful of the knee. In the MEXT test, free movement of the table due to the sliding motion enables all results to be expressed as positive values, and ankle movement keep free during measure to avoid knee stress.

Side Stepping

Side stepping has had a long tradition over many generations in Japan as being a measure of agility. From 1965 until the present, most Japanese students have participated in this test during school (Nishijima et al., 2003). For the test, three lines were placed 1 m apart. Participants were instructed to begin by standing on the center line with their feet apart. When instructed by a timer or a signal, the participants jumped to one side to stand with their feet apart on one line. After that, the participants jumped back to the center line to stand with their feet apart and then jumped to the other side of the line to stand with their feet apart. The movements were repeated as quickly as possible, without stopping, for 20 s. Total number of jumps are counted.

20-m Shuttle Run

The 20-m shuttle run has recently become a popular estimate of aerobic power. MEXT has administered the 20-m shuttle run as part of the nationwide physical fitness survey since 1998 (Matsuzaka et al, 2004). They adopted the same test protocol as that used by Leger and Lambert (1982). Participants were instructed to run in a straight line, to pivot upon completing the shuttle, and to pace themselves in accordance with the audio signals on a pre-recorded CD. Running speed increased by 0.5 km/h per min from a starting speed of 8.5 km/h. The test continued until the participant reached exhaustion or could not complete the laps twice continuously within the limited signal. The final lap of the test was measured as the aerobic capacity. The most important advantage of this test is that the results are not influenced by the ability of the participant to choose her running pace, which sometimes reduces the validity of distance-running tests (Matsuzaka et al., 2994).

50-m Sprint Run

The sprint run was begun from a standing position. Two participants stood on a straight line and started sprinting simultaneously at a signal. Regular stopwatches were used to record the time required to complete the sprint, and seconds were rounded off to the first decimal place. The purpose of the 50-m sprint run was to clarify the sprint/dash speed of participants.

Overhand Handball Throwing

For this test, the participants threw a handball at maximum power from one hand. The ball used was one authorized for official handball matches, with a 54–56-cm circumference, weighing 325–400 g. The participants were allowed to take 1–3 approach steps prior to throwing, ending with the foot opposite from the throwing arm in front. Participants were not allowed to move in front of the throwing line until the end of throwing. The distance between the throwing point and the drop point of the ball was measured and used as an assessment of throwing ability.

Standing Long Jump

For this test, participants were instructed to stand with both feet behind the starting line and then to jump forward forcefully as far as possible from the standing position, without a "run-up." Participants were allowed to swing their arms back and forth before the jump. The distance from the toes at the starting point to the nearest point where the heel touched the ground was measured. Results were recorded as the participants' explosive lower limb strength.

Statistics

Participants were divided into five groups based on their self-reported sports experience in childhood and adolescence, as follows: participants with no experience of regular exercises and sports (No experience group, NG; n = 18); and participants who exercised more than three times per week on a regular basis in one school category (low experience group, LG; n = 32); in two school categories (middle experience group, MG; n = 39); in three school categories (high experience group, HG; n = 42); or in all four school categories (super experience group, SG; n = 18). Japanese schools are divided sequentially into categories, from elementary school (ages 6–12), junior high school (ages 13–15), high school (ages 16–

18), and college or university (ages 18 and older). For example, the SG group associated with this research had regularly continued some kind of sports activity for over 13 years.

The values were expressed as mean and SDs. Levene's test was used to check equality of variance. ANOVAs were used to determine differences among the five groups for each test. Subsequent to the ANOVA analysis, the Tukey-Kramer's HSD post-hoc comparison was performed. The Pearson's correlation coefficient was used to determine the relationships among the results of the fitness tests. All statistical procedures were conducted with the JMP 12.0 statistical package (SAS Institute, Cary, NC, USA). The level of significance was set at p < 0.01 for all analyses.

RESULTS

The correlation coefficients among the tests are shown in Table 1. Most relationships among the test results were statistically significant (p < 0.01). Low to moderate correlation coefficients were found among the test results, with the exception of that for the 50-m sprint. Low to moderate negative correlations were found between the results of the 50-m sprint run and the results of the other tests.

The means and SDs for each test for each sports experience group are shown in Table 2. There were no significant differences among groups for handgrip strength, 50-m sprint results, and standing long jump results. The HG and SG tended to have higher test scores compared to those in the other groups in sit-up results, side stepping, 20-m shuttle results, and overhand handball throwing. The estimated VO2 max for each group, determined by using the prediction equation of Matsuzaka et al. (2004), were 38.4 mL/kg (NG), 40.5 mL/kg (LG), 41.8 mL/kg (MG), 43.5 mL/kg (HG), and 43.6 mL/kg (SG), respectively.

DISCUSSION

Socioeconomic transformation over the previous decades has induced a decline in fitness level for young adolescents in many countries. Volbekiene and Griciute (2007) reported a marked decrease in aerobic fitness and flexibility among Lithuanian schoolchildren. Przeweda and Dobosz (2003) reported that the physical fitness levels of Polish school children had decreased significantly in this decade compared to levels of 20 years ago. Nader et al. (2008) reported that the mean moderate-to-vigorous physical activity decreased by about 120 minutes from that at 9 years old to that at 15 years old in both boys and girls.

In Japan, the physical fitness of youth has been decreasing in recent decades. Total physical fitness test scores of young students have decreased dramatically, regardless of physical activity level, in the past 25 years (Nishijima et al., 2003). To establish the health-related fitness of young adolescents, determining the relationships between fitness level and profiles of exercise history is very important. The purpose of this study was to clarify the relationship between profiles of exercise history and performance on a Japanese fitness test for female university freshmen in Japan.

Table 1. Correlation Matrix Table for Result of MEXT Test

	HS	SU	SR	SS	20S	50S	SLJ	HT
Handgrip Strength	----	0.218 *	0.031	0.292 *	0.295 *	-0.284 *	0.292 *	0.272 *
Sit Up	0.218 *	----	0.174	0.546 *	0.525 *	-0.383 *	0.470 *	0.414 *
Sit and Reach	0.031	0.174	----	0.333 *	0.289 *	-0.267 *	0.267 *	0.154
Side Step	0.292 *	0.546 *	0.333 *	----	0.539 *	-0.572 *	0.527 *	0.470 *
20m Shuttle Run	0.295 *	0.525 *	0.289 *	0.539 *	----	-0.533 *	0.473 *	0.546 *
50m Sprint Run	-0.284 *	-0.383 *	-0.267 *	-0.572 *	-0.533 *	----	-0.498 *	-0.334 *
Standing Long Jump	0.292 *	0.470 *	0.267 *	0.527 *	0.473 *	-0.498 *	----	0.365 *
Overhand Handball Throw	0.272 *	0.414 *	0.154	0.470 *	0.546 *	-0.334 *	0.365 *	----

*: $p < .01$.

Table 2. MEXT Test Results for Each Group

	NG (n = 18)		LG (n = 32)		MG (n = 39)		HG (n = 42)		SG (n = 18)	
	Mean	SD	Mean	SD	Mean	SD	Mean	SD	Mean	SD
Handgrip Strength (kg)	22.8	3.4	23.7	4.5	24.8	4.5	24.1	4.7	24.7	4.7
Sit Up (times)	17.8	4.0	19.5	4.2	19.4	5.3	23.3 [ac]	5.5	24.4 [ac]	6.2
Sit and Reach (cm)	38.5	8.9	43.6	8.9	47.0	9.4	47.2	9.8	50.8 [a]	9.4
Side Step (s)	39.8	6.3	43.4	6.3	44.9	6.7	49.2 [ab]	5.9	48.2 [a]	8.1
20m Shuttle Run (times)	37.7	11.0	45.2	10.4	46.3	14.6	56.0 [a]	16.2	56.7 [a]	19.3
50m Sprint Run (s)	9.4	0.7	9.2	0.8	9.1	0.8	8.9	1.2	8.9	1.2
Standing Long Jump (cm)	151.8	25.1	159.2	29.8	160.6	17.0	173.2	17.6	170.0	27.9
Overhand Handball Throw (m)	11.8	2.0	14.0	3.0	14.1	2.7	16.9 [abc]	3.6	17.1 [abc]	3.6

a: vs NG p <.01; b: vs LG p < .01; c: vs MG p <.01.

Despite the low to moderate correlation coefficients, our results showed that many test results were significantly correlated. These results were similar to those reported by Suzuki et al. (1999). Side stepping was more highly correlated with sit-up results ($r^2 = 0.546$), 20-m shuttle running ($r^2 = 0.539$), 50-m sprint running ($r^2 = -0.572$), and standing long jump results ($r^2 = 0.572$) than it was to hand grip strength (r2 = 0.292), sit and reach results ($r^2 = 0.333$), and overhand handball throwing ($r^2 = 0.470$). The 20-m shuttle run results were more highly correlated with sit-up results ($r^2 = 0.525$) and the 50-m sprint results ($r^2 = -0.533$) than it was with other test results. The use similar skeletal muscle areas during these tests may explain the higher correlations. However, the higher correlation of overhand handball throwing with the 20-m shuttle run results ($r^2 = 0.546$) is difficult to clarify. Further investigation is needed to clarify that relationship.

It is interesting to note that the groups with longer sports experience showed higher scores for sit-ups, side stepping, 20-m shuttle running, sit and reach results, and overhand handball throwing compared to those scores in the groups with less sports experience. However, there were no significant differences among these groups in handgrip strength, 50-m sprint results, and standing long jump results.

It is well known that training and detraining affect the change in muscle fiber type area. Staron et al. (1991) clarified that a detraining period of 30–32 weeks after 20 weeks of training caused significant decreases in the type IIab + IIb fiber area (14.2%) and non-significant decreases in the area of type IIa (9.8%) and type I (1.4%) fibers. In the present research, the group with longer sports experience may have retained slow-twitch muscle fibers and aerobic capacity, which may led to the higher results for the sit-up test and side stepping.

Excluding the NG, most participants in the present research participated in some kinds of sports requiring regular shoulder movement, for example, basketball, tennis, volleyball, and badminton. Suzuki et al. (1999) reported that the score of overhand handball throwing was affected by the sports habits from elementary school to high school. A long duration of overhand shoulder movement in their exercise histories may be reflected as muscle memory underlying the significant differences in overhand handball throwing among the groups.

The score of the 20-m shuttle run test describes the aerobic capacity of each participant. Aerobic capacity is acquired after a long-term aerobic training history. Mujika and Padilla (2000) summarized that the maximum VO2 of athletes declines markedly but remains above control values during long-term detraining. The high score for the 20-m shuttle run for the SG reflects the effect of their training and exercise habits for over a decade. The inverse relationship between aerobic fitness and adult disease, including obesity, hypertension, and cardiac disease, are thus indicated (Franks et al., 2004; Katzmarzyk et al., 2005). It may be suggested that regular exercise and sports activities will prevent such diseases after the entrance of the SG into university. Itaki et al. (2001) reported that 21-year-old university students with long-term regular exercise habits (2 times per week for more than 6 months) had lower total cholesterol, lower LDL cholesterol, and higher HDL cholesterol compared to individuals without long-term regular exercise habits.

There was a significant difference in flexibility only between the NG and the SG. Stretching before participation in athletic activities is standard practice for all levels of sports, competitive or recreational (Thacker et al., 2004). Bandy et al. (1994) reported that 30 s and 60 s of static stretching of the hamstring muscles were more effective for increasing muscle flexibility than was stretching for 15 s or no stretching. Thus, it may be that stretching over a long-term sports history enabled the maintenance of flexibility in the SG.

Kuribayashi et al. (2007) reported that female university student with lower fitness test scores also had lower functional fitness test scores, which were developed for the assessment of middle-aged and older age groups. Habitual exercise is effective not only for preventing lifestyle-related illness but also for strengthening immunity. Takahashi et al. (2008) suggested that 8 weeks of resistance training improved physical fitness, muscle strength, and natural killer cell activity in young female participants.

People who participate in sports during the university era may continue to do so after their graduation. Okada et al. reported that people who are active in sports (participating 5.7 days per week for 3.8 hour per day) have the following tendencies: 1) 76.8% will continue regular sports activities after graduation, and 2) 88.1% have a good self-diagnosis of their own health. Nishijima et al. (2003) suggested that participation in exercise and sports and time spent in exercise and sports in daily life significantly prevented a decrease in physical ability over the years.

CONCLUSION

This study demonstrated that there were no significant differences among female university students based on their sports experience from childhood and adolescence with respect to handgrip strength, 50-m sprinting, and standing long jump scores. However, the group with longer sports experience showed higher test scores compared to those in the other groups with regard to sit-ups, side stepping, 20-m shuttle running, and overhand handball throwing. Long-term participation in sports might have affected their slow deterioration of muscle strength, muscle flexibility, and aerobic capacity.

REFERENCES

Bandy, W. D. and Irion, J. M. (1994). The effect of time on static stretch on the flexibility of the hamstring muscles. *Physical therapy*, *74*(9), 845-850.
Cavill, N., Biddle, S. and Sallis, J. F. (2001). Health enhancing physical activity for young people: Statement of the United Kingdom Expert Consensus Conference. *Pediatric exercise science*, *13*(1), 12-25.
Council of Europe, Committee of Experts on Sports Research. (1993). EUROFIT: Handbook for the EUROFIT tests of physical fitness (2nd ed.). Strasbourg: Council of Europe.
Franks, P. W., Ekelund, U., Brage, S., Wong, M. Y. and Wareham, N. J. (2004). Does the association of habitual physical activity with the metabolic syndrome differ by level of cardiorespiratory fitness?. *Diabetes Care*, *27*(5), 1187-1193.
Government of Canada, Fitness and Amateur Sport. (1987). Canadian standardized test of fitness: CSTF: (interpretation and counseling manual: a joint project of the Canadian Association of Sport Sciences Fitness Appraisal Certification and Accreditation Program and Fitness Canada). Ottawa: Government of Canada, Fitness and Amateur Sport.

Hall, G.L., Hetzler, R.K., Perrin, D. and Weltman, A. (1992). Relationship of timed sit-up tests to isokinetic abdominal strength. *Research quarterly for exercise and sport, 63*(1), 80-84.

Itaki, C., Momma, M., Kyo, E., Oda, S., Moriya,K., and Takeda, H.(2001). Effect of NK cell activity and blood component owing to Exercise habits in university students. *Sapporo Medical University Bulletin of School of Health Sciences, 4*, 23-27. (in Japanese).

Kuribayashi, T., Kamada, Y., Iwama, M., Takahashi, H., Sawamura, S., Kamihama, T., Shimizu,S., Yamashita, Y., Ogasawara,Y. and Kurokawa, K. (2007). The relationship between physical fitness test and functional fitness test among female college students. *Bulletin of Clinical Research Center for Child Development and Educational Practice, Iwate University, 6*, 85-90. (in Japanese).

Katzmarzyk, P. T., Church, T. S., Janssen, I., Ross, R. and Blair, S.N. (2005). Metabolic syndrome, obesity, and mortality impact of cardiorespiratory fitness. *Diabetes care, 28*(2), 391-397.

Leger, L.A. and Lambert, J. (1982). A maximal multistage 20-m shuttle run test to predict VO2 max. *European journal of applied physiology and occupational physiology, 49*(1), 1-12.

Matsuzaka, A., Takahashi, Y., Yamazoe, M., Kumakura, N., Ikeda, A., Wilk, B. and Bar-Or, O. (2004). Validity of the multistage 20-m shuttle-run test for Japanese children, adolescents, and adults. *Pediatric exercise science, 16*, 113-125.

Ministry of Education, Culture, Sports, Science and Technology. (2000). New Fitness Test: Beneficial Application, Tokyo, Gyosei. (in Japanese).

Ministry of Education, Culture, Sports, Science and Technology-Japan.(2012) Results of the FY2012 Physical Fitness Survey, http://www.mext.go.jp/english/topics/1343347.htm.

Minkler, S., and Patterson, P.(1994). The validity of the modified sit-and-reach test in college-age students. *Research quarterly for exercise and sport, 65*(2), 189-192.

Mountjoy, M., Andersen, L. B., Armstrong, N., Biddle, S., Boreham, C., Bedenbeck, H. P. B. and van Mechelen, W. (2011). International Olympic Committee consensus statement on the health and fitness of young people through physical activity and sport. *British Journal of Sports Medicine, 45*(11), 839-848.

Mujika, I. and Padilla, S. (2000). Detraining: loss of training-induced physiological and performance adaptations. Part II. *Sports Medicine, 30*(3), 145-154.

Nader, P. R., Bradley, R. H., Houts, R. M., McRitchie, S. L. and O'Brien, M. (2008). Moderate-to-vigorous physical activity from ages 9 to 15 years. *Jama, 300*(3), 295-305.

Nishijima, T., Nakano, T., Takahashi, S., Suzuki, K., Yamada, H., Kokudo, S. and Ohsawa, S. (2003). Relationship between changes over the years in physical ability and exercise and sports activity in Japanese youth. *International Journal of Sport and Health Science, 1*(1), 110-118.

Okada, J., Onozawa, K., Seki, K., Yajima, T., Ichinohe, S. and Kato, K.(1996). A report on the health and physical activity conditions of middle and old aged men belonged to the university sports club. *Waseda Studies in Human Sciences, 9*(1), 171-182. (in Japanese).

Przeweda, R. and Dobosz, J. (2003). Growth and physical fitness of Polish youths in two successive decades. *Journal of Sports Medicine and Physical Fitness, 43*(4), 465-474.

Staron, R. S., Leonardi, M. J., Karapondo, D. L., Malicky, E. S., Falkel, J. E., Hagerman, F. C. and Hikida, R. S. (1991). Strength and skeletal muscle adaptations in heavy-resistance-trained women after detraining and retraining. *Journal of Applied Physiology, 70*(2), 631-640.

Steele, R.M., Brage, S., Corder, K., Wareham, N. J. and Ekelund, U. (2008). Physical activity, cardiorespiratory fitness, and the metabolic syndrome in youth. *Journal of Applied Physiology*, *105*(1), 342-351.

Suzuki, K. and Nishijima, T. (2005). Effects of sports experience and exercise habits on physical fitness and motor ability in high school students. *School health*, *1*, 22-38.

Suzuki, H., Ninomiya, K., Miura, T., Kajigaya, N., Tokunaga, T., Obara, N., Araki, I., Kaga, M. and Takahishi, K.(1999). Relationship between physical characteristics, lifestyle and physical fitness in a new sports test of the Ministry of Education. *Bulletin of Faculty of Education, Okayama University, 111*, 139-144. (in Japanese).

Takahashi, T., Arai, Y., Hara, M., Ohshima, K., Koya, S. and Yamanishi, T. (2008). Effects of resistance training on physical fitness, muscle strength, and natural killer cell activity in female university students. *Japanese Journal of Hyglene, 63*, 642-650. (in Japanese).

Thacker, S. B., Gilchrist, J., Stroup, D.F. and Kimsey Jr, C.D. (2004). The impact of stretching on sports injury risk: a systematic review of the literature. *Medicine and Science in Sports and Exercise*, *36*(3), 371-378.

Volbekiene, V. and Griciute, A. (2007). Health-related physical fitness among schoolchildren in Lithuania: a comparison from 1992 to 2002. *Scandinavian Journal of Public Health, 35*(3), 235-242.

In: Physical Activity Effects on the Anthropological Status ...   ISBN: 978-1-63484-782-7
Editors: Fadilj Eminović and Milivoj Dopsaj   © 2016 Nova Science Publishers, Inc.

Chapter 7

EFFECTS OF APPLIED PHYSICAL EXERCISE ON THE MOTOR ABILITIES OF PEOPLE WITH SPINAL CORD INJURY

Fadilj Eminović[1] and Dragana Kljajić[2]*
[1]Faculty for Special Education and Rehabilitation,
University of Belgrade, Belgrade, Serbia
[2]High Health School of Professional Studies, Belgrade, Serbia

ABSTRACT

Spinal cord injury affects physical, psychological, social and professional functioning, and often occurs suddenly and completely changes life. Sports activities affect motivation but also improve motor and functional abilities. Application of sports activities must be dosed, respecting the principles of training and physical abilities of people with spinal cord injury. The aim of this study was to determine whether application of sports activities improves level of some motor abilities (upper extremity) - maximal muscle hand grip force, flexibility of shoulders, speed (speed of reaction and frequency of movements) and precision. The study included 44 participants of both gender with spinal cord injury – paraplegia, 26 participants were athletes and 18 were non-athletes. A specially designed questionnaire, medical documentation and tests for motor abilities were used for this study. For testing difference between groups χ^2- test was used, and for determination of difference between groups of variables multivariate analysis of variance (MANOVA) was used. Within the group of males, athletes had significantly higher levels of motor abilities compared to non-athletes (maximal muscle hand grip force p = 0.000; flexibility of shoulders-absolute p = 0.027 and relative p=0.038; speed of reaction p = 0.000 and frequency of movement p = 0.025). Within the group of female, athletes were significantly different from non-athletes in relation to maximal muscle hand grip force (p = 0.023), speed of reaction (p = 0.000), frequency of movements (p = 0.000) and precision (p = 0.026). Application of sports activities for 2-3 times a week significantly improves motor abilities in people with spinal cord injury after rehabilitation.

---

* Corresponding author: Email: eminovic73@gmail.com.

Keywords: spinal cord injury, motor abilities, applied physical exercise

INTRODUCTION

According to the report on disability - World report on disability (the World Health Organization) in 2011, more than a billion people live with some form of disability, or about 15% of the total population. Data from the NSCISC (National Spinal Cord Injury Statistical Center, Birmingham, Alabama, USA), published in 2013, showed that the incidence of spinal cord injuries (SCI) in the United States is 40 cases per million people, or 12 000 new cases per year. Prevalence in the USA is between 236-327000 persons with spinal cord injury. The average age of people who have suffered spinal cord injuries in the seventies was 28.7 years, and from 2005 to 2012 the average age is 41 years. The most common causes of SCI are: injuries in traffic accidents (39.2%), falls (28.3%), violence (14.6%), injuries in sports (8.2%).

According to a 2006 study, one third of the total number of persons with SCI has tetraplegia, and two thirds have paraplegia. The average age of the patients at the time of injury is 33 years, and the distribution of injuries in relation to the male/female gender is 3.8-4.8/1 (Wyndaele and Wyndaele, 2006). Within the total number of people with SCI from 2005 to 2012 the largest percentage is in persons with incomplete tetraplegia (40.8%); this percentage is followed by persons with complete paraplegia (21.6%), incomplete paraplegia (21.4%) and complete tetraplegia (15.8%) (NSCISC, 2013).

However, SCI affects the physical, psychological, social and professional functioning, often occurs suddenly and completely changes life. SCI rehabilitation is a complex and integrative. Its goal is to restore people with SCI within the family and social environment. The starting point of rehabilitation is the readjustment with a focus on medical, educational, sports and scientific, psychological and sociological fields, which assume the cooperation of a multidisciplinary team of experts (Trgovčević et al., 2011; Kljajić et al., 2013).

Application of physical exercises during and after the rehabilitation process has multiple effects on the person with SCI. These persons can practice only certain forms of exercises and in work with this population we use specifically applied methods of exercise which are allowed by their damage. Applied physical exercises are important in order to prepare for sports activities.

It is well known that sport is very suitable for the promotion of self-esteem, confidence, determination, team spirit, improve interpersonal relationships, positive characteristics in people with disabilities, which are easy to be lost, and no other method of rehabilitation can effectively restore them (Figoni, 2002; Dowling et al., 2010; Eminović et al., 2011b; Eminović, 2014).

Application of sports activities helps a person with SCI to rely on the remaining healthy power to initiate its potential reserves and overcome the disability (van Langenveld et al., 2011; Kawanishi and Greguol, 2013; Kljajić et al., 2013). However, the choice of sports activities that can be practiced by people with SCI is limited, and there are a large number of organized competitions which often have more "fighting spirit" than the competition of athletes without disabilities. Sports in persons with SCI is considerably changed from the beginning, actually from the first, but the most important steps made by professor Sir Ludwig

Guttmann in the forties of the twentieth century (Rogan and Rogan, 2010; Otašević and Kljajić, 2013).

Spinal Cord Injury

In its function the spinal cord is conveyor of upstream and downstream impulses that connect the higher centers of nervous system with the periphery. The spinal cord is also the centre of the relatively simple reflexes (a reflex to stretching, the Golgi tendon reflex, reflex of flexor and cross extensor). Spinal cord injuries are divided into two broad categories: tetraplegia and paraplegia, complete or incomplete.

Terms which were used to indicate partial spinal cord injury - paraparesis and quadriparesis due to their imprecision of defining are not recommended any more. Tetraplegia indicates impairment or loss of motor and sensory functions in the cervical segments of the spinal cord due to lesions of neurons in the spinal canal. Tetraplegia results in impaired function of upper limbs, trunk, lower limbs and pelvic organs. Paraplegia indicates impairment or loss of motor or sensory function in the thoracic, lumbar or sacral segments of the spinal cord due to lesions of neurons in the spinal canal. In paraplegia upper limb function is preserved, and depending on the level of the lesion hull function, lower extremities and pelvic organs can be impaired. This term is also used for impairment of cauda equina and conus medularis, but not for the lumbosacral plexus lesions or injury to peripheral nerves outside the spinal canal. The syndrome cauda equina involves impairment of lumbosacral roots in the spinal canal which leads to impairment of the function of the bladder, bowel and lower extremities. The syndrome conus medularis indicates conus medularis lesion and sacral roots in the spinal canal causing impairment of the function of the bladder and bowel (Jović, 2011; Kirshblum et al., 2011; Verhaagen and McDonald, 2012).

Completeness SCI

Evaluation of patients with spinal cord injury involves assessing the levels of neurological damage, the degree of completeness of spinal cord lesions and determination of motor and sensory scores. Axons of sensory neurons of the spinal input into spinal cord and motor neurons output from the spinal cord through the spinal roots. Each dorsal root receives information from a certain part of human skin, which is called a dermatome. Motor fibers of each ventral root innervate group of muscles that make a *myotome*. Implementation of the motor and sensitive information is compromised on the spot of spinal cord lesions. If the dermatomes and myotome are systematically examined, the level (segment) which has been damaged in spinal cord can be determined. Damage to the spinal cord presents neurological level of the lesion and the degree of completeness of spinal cord lesions. The neurological level of the lesion indicates the lowest segment of the spinal cord with normal motor function and sensitivity on both sides of the body. Skeletal level refers to the level at which only with the help of X-rays the biggest injury of the spinal cord is seen. Sensitive and motor scores represent the sum of the numerical test results, which reflects the degree of neurological impairment due to spinal cord lesions (Jović, 2011; Kirshblum et al., 2011; Verhaagen and McDonald, 2012).

Firstly, complete spinal cord injury exists in conditions when there is not preserved neither sensitive nor motor function in the lowest sacral segments of the spinal cord (S4, S5). Sacred sensitivity is a present feeling in the area mucocutaneous compound, as well as deep anal feeling. Test motor preservation makes the presence of voluntary contraction of the external anal sphincter to digital examination. Incomplete lesion is characterized by the existence of any preservation of sensitive or motor function below the neurological level, which includes the lowest sacral segments (S4, S5). To assess the completeness or incompleteness of spinal cord injury Frenkel scale damage was first applied (Frenkel et al., 1969). Because of the lack of reliability of this scale, the *American Association for spinal cord injury* in 1982 gave the proposal for new and more precise standards that clearly define the level and completeness of spinal cord injury. These standards were adopted in 1992 by the International Medical Society of Paraplegia (IMSOP). ASIA Impairment Scale - AIS, in accordance with International standards for neurological classification of spinal cord injuries (ISNCSCI) has so far had few revisions - 2000, 2006, 2011 and 2013 (Waring et al., 2010; Kirshblum et al., 2011).

The levels of completeness/incompleteness of spinal SCI to the ASIA standards are: A - complete impairment (there is no preservation or motor or sensory function in sacral segments S4 - S5); B - incomplete injury (preserved only sensibility below the neurological level including the last sacral segments S4-S5); C - incomplete injury (motor function is preserved below the neurological level), the majority of key muscles below the lesion is below the grade of 3 to the manual muscle test - MMT); D - incomplete injury (motor function is preserved below the neurological level, most key muscles below the neurological level of the MMT for grade 3 or higher; E - normal finding (motor and sensitive functions are normal). Zone of partial preservation refers to the dermatome (the 28 dermatomes on the left and the right - to detect sensitivity to pinprick and light touch) and myotomes (testing 10 pairs of key muscles whose strength is measured according to MMT) below the level of neurological lesions that are partially innervated. The exact number of partial innerved segments on each side of the body is determined (Kirshblum et al., 2011).

Etiology SCI

In relation to etiology, spinal cord injuries are classified as traumatic and non-traumatic (Crisp et al., 2011; New et al., 2014). Traumatic spinal cord injuries occur most often in people between the age of 16 and 30, more in males (80%) (Osterthun et al., 2009). From non-traumatic, tumors are the most common causes of spinal cord injury in Europe (33%), South Africa (28%) and Australia (27%), a degenerative disease of the spinal column in East Asia (59%) and North America (54%) (New et al., 2014).

Spinal cord lesions are usually consequence of the indirect forces caused by movements of the head and trunk and less direct spine injuries. Common mechanisms of spinal cord injury include flexion, compression, hyperextension and flexion - rotation. These forces result in the fracture and/or dislocation. The intensity and combination of imposed forces have a direct impact on the type and location of the fracture, dislocation degree and extent of soft tissue damage. The spine shows a distinct preference to injuries: some areas are more vulnerable because of the higher mobility and the lack of stability compared to other segments of the spine (e.g., a rigid thoracic region). The most frequently damaged parts are between C5 and C7 in the cervical region and between Th12 and L2 in thoracolumbar region. Two contributing mechanisms of spinal cord injuries are shearing and stretching. Shearing is happening during the action of horizontal forces to the surrounding segments. Shearing tears ligaments and often is associated with dislocation fracture thoracolumbar region. Stretching means traction force and it is the rarest mechanism of spinal cord injury (Bryce, 2009; Jović, 2011; Verhaagen and McDonald, 2012).

Medical Rehabilitation SCI

The basis rehabilitation of people with SCI is based on the application of bio-psycho-social model, which includes the physical, social and psychological components and their interaction (Cohen and Napolitano, 2007; Dorsett and Geraghty, 2008). The essence of this approach also applies to the participation of patients in decision-making regarding the development and implementation of the plan of the rehabilitation process (Duff et al., 2004; Byrnes et al., 2012), with the aim of returning lost skills and acquiring new ones and abilities (Wade, 2009). Studies show that the impact of the patient in the setting up and implementation of rehabilitation goals significantly contributes to increasing self-esteem, physical abilities and personal satisfaction (McGrath et al., 1995; Orbell et al., 2001).

Possibility of recovery after spinal cord injury depends on the extent of the lesion cord and its roots. In complete lesions improvements are not expected, except for one which is the consequence of the recovery of the nerve roots. In the incomplete lesions some degree of sensory or motor function is registered below the level of the lesions after the withdrawal of spinal shock (Milićević et al., 2012a). The dynamic recovery is highest in the first few months, after which the dynamics is maintained or it slows down. After that, newly recovered muscular activity is not usually expected within following several weeks and months. Further recovery is not expected (Cohen et al., 2012; Verhaagen and McDonald, 2012). In the acute phase, people with SCI are indicated by a respiratory treatment, targeted maintenance of mobility and positioning, selective muscle strengthening and directing to a vertical position. In the next phase - the phase of mobilization, treatment focuses on training the patient to self-inspection skin, and when one reaches the level of a wheelchair it is important to evaluate cardiovascular capacity with load tests (fatigue upper extremities or drive a wheelchair). During the mobilization phase, in addition to therapeutic activity in the previous stages, the patient will be included in a program of exercises to strengthen the muscle strength (PNF, manual resistance, wall reel, suspension, group exercises), postural control and balance by substituting the upper limbs and vision (for damaged proprioception). The treatment plan at this stage include: patient relaxation training, breathing exercises, training and mastering transfers, exercises to reduce spasticity, master new motor patterns, balance exercises, activities on the mat, activity in a wheelchair and with the wheelchair, exercises in the parallel bars, standing and walk out looms, training using of crutches and sporting activities. Furthermore, for improving mobility and physical performance in people with spinal cord injury application of physical, occupational therapy and sporting activities significantly important (Noreau and Shephard, 1995; Jović, 2011; van Langenvelt et al., 2011; Jones et al., 2012).

Nevertheless, in the last 60 years development of medicine and a healthcare, significantly increased the life expectancy of people who have experienced spinal cord injury (Strauss et al., 2000; Imai et al., 2004). The most common secondary health conditions relate to the presence of pain, ulcers, bowel and bladder regulation problems, muscle spasms, fatigue, symptom of esophageal, kidney and urinary infections and osteoporosis (Krassioukov et al., 2010; D'Hondt and Everaert, 2011; Milićević et al., 2012b). In older people with SCI, often occur secondary health conditions, as well as cardiovascular disease, diabetes, bone mineral density loss, fatigue and respiratory complications or infections (Garshick et al., 2005; Jensen et al., 2013).

Besides, in a prospective study conducted by Krause and Kjorsvig (1992) several predictors of mortality after spinal cord injury are documented: reduced social and work activities, increased time spent in bed, perceived lower quality of life, lack of employment or involvement in education. An important aspect of long-term rehabilitation plan is to train patients to take care of their impairments during their lifetime. This requires re-integration into the community and maintenance of optimal health levels during rehabilitation. Aspects are numerous: housing, food, transportation, finance, maintenance of functional skills and further training, participation in social and recreational activities. These issues should be treated early in the course of rehabilitation in collaboration with the patient, families, and rehabilitation teams (Taylor-Schroeder et al., 2011; Hammond et al., 2011; Tomasone et al., 2013; Trgovčević et al., 2014).

SPORTS ACTIVITIES IN PERSON WITH SCI

Application of Physical Activity in People with SCI - Paraplegia

Process of training is systematic and planned activity based on objective regularities of functioning of man as a biological being. In the process of training the characteristics, needs and abilities of participants are taken into account; and the process of exercise is characterized by the structure, content, scope, intensity, resources and nature of the work, which cause certain effects on body and allow for appropriate adaptation, in accordance with the set plans (Kukolj, 2006; Kenney et al., 2011).

Regular application of physical activity in people with SCI influences on prevention, as well as on reduction and slowing down the symptoms of chronic diseases. Among the sedentary population and those who have developed a specific chronic health conditions (hypertension, heart disease, diabetes, arthritis, etc.) undertaking some physical activity contributes to improving the general health, cognitive functioning, reduces symptoms of stress; and all these contribute to a better quality of life (Anneken et al., 2010; Martin Ginis et al., 2010; Ravenek et al., 2012; Geyh et al., 2013; Omorou et al., 2013). During the physical exercise physiological processes occur in the body and these contribute to the optimization of physical performance, whereby they increase the efficiency and capacity, thus contributing to the reduction of cardiovascular risk (Tasiemski and Brewer, 2011; Kawanishi and Greguol, 2013). According to research by Heath and Feltem (1997) the level of fitness is correlated with reduced time spent in bed, increased social interaction and overall life satisfaction.

However, only 13-16% of people with spinal cord regularly practice physical activity (Washburn and Hedrick, 1997), and some studies show that approximately 50% is physically inactive (Tasiemski et al., 2005; Anneken et al., 2010). The beginning of "conditioning" of people with SCI is achieved in the first phase of rehabilitation in order to maintain an active lifestyle and improve functional ability (Bizzarini et al., 2005; Haisma et al., 2006; Hicks and Martin Ginis, 2008). The primary function of sport as therapy is to develop neuromuscular mechanisms in intact parts of the body to compensate lost function parts that are not under the control of the CNS. In the case of complete spinal cord, function of all voluntary muscles is lost, as well as all aspects of sensitivity, including deep sensibility which is responsible for maintenance of static and dynamic postural stability. However, even with complete spinal cord injury, paralyzed body parts still remain associated with central nervous system thanks to the anatomical distribution of certain muscle groups (Verhaagen and McDonald, 2012).

For example, in impairment of the spinal cord above the sixth dorsal segment (Th6), when abdominal and distal spinal muscles are paralyzed, *m. latissimus dorsi* with its connections to the pelvis, and *m.* trapesius which reaches up to the twelfth dorsal vertebra (Th12), are still capable to function due to this connection and thanks to their innervations in the cervical spinal cord. The training ensures that these muscles of the back and trunk are developed into a kind of physiological corset, which allows a person with SCI to maintain an upright position without the aid of tools. Swimming, weightlifting, rope-climbing and archery in particular proved, proved to be an ideal sports in this respect (Bhambhani, 2002; Bryce, 2009; Jović, 2011).

Participating in physical activities for people with SCI decreases the frequency of urinary, respiratory infections, severe spasticity and pressure ulcers (Noureau and Shephard, 1995; Huonker et al., 1998). Physical activity also affects the level of triglycerides, body fat, insulin resistance and the regulation of blood pressure (Noreau and Shephard, 1995; Nash et al., 2001; Nash and Mendez, 2009).

The Principles of Training for People with SCI – Paraplegia

In order to participate actively in physical or sporting activities for persons with SCI, following diagnostic tests are recommended: Exercise Stress Test, Bone Mineral Density – BMD Scan, Blood Work (cholesterol - often due registered atherogenic lipid profile, and glucose) and Pulmonary Function Test - PFT (Jacobs and Nash, 2004).

For the application of physical activity in people with SCI the basic principles of training for people without disabilities are used: load, specificity, individuality, reversibility. The principle of the load based on the training that is of greater intensity, specific to the activity which is being applied in order to achieve physiological improvements. Combination of frequency, intensity and duration is achieved by proper load during training. The load is correlated with the specifics prescribed exercises and specificity refers to the adaptation of metabolic and physiological functions that depend on the applied loads. Specific exercises induce specific adaptations and thus lead to the specific effects of training. Outcome of the exercises is specific for the muscles and energy, but also for the type of training. Individuality is related to individual variation in response to training. For this principle, the condition in which a person is found and other specific factors to the prescribed exercises, according to the needs and capacities of person, is taken into consideration. For people with SCI the degree of disability is also taken into account. Individuality focuses on interventions for persons trained to exercise safely and to prevent injuries or adverse effects during exercise. The reversibility refers to the response after training; after finishing the training improvement achieved by the systematically dosed exercises is irretrievably lost (Myslinski, 2005; Kenney et al., 2011).

Application of physical activity, training or sporting activities of people with SCI should be based on the principles of training and the load:

a) Aerobic training (intensity) refers to maintaining a target heart rate and pulse rate (target heart rate - THR). It is 40% to 80% of maximum heart rate reserve (HRR). It is calculated by Karnoven's formula: THR = [(MHR-RHR) x 40-80%] + RHR, where MHR (maximum heart rate) maximum heart rate on exercise stress test, RHR (resting heart rate), heart rate at rest (value morning pulse), percentage (%) which shows the dosage of the training load. If a load test is not applied, then the target heart rate is calculated - THR = (20-30) + RHR; or 20-30 plus the value of the morning heart pulse (Durán et al., 2001; Hicks et al., 2003).

It is recommended that duration of aerobic training should be 30 minutes of continuous aerobic exercise, 2-3 times a week using the hand ergo meter, the wheelchair trainer, free trolley rides, seated aerobics, swimming, riding an ergo meter bike by applying electrical stimulation, exercise with weights by method of circuit training (methods of work per cell) (Durán et al., 2001; Figoni, 2002; Ditor et al., 2003; Hicks et al., 2003; Jacobs and Nash, 2004; Nash, 2005).

b) Anaerobic training - intensity - 50% to 80% of 1RM (Repetitio maximum), duration - 2 to 3 sets of 10 repetitions, frequency - twice a week, lifting weights and using the tape T (Durán et al., 2001; Tordi et al., 2001; Ditor et al., 2003; Hicks et al., 2003; Jacobs and Nash, 2004; Myslinski, 2005).

Application of exercises for increasing the strength can increase and aerobic capacity, and also contributes to efficiency of program of physical activity in people with SCI. Jacobs et al., (1997) state that after applying FNS (functional neuromuscular stimulation), there is an increase in VO_{2max}, strength and endurance in wheelchair trainer. Aerobic training, in people with SCI, increases the endurance of respiratory muscles (Silva et al., 1998).

There are several studies comparing athletes with SCI and athletes without SCI, documenting objective physiological changes that occurred after the injury (Bhambhani, 2002). In studies that compared people with SCI within athletes and non-athletes it is determined that there is a difference in aerobic power or performance concerning endurance. There is evidence that the endurance can be achieved by the continuous training (Bhambhani, 2002). Aerobic capacity (VO_{2max}) is higher in people with paraplegia in relation to the quadriplegia, and in persons with incomplete paraplegia with respect to the entire lesion of the spinal cord. This difference can be explained by a reduced active muscle mass, which produces the extraction of oxygen from the blood, and also decreased response to catecholamines in patients with quadriplegia (Frey et al., 1997).

In a study in which participated canoeists without injury and canoeists with paraplegia participated, it was determined that those with no injuries have a higher aerobic capacity by 41% (Huonker et al., 1998). Athletes with paraplegia and quadriplegia who participated in endurance trainings, showed significantly greater aerobic power measured VO_2 maximum, compared to those who were leading a sedentary lifestyle (Price and Campbell, 1999). Anaerobic power is inversely proportional to the level of SCI and completeness of spinal cord lesions (Davis and Shepherd, 1988). In a study in which *Wingate test* with trolley was used for 30 seconds, a significant difference in anaerobic power was not shown in people without injuries compared to people with SCI below levels Th8 (Hutzler et al., 2000).

Motor Abilities and Sports Persons with SCI

Motor abilities are a set of internal characteristics of a person on which depends the success of movement. They are the result of complex abilities of a person for the manifestation of motor structures in certain activities that combine physical characteristics, biochemical processes and functional changes (Kukolj, 2006; Kenney et al., 2011). Studies of motor abilities are extremely responsible and complex processes of applying the procedures, methods and tools in order to determine the effectiveness of implementation of various program contents (Eminović et al., 2011b; Kljajić et al., 2012; Dopsaj et al., 2013; Dopsaj et al., 2015).

Motor abilities are changing under the influence of systematic physical exercise, with set goals and specified procedure of applying exercises, not only in healthy population and athletes, but also in various pathological conditions and disabilities (Dopsaj et al., 2010; Adamović et al., 2014; Arsić et al., 2014; Eminović and Arsić, 2014; Arsić et al., 2015a; Arsić et al., 2015b).

Definition of objective characteristics of human abilities involves an assessment of strength, endurance, agility and flexibility. In relation to the anatomical and physiological characteristics, the level of motor abilities is associated with the state of the musculoskeletal system, and in relation to biomechanical characteristics, abilities are analyzed on the basis of dynamic and kinematic characteristics of movement (Ivanović et al., 2009; Dopsaj et al., 2011; Kljajić et al., 2012).

Besides, in relation to the basic motor abilities, contractile ability represents the basic abilities responsible for the movement in humans because with no muscle contraction there is no movement (in dynamic conditions) or attempted movement (in static conditions). From the aspect of metrology procedures in sport, i.e., procedures of analytics and diagnostics of physical capabilities, measurement of muscular force is conducted by means of dynamometry and isometric (Sisto and Dyson-Hudson, 2007; Larson et al., 2010; Eminović, 2011a).

The term *speed* means the ability to perform movements or movement maximum possible speed for the given conditions. To perform the movement at high speed rapid muscle contraction is essential, where the main role is on fast contracting muscle fibers. The percentage of fast muscle fibers in the muscle is genetically predetermined and cannot be significantly changed by any training. Speed of reaction is highly genetically conditioned, i.e., depends on innate characteristics (85-95%). Frequency of movement is ability to perform cyclic movements in maximum speed, i.e., those movements which are repeated. The ability to run a maximum of rapid repetitive movements (cyclical) depends on the inner muscular coordination (synchronized action of all muscle fibers in a muscle), coordination between muscles (synchronized action of all the muscles involved in a given movement) and movement techniques. Accuracy is often defined as motor ability of accurately targeted and dosed movements and motion. Accuracy is the ability to hit some static or moveable target, which is located at a certain distance, by shooting or targeting. Results in this motor ability vary a lot depending on the emotional state and are genetically determined to a large extent (Zaciorsky, 1975; Kenney et al., 2011).

During rehabilitation sport activities that can be applied in people with SCI and are selected with special attention. Sports activities have a positive effect on the locomotors apparatus (develop strength, speed, agility, endurance, flexibility), as well as the motivation of patients (Bhambhani, 2002; van der Berg Emons et al., 2008; Visers et al., 2008). In order to have the most favorable effect of sports activities, it is necessary to assess condition of the person (medical evaluation) and make proper selection methods (sport) and volume of the load of the body. Important factors for these are: state of cardiovascular and respiratory systems, proper selection of starting position, speed and range of movements (ROM), rest breaks and their distribution, complexity and precision of movement performance, use of tools to perform the movement, terrain, and other devices. Furthermore, gymnastics (parterre and exercises on the mat), athletics, sports dry, water sports, winter sports and sports games (basketball sitting, sitting volleyball, table tennis, bowling) are used (Tordi et al., 2001; Wu and Williams, 2001; Elfström et al., 2005; Bernardi et al., 2010; Gassaway et al., 2011; Uzunković et al., 2011; Jovanović et al., 2013).

Most authors believe that people with SCI can improve the level of functional ability, self-care and activities of daily living if regularly apply physical activity (Heath and Fentem, 1997; Tasiemski et al., 2005; Haisma et al., 2006; van den Berg Emons, 2008; Vissers et al., 2008). Muraki et al., (2000a and 2000b) indicate that the psychological benefits of sport for people with SCI exist if the frequency of training at least 3 times a week.

As with persons without disabilities (Sibilio and Aiello, 2010), and people with SCI may also apply recreational, amateur and professional motor and sports activities. Recreational and sports activities are implemented through the associations of persons with disabilities and a variety of sports clubs. Amateur sport means a systematic and organized implementation of sport activities.. Athletes with SCI do not have a professional contract, but have a chance of winning prizes in competitions. Professional sport person with SCI provides professional contract in accordance with sport event and organization of sport clubs. The most important competition is the *Paralympics Games* that bring together top athletes from around the world. According to the official website of the Paralympics movement in summer Paralympics Games athletes compete in: archery, canoe, soccer (5 players), dance in a wheelchair, rowing, sitting volleyball, triathlon, wheelchair rugby, athletics, cycling, football (7 players), judo, sailing, swimming, wheelchair basketball, wheelchair tennis, bowling, horseback riding, goal ball, weightlifting, shooting, fencing and table tennis in a wheelchair. In winter Paralympics Games a smaller number of sports are represented: alpine skiing, biathlon, cross country skiing, ice skating and curling in a wheelchair (Official website of the Paralympics Movement, 2015).

METHODS

In people with SCI need for physical activity through sport is crucial in rehabilitation and after it. It helps re-formation of the whole personality of persons with disabilities whose integrity was compromised through re-adaptation and re-socialization (McVeigh et al., 2009; Kasum et al., 2011). Playing sports contributes to the feeling of satisfaction and a series of positive changes in mood and emotional state, makes it easy to navigate numerous psychological and other conflict situations in the family and at the workplace (Hicks et al., 2003; Martin Ginis et al., 2003; Tasiemski et al., 2005; Valtonen et al., 2006). In addition to confirmation of its own power and physical condition, by engaging the remaining abilities, sport contributes to improvement and establishment of normal human relationships, better adaptation to disability, facilitating the integration of newly created body scheme in the idea of body (Silva et al., 2005; Martin Ginis et al., 2010; Hicks et al., 2011).

Motor abilities themselves, are determined by unstable communication systems, resulting in synchronized interactions between body functions (physiological, biochemical, biomechanical, etc.). As part of interaction of certain functions of body, more or less variable, latent characteristics are formed, as a basis for the manifestation of different modalities and abilities as a factor in explaining function of efficiency of the activities of a man (Huonker et al., 1998; Hutzler et al., 2000; Hicks and Martin Ginis, 2008). In periods of 1 to 3 months, 1 year or 2 to 4 years, there are real opportunities to achieve functional morphological, biochemical and neuromuscular changes, and there are no conditions for harmonization and building a kinematic and dynamic structure of movement, habits and condition of "experiencing themselves" (Kukolj, 2006; Kenney et al., 2011; Cohen et al., 2012).

Besides, motor abilities are largely shaped by individual set of endogenous and exogenous factors. Improving of exogenous factors is particularly present in the sport as it is a specific activity, which has its own specific characteristics (competition, many years of preparation in training, a lot of emotional discharge, a special sport mode of life) and is a significant factor in forming of athletes. Science has achieved significant results in the discovery, study and training opportunities for persons with disabilities. Progress of science and interdisciplinary approach sport increased level of expertise of trainers and other professionals, who work on development of sport for disabled persons.

Participants of this research are people with SCI - paraplegia, which have undergone rehabilitation, and who are actively involved or not involved in sports activities. The aim of the research was to determine the difference between a person with SCI – paraplegia who are actively involved in sports and those who do not train in relation to motor abilities that relate to the maximum power grip, flexibility of the shoulders, speed (speed of reaction and frequency of movements) and precision.

Participants

From a total of 80 available participants with SCI, at the age of 20-60, only 44 met the criteria - minimum 2 years have passed from spinal cord lesions; a spinal cord injury at the level of the thoracic, lumbar or sacral region (paraplegia); and athletes who actively practice minimum of 2-3 times a week in the last two years.

The experimental group consisted of 26 participants who are actively involved in sports minimum 2-3 times a week, and a control group of 18 participants who do not do sports. All participants have declared that their right hand is dominant. The groups were formed according to the level of spinal cord injury determined by ASIA impairment scale (Waring et al., 2010; Kirshblum et al., 2011), which is taken from the medical records documentation of participants.

The research was conducted during 2013 at the Home for Adult Persons with Disabilities in Belgrade, Association of paraplegics and quadriplegics "Dunav" in Belgrade, Athletic club "Pogledi" from Belgrade, Wheelchairs basketball club "Dunav" from Belgrade, Table tennis club of persons with disabilities Belgrade "STIB" and Sports and Recreational Association "Sve je moguće" from Belgrade.

Instruments and Statistics

The basic methodological principle of this research is based on the comparison of results between participants with SCI – paraplegia who are involved in sports activities as compared to participants who are not involved in sports activities, with the aim of determining the differences between the given research variables. Basic measures of central tendency of the results were represented by arithmetic mean (M) and standard deviation (SD). Differences between individual groups were tested by χ^2- test. Multivariate analysis of variance (MANOVA) was used to determine differences between the sets of variables between the experimental and control group, while Bonferroni criterion was used to test differences between pairs of individual variables.. Statistical analysis was carried out by software package Excel 2003 (Microsoft®Office Excel 2003) and SPSS Win 17.0.

For the purpose of the study were used medical documentation of participants was used and specially designed questionnaire which is completed by athletes referring to the type of sport, the number and frequency of training. Among the tests for motor abilities the following were applied:

1. Maximal muscle hand grip force - the method of isometric dynamometry, a standardized test was used - hand grip (Dopsaj et al., 2009a; Dopsaj et al., 2011; Eminović et al., 2011a; Kljajić et al., 2012). Testing procedure: after warming up for 5 minutes, participants were instructed testing procedures, after which the participants performed two trial attempts grip (left and right hand) for specific warming. After a rest period of 5 minutes the participants started the test protocol: two trial measurements maximum grip both hands (first dominant and non-dominant hand) are performed, with a pause between each attempt to test one arm for at least 1 minute. Testing was conducted in a sitting position in a wheelchair (Figure 1).

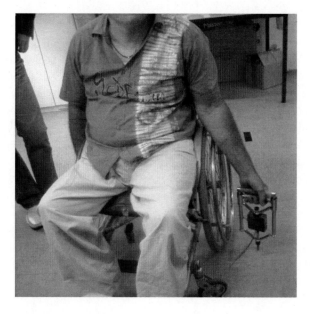

Figure 1. Outline of isometric dynamometry.

Variables covered are:

- Maximum muscle hand grip force of left and right hand expressed in dekanewton (daN) - $F_{max}L$ and $F_{max}R$;
- Sum maximal muscle hand grip force of left and right hand expressed in dekanewton (daN) - $F_{max}SUM$, where: $F_{max}SUM = F_{max}L + F_{max}R$.

2. Test for the assessment of flexibility of shoulders – The stick turn (Kukolj, 2006, p. 255). Testing is done in a sitting position in a wheelchair, where the participant holds a stick (150 cm long and 3 cm in diameter, on which a centimeters ribbon is glued, from grips on one end to the other end of the stick) and one hand is on the grip of the stick and the other hand is set next to it. A participant tries to move the stick straight up over his head and roll behind his back with the smallest distance between the hands. The minimum distance (in cm) between hands after completing the movement is measured. Among the two attempts better (smaller) result is registered.

Included variables are:

- Absolute indicator of shoulders flexibility, expressed in centimeters (cm) - SF_{abs};
- Relative indicator of shoulders flexibility (defined as the relation of absolute indicators index supple shoulders and shoulder width biacromial-ratio) - SF_{rel}.

Shoulder Width (biacromial ratio) was measured anthrop meter by Martin and is expressed in cm.

3. Test for assessing speed (Oja and Tuxworth, 1995; Kukolj, 2006, p. 245).

- Speed of reaction (Karar's stick) left and right hands, expressed in centimeters (cm) - SR_L and SR_R and summation (sum) of the speed of reaction of the left and right hands - SR_{SUM}, where $SR_{SUM} = SR_L + SR_R$;
- Frequency of movement - Hand tapping - tapping left and right hand - HT_L and HT_R and the mean value of tapping left and right hand – $HT_M = (HT_R + HT_L)/2$.

Assessment of speed of reaction (Karar's stick) is implemented in a sitting position in a wheelchair, while a participant's hand is in semi-flexed position, palm facing inward, fingers extended. An examiner holds the stick over fist in vertical position. Centimeters are marked on a stick. The mark "0" on a stick is in a level of the upper edge of a hand. When the examiner drops the stick, the participant tries to cover the stick with fingers quickly. The number above the upper edge of the hand is registered as speed reaction (in cm) (Kukolj, 2006). The first testing of a dominant and non-dominant hand is a trial, and is followed by the first and second measurement, while the better (smaller) result is recorded.

A hand tapping participant performs in a sitting position in a wheelchair, which are secured with their own brakes, and additional assistance is also provided (Figure 2). There are two circles of 20 cm in diameter at a distance of 61 cm in front of the participants on the table. The hand which is not examined is set on the central line (circle) between the laps, and the hand which is examined is set on the opposite circle. At the signal of an instructor a participant tries to as quickly as possible alternately continue touching the circles. The even numbers of properly carried out touches for a time of 10 seconds (s) are measured, first by a dominant and then by a non-dominant hand. The first attempt is a trial, then follows first and second measurement and better (higher) scores are recorded.

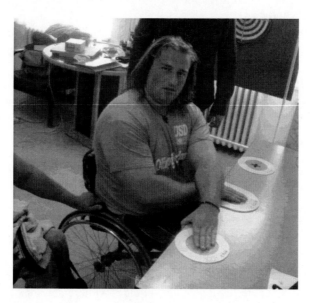

Figure 2. Hand tapping.

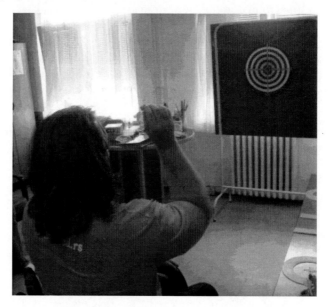

Figure 3. Darts.

4. Test for evaluation of precision - Darts (Kukolj, 2006 p. 254) - which are covered by variables:

- Precision of left and right hand - D_L and D_R;
- Summation (sum) of those parameters - D_{SUM}, where $D_{SUM} = D_L + D_R$.

The participant sits in a wheelchair which is on the distance of 250 cm from the target. The goal has five circles and their value from 1 to 10 from the periphery to the center. Participant has three trial test firing target, then shoot the target five times, first by dominant and then by non-dominant hand. Edges which are hit between two rounds counts as a better result. Record the total number of hits is registered, the mean value in relation to the number of shooting (five) is documented.

Ethical Notes

The research was realized in accordance with the terms "Declaration of Helsinki for recommendations guiding physicians in biomedical research involving human subjects" (http://www.cirp.org/library/ethics/helsinki/), with the approval and consent of the Ethics Committee of the Faculty of Sport and Physical Education, University of Belgrade.

RESULTS

The study included a total of 44 participants with SCI-paraplegia, who underwent rehabilitation. The experimental group (E group) was composed of composed of people who are systematically involved in some kind of sports activities, a total of 26 (59.09%) participants, 19 (73.08%) were male and 7 (26.92%) were female. The control group (C group) consisted of 18 (40.91%) participants who do not apply sports activities, 13 (72.22%) male and 5 (27.78%) female participants (Table 1). According to the results of the chi-square test, E and C groups did not differ statistically in relation to gender, $\chi^2 = 1.45$, $p = 0.228$, which means that the groups are equal in terms of the number of female or male.

Table 1. Structure of participants in E and C groups in relation to gender

E group-athletes			C group-non-athletes		Total	
Sex	N	%	N	%	N	%
Male	19	73.08	13	72.22	32	72.73
Female	7	26.92	5	27.78	12	27.27
Total	26	59.09	18	40.91	44	100

Experimental and control groups were matched with respect to completeness injuries/lesions of the spinal cord. Of the total sample of participants, complete spinal cord injury (ASIA A) had 27 (61.36%) participants, and incomplete injury (ASIA B, C) had 17 (38.64%) participants. Incomplete spinal cord injury ASIA D and E had none of the participants (Table 2). According to the results of the chi-square test, E and C groups are equal or statistically do not differ in terms of completeness of spinal cord injury, $\chi^2 = 2.27$, $p = 0.132$.

Table 2. Structure of participants in E and C groups in relation to the completeness of the spinal cord injury and level of injury

	E group-athletes		C group-non-athletes		Total	
	N	%	N	%	N	%
ASIA A	16	36.36	11	25	27	61.36
ASIA B	4	9.09	3	6.82	7	15.91
ASIA C	6	13.64	4	9.09	10	22.73
Total	26	59.09	18	40.91	44	100
Level of injury, n (%)						
thoracic	15	57.7	10	55.6	25	56.82
lumbar	11	42.3	8	44.4	19	43.18

Table 3. Age and time after injury in participants in group E

E group-athletes					
Age	M	SD	cV%	Min	Max
Male (N = 19)	35.95	6.55	18.22	23.5	46.3
Female (N = 7)	43.2	8.55	19.78	31.1	56
Time after injury					
Male (N = 19)	14.22	6.67	46.85	3.5	23.2
Female (N = 7)	19.77	0.46	2.31	19	20.3

In relation to the age youngest male athletes was 23.5 years, and the oldest was 46.3 years, while females this ratio was 31.1 vs. 56 years respectively. Table 3 shows that the average age of the group E 35.95±6.55 (males), and 43.2±8.55 years (females). Time after injury for male participants ranged 14.22±6.67 years and female 19.77±0.46 years.

Table 4 shows that the average age of male athletes were 48.77±6.96 years and of female athletes 43.37±13.22 years. Time after injury is the male participants was 22.54±8.76 years, while the female 24.5±16.67 years.

Table 4. Age and time after injury in participants in group C

C group-non-athletes					
Age	M	SD	cV%	Min	Max
Male (N=13)	48.77	6.96	14.28	35.6	59.9
Female (N=5)	43.37	13.22	30.48	29.5	59.1
Time after injury					
Male (N=13)	22.54	8.76	38.86	12.3	44
Female (N=5)	24.5	16.67	68.03	5.2	47.1

MANOVA results, shown in Table 5, show a statistically significant difference in variables - age and the time after injury in relation to gender and affiliation E and C group. The results showed that the participants males, athletes and non-athletes, significantly differ by age (p = 0.000) and time after injury (p = 0.005), while female participants were not statistically different by the given variables.

Table 5. The results of MANOVA of variables - in relation to gender and belonging to a group of athletes/non-athletes

athletes/ non-athletes	Type III Sum of Squares	df	Mean Square	F	Sig.
Age					
Male	1266.837	1	1266.837	28.049	0.000
Female	0.089	1	0.089	0.001	0.978
Time after injury					
Male	534.239	1	534.239	9.319	0.005
Female	65.346	1	65.346	0.587	0.461

Table 6. Structure of participants in E-group - athletes in relation to gender and type of sport they train

| | E group-athletes | | | | Total | |
	Male		Female			
Type of sport:	N	%	N	%	N	%
Athletics	7	26.92	-	-	7	26.92
Basketball wheelchair	9	34.61	-	-	9	34.61
Shooting	-	-	3	11.54	3	11.54
Bicycling	1	3.85	-	-	1	3.85
Archery	1	3.85	2	7.69	3	11.54
Table tennis	-	-	2	7.69	2	7.69
Body building	1	3.85	-	-	1	3.85
Total	19	73.08	7	26.92	26	100

Table 7. Structure of participants in E-group - athletes in relation to gender, number on the level of weekly trainings and the total number of years of training

| | E group-athletes | | | | Total | |
	Male		Female			
Number of training sessions/weekly:	N	%	N	%	N	%
2-3 x (basketball wheelchair, table tennis, bicycling)	10	38.4	2	7.7	12	46.15
4-5 x (archery, shooting)	1	3.8	5	19.2	6	23
6-7 x (body building)	1	3.8	-	-	1	3.8
8-12 x (athletics)	7	26.9	-	-	7	26.9
Total	19	72.98	7	26.92	26	100
Years of training:	M	9.25	M	9.92	M	9.42
	SD	5.04	SD	3.06	SD	4.54
	min	2	min	5	min	2
	max	20	max	15	max	20

In relation to sport training (Table 6) the highest percentage of male participants trained basketball in a wheelchair (34.61%), and the highest percentage of female participants trained archery (11.54%). Other sports are athletics, cycling, archery, table tennis and body building.

From Table 7 shows that the largest number of participants, a total of 12 (46.15%), train 2-3 times a week, 7 (26.9%) participants train 8-12 times a week, 6 (23.1%) participants train 4-5 times a week and 1 participant trains 6-7 times a week. The average number of years of training for all participants group E was 9.42±4.54 years, and for males was 9.26±5.04 years, and for females was 9.92±3.06 years.

The following tables show the results of descriptive statistics in relation to motor abilities.

Table 8. Results of basic descriptive statistics variables maximal muscle hand grip force participants of both gender in E and C groups

| | E group-athletes | | | |
| | Male | | Female | |
	$F_{max}L$ (daN)	$F_{max}R$ (daN)	$F_{max}L$ (daN)	$F_{max}R$ (daN)
M	58.92	59.46	41.62	43.21
SD	9.81	10.04	6.2	8.13
cV%	16.65	16.89	14.9	18.82
Min	39.6	31.6	32.4	32.2
Max	74.6	76.5	51.21	54.22
C group-non-athletes				
M	43.55	47.7	33.3	34.27
SD	8.5	7.7	1.23	0.82
cV%	19.5	16.15	3.68	2.4
Min	25.8	28.4	32.2	33.2
Max	63.7	63.9	35.3	35.3

Table 9. Results of basic descriptive statistics variables of flexibility of shoulders for participants in E and C groups in relation to gender

| | E group-athletes | | | | C group-non-athletes | | | |
| | Male | | Female | | Male | | Female | |
	SF_{abs} (cm)	SF_{rel}	SF_{abs} (cm)	SF_{rel}	SF_{abs} (cm)	SF_{rel}	SF_{abs} (cm)	SF_{rel}
M	111.44	2.37	104	2.54	122.58	2.6	104.62	2.64
SD	13.57	0.29	7.77	0.14	12.96	0.31	5.04	0.06
cV%	12.18	12.36	7.47	5.69	10.58	12.07	4.82	2.12
Min	96	2.05	94	2.35	106	2.08	98	2.55
Max	145	3.02	117	2.72	150	3.4	110	2.69

This table shows that the maximal muscle hand grip force of the dominant hand (right) for male athletes was 59.46 ± 4.10 daN and female athletes was 43.21 ± 8.13 daN, while for the non-athletes was 47.7 ± 7.7 daN for male, and 34.27 ± 0.82 daN female participants. Table 9 shows the absolute and relative values of flexibility of shoulder E and C groups. The absolute value of flexibility of shoulders for participants E group males was 111.44 ± 13.57 cm and for female was 104 ± 7.77 cm, and for group C males was 122.58 ± 12.96 cm and females was 104.62 ± 5.04 cm.

The average speed of reaction for male athletes for left hand was 4.59 ± 1.72 cm and for right hand was 2.89±1.42 cm, and the female for left hand was 3.6 ± 0.45 cm and for right hand was 2.87 ± 1.04 cm. The average speed of reaction of male non-athletes was 7.54 ± 1.41 cm (left hand) and 5.92±1.86 cm (right hand) and for female non-athletes was 8.82 ± 0.77 cm (left arm) and 7.6 ± 0.67 cm (right hand) (Table 10).

Table 11 presents the results obtained from the value of the hand tapping test in relation to the left and right hand, and in relation to gender and affiliation E and C group.

Table 10. Results of basic descriptive statistics variables of speed of reaction for participants in E and C groups in relation to gender

| | E group - athletes C group - non-athletes | | | | | | | |
| | Male | | Female | | Male | | Female | |
	SR_L (cm)	SR_R (cm)	SR_L (cm)	SR_R (cm)	SR_L (cm)	SR_R (cm)	SR_L (cm)	SR_R (cm)
M	4.59	2.89	3.60	2.87	7.54	5.92	8.82	7.60
SD	1.72	1.42	0.45	1.04	1.41	1.86	0.77	0.67
cV%	37.45	49.23	12.42	36.4	18.7	31.37	8.72	8.87
Min	1.5	1	3	1	5	2.6	8	6.9
Max	7.1	6	4	4	9.1	8.5	10	8.5

Table 11. Results of basic descriptive statistics of variables of hand tapping in participants in E and C groups in relation to gender

| | E group - athletes C group - non-athletes | | | | | | | |
| | Male | | Female | | Male | | Female | |
	HT_L	HT_R	HT_L	HT_R	HT_L	HT_R	HT_L	HT_R
M	15.3	15.1	17	18.4	14.2	12.7	13.7	13.3
SD	2.1	2.9	1.2	1.2	2.1	2.2	1.9	1.8
cV%	14	19.3	6.5	6.3	15.2	16.9	13.9	13.5
Min	12	10	16	16	11	9	11	11
Max	19	19	20	20	19	17	16	16

Table 12. Results of basic descriptive statistics variable precision - Darts in participants in E and C groups in relation to gender

| | E group - athletes C group - non-athletes | | | | | | | |
| | Male | | Female | | Male | | Female | |
	D_L	D_D	D_L	D_D	D_L	D_D	D_L	D_D
M	4.28	7.28	4.93	6.93	4.07	6.53	3.32	4.17
SD	1.61	1.28	1.53	2.05	0.98	1.44	0.19	1.02
cV%	37.54	17.65	30.93	29.54	24.20	22.12	5.77	24.56
Min	1.2	3.4	1.6	2.4	3	4.4	3.1	3.1
Max	6.8	9	6.2	8.2	5.8	8.6	3.6	5.2

Results of descriptive statistics for E and C group test darts are shown in Table 12. The average value of the participant E group was for males 4.28 ± 1.61 (left hand) and 7.28±1.28 (right hand) and for females 4.93 ± 1.53 (left arm) and 6.93±2.05 (right hand), while in C groups for males was 4.07 ± 0.98 (left hand) and 6.53 ± 1.44 (right hand), and for females was 3.32 ± 0.19 (left hand) and 4.17 ± 1.02 (right hand).

Table 13. Results of the MANOVA examined variables for male participants in relation to affiliation to E (athletes) and C (non-athletes) group

athletes/ non-athletes	Type III Sum of Squares	df	Mean Square	F	Sig.
Male					
F_{max}SUM	5574.873	1	5574.873	18.065	0.000
SF_{aps}	957.703	1	957.703	5.387	0.027
SF_{rel}	0.427	1	0.427	4.696	0.038
SR_{SUM}	276.333	1	276.333	34.145	0.000
HT_M	28.917	1	28.917	5.576	0.025
D_{SUM}	7.048	1	7.048	1.344	0.255

Table 13 shows the results of the MANOVA examined variables, the partial basis for male participants in relation to affiliation E and C group. Participants male athletes and non-athletes were statistically significant differences in favor of male athletes, compared to the values of the maximum hand grip force (p = 0.000), flexibility of shoulders - absolute and relative value (SF_{abs}, p = 0.027, SF_{rel}, p = 0.038), speed of reaction (SR_{SUM}, p = 0.000) and hand tapping (HT_M; p = 0.025). The participants from both groups of male were not statistically significantly different in relation to the accuracy (precision in target - Darts-D_{SUM}).

Female participants in E and K groups differed significantly in favor of the athletes, compared to the values of the maximum hand grip force (p = 0.023), speed of reaction (p = 0.000), hand tapping (p = 0.000) and the precision (p=0.026). In statistic they did not differ in relation to flexibility of shoulders-absolute and relative value (Table 14).

Table 14. Results of the MANOVA examined variables for the participants of the female gender in relation to affiliation to E (athletes) and C (non-athletes) group

athletes/ non-athletes	Type III Sum of Squares	df	Mean Square	F	Sig.
Female					
F_{max}SUM	868.729	1	868.729	7.134	0.023
SF_{aps}	1.139	1	1.139	0.025	0.879
SF_{rel}	0.029	1	0.029	2.129	0.175
SR_{SUM}	289.241	1	289.241	281.889	0.000
HT_M	69.732	1	69.732	37.276	0.000
D_{SUM}	55.614	1	55.614	6.789	0.026

DISCUSSION

Within the total sample - 44 participants, 72.73% were male and 27.27% were female. This proportion of participants is in line with the existing data from the National Statistics Centre - NSCISC published in 2012, as well as comprehensive research Tasiemski and Brewer (2011) which states that men more often than women experience a SCI, in fact even 80.6% of the total number of persons with SCI are men.

Our participants have SCI in the thoracic (56.82%) or lumbar region (43.18%). In order to obtain valid research, experimental and control groups had to be equal in relation to the ASIA scale (Waring et al., 2010; Kirshblum et al., 2011). The largest number of participants had a complete spinal cord injury (61.36%), while15.91% had incomplete spinal cord injury ASIA B and 22.73% were ASIA C patients (Table 2). The chi-square test indicates that the groups are equal in relation to the level of injuries/spinal cord lesions ($\chi^2 = 2.27$, p = 0.132).

The largest percentage of athletes has played basketball in a wheelchair (34.61%), this is followed by athletics (26.92%), shooting (11.54%), archery (11.54%), table tennis (7.69%), cycling (3.85%) and body building (3.85%) (Table 6). The average number of years of training for male participants was 9.25 ± 5.04 years and for female participant was 9.92 ± 3.06 years, while the largest percentage of participants practiced 2-3 times a week (46.15%), 8-12 times a week (26.9%), 4-5 times a week (23.1%) and 6-7 times a week (3.8%) (Table 7).

Motor abilities are defined as indicators of the level of development of basic movement dimension of man. Zaciorsky (1975) singled out seven basic characteristics of athletes, such as strength, speed, endurance, coordination, balance, precision and flexibility, and in this study the focus in on the impact of sports for people with SCI on the strength, speed, flexibility and precision. In studies in the general population, especially among athletes, the measurement of muscular force dynamometry method is applied, in isometric conditions, in the field of analytics and diagnostics physical abilities (Dopsaj et al., 2009a; Dopsaj et al., 2010; Eminović et al., 2011a; Kljajić et al., 2012). Dynamometric method of testing muscle strength is applied in people with SCI to test postural muscle strength (Larson et al., 2010), as well as a loss of prevention and measure for monitoring and improving muscle strength in the upper extremities (Sisto and Dyson Hudson, 2007). Reduced working capacity and low muscle mass of the upper extremities increases physical exertion during activities of daily living, causing fatigue, discomfort and possible injury to the upper extremity (Hjeltnes and Janssen, 1990; Sie et al., 1992; Janssen et al., 1996). This situation in people with SCI is getting worse over time during the aging process, because physical capacity decreases significantly both in people with disabilities and in people without disabilities (Sawka et al., 1981). Reduced muscle strength in persons with SCI limits functional ability of performing activities of daily life, especially in people with a higher level of the lesion (Marciello et al., 1995). In relation to the maximum muscle hand grip force (F_{max}), our male participants - athletes had an average value of 58.92 ± 9.81 daN (left hand) and 59.46 ± 10.04 daN (right hand) and non-athletes 43.55 ± 8.5 daN (left arm) and 47.7 ± 7.7 daN (right hand). If we compare this with previously published results (Kljajić et al., 2012) with the participant who did not systematically practiced sport, we see that our participants with paraplegia – male non- athletes had lower levels of maximal hand grip force to 33.54% for the left hand and 30.4% for the right hand. Compared to top athletes who participated in the research group of authors (Ivanović et al., 2009), and whose maximum grip force of the left and right hand was 591.06 ± 118.91 N and 632 ± 125.67 N, our participants - athletes were weaker, only 2.92% for the left hand and 8.38% for the right hand. The female participants with SCI - paraplegia, who were not involved in sports, had a maximum hand grip force for the left and right hand 33.3 ± 1.23 daN and 34.27±0.82 daN, and participants who played sports 43.21 ± 6.2 daN and 43.21±8.13 daN for left and right hand. When we compare these values with the defined standards of motor abilities of healthy and trained young persons (Dopsaj et al., 2010b) our female participants (non-athletes) belong to a group that is developing the "average," i.e., "below average" (left/right hand) for maximum strength, while participants athletes belong to the group that develops a maximum power as a "great power," i.e., force "above average" (left/right arm). When comparing the values obtained from participants in E and C groups, we see that the results show a significantly higher maximum power grip force of the left and right hand both compared to male participants (p = 0.000) and compared to those of female (p = 0.023) (Tables 13 and 14). These data suggest that the use of sports activities significantly influenced the increase in maximum output force in our participants. Similar information can also be found in other studies, where the authors state that the application of mixed exercise program (exercise of power, aerobic exercises and exercises to increase mobility) significantly increases maximum power output after 16 weeks of resistance training (Durán et al., 2001), as well and after 3, 6 and 9 months of training (which is applied 2 times per week) (Hicks et al., 2003). Other authors who studied the effects of using hand ergo meter in the research, got the results that during the rehabilitation the maximum output strength of its application is increased (Hicks et al., 2003), as well as after 6-8 weeks of training after rehabilitation, regardless of the intensity of training (de Groot et al., 2003, Sutbeyaz et al., 2005).

Female athletes compared to those of female non-athletes had significantly higher maximum output force (F_{max}) (p = 0.023). This result can also explain the kind of sport that the participants train, approximately in average 9.92 ± 3.06 years, usually 4-5 hours per week (Table 7), such as table tennis, shooting, archery. These results can be linked to the fact that training improves the efficiency of the realization of the potential of the muscle, which is obvious in maximal muscles contraction. A trained person is able to recruit the entire motor units, while a not trained person is not. Direct indication of the general (aerobic) endurance is the maximum oxygen consumption that the participant accomplishes with his work of maximum possible intensity for one minute; and different kinds of sports activities have a different oxygen consumption over a certain age (Kukolj, 2006; Kenney et al., 2011).

In order to examine the impact of sports activity on motor abilities – flexibility of shoulders, we applied the test of "The stick turn," as described above. This test is, in our participants, performed in a sitting position in a wheelchair. The test results are shown in Table 9, and the absolute values show that female participants had greater mobility of the shoulder compared to male participants for 12.17%. Other studies also show that females with SCI have a greater range of motion (ROM) of the shoulder in comparison to the males with SCI (Wessels et al., 2013). This result was expected, since there is evidence that women have greater flexibility in relation to men. Furthermore, as well as women achieve the same effect with 10-15% lesser volume of effort (Kukolj, 2006). However, the involvement in sports activities did not significantly contribute to improving the flexibility of shoulders in female participants (p = 0.879 for absolute and p = 0.175 for the relative value). Based on these, it can be concluded that the type of sports (table tennis, archery and shooting) female athletes were involved in, did not significantly affect this motor ability. Uniformity of this motor ability between the female participants can be justified and by possible greater involvement of non-athletes in terms of daily activities - performance with a wheelchair, or that they do self-applied stretching exercises, because it is known that activity in conditions of maximum range of motion in the joints resulting in flexibility (Kukolj, 2006). Unlike the female participants, the male athletes had significantly better mobility of the shoulders (and in relation to the absolute and relative to relative values) compared to those in non-athletes (SF_{abs}, p = 0.025 and SF_{rel}, p = 0.038). Furthermore, this means that the involvement in sports of 84.21% of male participants who practiced athletics and basketball had significant increase in the level of specified motor abilities.

To test the motor abilities relate to speed, we applied the test participants in terms of speed of reaction and frequency of movement (hand tapping). This indicates the frequency of movement per time unit and includes the ability to quickly switch-on and switch-off antagonistic muscle groups (Tables 10 and 11). Participants in E groups in both tests were significantly more successful than in group C, and in relation to the male gender (p = 0.000 and p = 0.025) and in relation to the female gender (p = 0.000 and p = 0.000) (Table 13 and 14). This means that the involvement in sports activities significantly contributed to improvement of motor abilities. Besides, applied training in participants athletes included a component of application of maximum effort in conditions of a small external resistance. This resulted in an increase in motor abilities-speed, as shown in other studies (Rahimi et al., 2006).

Precision was tested by shooting darts at the target, and the results indicate that the male participants were equal. This was calculated by the multivariate analysis of variance (Table 13 and Table 14; p = 0.255). In relation to the tested sample in our study, the involvement in sports activities such as of wheelchair basketball and athletics in the majority of participants did not contribute to improvement of precision. However, female athletes participants were significantly more successful on this test than the non-athletes participants (p = 0.026), indicating that the use of sports activities such as table tennis, shooting and archery in female participants significantly contributed to improving the precision. Since the high-precision is genetically determined ability, it still may be affected, as shown by other studies (de Oliveira et al., 2008; Menez et al., 2009).

Researching the problem of motor abilities was extremely complicated by the fact that the efficiency of humans, based on body activities actually result in total capacity and characteristics of man's biological and psycho-social agenda, as well as the specific features of certain activities. Therefore, some sports results in different disciplines may be explained by the participation of motor abilities in the range of 35-70% (Kukolj, 2006).

CONCLUSION

In terms of motor abilities the male athlete participants were more successful than male non-athletes participants in comparison to maximum muscle hand grip force of left and right hand, flexibility of shoulders, speed of reaction and hand tapping. Female athletes participants were more successful than female non-athletes participants in comparison to maximal muscle hand grip force of left and right hand, speed reaction, frequency of movement (hand tapping), and precision. Male participants in E and C groups were not statistically different in the precision. Female participants were not different in flexibility of shoulders (absolute and relative). Based on these results we can conclude that sporting activities, which are applied minimum 2-3 times a week, contribute to improvement of level of motor abilities in relation both to male and female gender.

Complexity of disability that carries spinal cord on one hand and positive effects of sport application on the other hand is the topic of modern research in order to improve and advance health and social integration. Organization and implementation of sport activities in persons with SCI-paraplegia, whether it is a recreational or systematically enforced by training, should be supervised by a multi-disciplinary team of experts: doctors, physical therapists, special education teachers, coaches, and others.

Limitations

Influence of sports activities on motor skills of people with SCI is a very important issue, because it provides insight in positive effects of sport on functioning and physical condition. The study limitations primarily relate to the information that the participants filled in a questionnaire themselves. This can be a subject to non objective evaluation of situation or bias (concerning the type of training, frequency and pauses in training). Furthermore, the limit of the study might be relatively small number of participants who took part in the survey, as well as the individual characteristics among them which were not unified. Future research should include a larger number of participants of both genders.

ACKNOWLEDGMENTS

This study was a part of the program projects funded by the Ministry of Science and Technology Development of the Republic of Serbia (No. III47015, 2011-2014).

REFERENCES

Adamović, M., Eminović, F., Mentus, T. and Stošljević, M. (2014). *Determining functional abilities of lower extremities in elderly as a predictor of falls in relation to the expected norms.* In M., Kulić et al. (eds.), International thematic collection "Education and rehabilitation of adult persons with disabilities." (pp. 75-86). Belgrade: University of East Sarajevo, Faculty of Medicine, Foča; University of Belgrade, Faculty of Special Education and Rehabilitation.

Anneken, V., Hanssen Doose, A., Hirschfeld, S., Scheuer, T. and Thietje, R. (2010). Influence of physical exercise on quality of life in individuals with spinal cord injury. *Spinal Cord, 48,* 393–399.

Arsić, S., Eminović, F., Konstantinović, L. J., Pavlović, D., Kljajić, D. and Despotović, M., (2015). Correlation of functional independence and quality of executive functions in patients after a stroke. *Turkish Journal of Physical Medicine and Rehabilitation*, (in Press), DOI: 10.5152/tftrd.2015.25932.ISSN 1302-0234.

Arsić S., Eminović, F., Konstantinović, LJ., Pavlović, D., Popović, M. and Arsić, V. (2014). Interaction of the ability of planned behavior and motor functioning of patients after stroke. *International Journal of Sciences: Basic and Applied Research, 14*(1), 519-529.

Arsić, S., Konstantinović, LJ., Eminović, F., Pavlović, D., Popovic, M. and Arsic, V. (2015). Correlation between the quality of attention and cognitive competence with motor action in stroke patients. *BioMed Research International,* Article ID 823136, DOI:10.1155/2015/823136. ISSN 2314-6141.

Arsić, S., Eminović, F., Stanković, I., Janković, S. and Despotović, M. (2012). The role of executive functions at dyscalculia. *HealthMed Journal, 6*(1), 314-319.

Bernardi, M., Guerra, E., Di Giacinto, B., Di Cesare, A., Castellano, V. and Bhambhani, Y. (2010). Field evaluation of paralympic athletes in selected sports: implications for training. *Medicine and Science in Sports and Exercise, 42*(6), 1200–1208.

Bizzarini, E., Saccavini, M., Lipanje, F., Magrin, P., Malisan, C. and Zampa, A. (2005). Exercise prescription in subjects with spinal cord injuries. *Archives of Physical Medicine and Rehabilitation*, *86*, 1170–1175.

Bhambhani, Y. (2002). Physiology of wheelchair racing in athletes with spinal cord injury. *Sports Medicine*, *32*, 23–52.

Bryce, T. (2009). *Rehabilitation Medicine Quick Reference: Spinal Cord Injury*. New York: Demos Medical Publishing.

Byrnes, M., Beilby, J., Ray, P., McLennan, R., Ker, J. and Schug, S. (2012). Patient-focused goal planning process and outcome after spinal cord injury rehabilitation: Quantitative and qualitative audit. *Clinical Rehabilitation*, *26*(12), 1141–1149.

Cohen, J. T., Marino, R. J., Sacco, P. and Terrin, N. (2012). Association between the Functional Independence Measure following spinal cord injury and long-term outcomes. *Spinal Cord*, *50*(10), 728-733.

Cohen, C. B. and Napolitano, D. (2007). Adjustment to disability. *Journal of Social Work in Disability and Rehabilitation*, *6*, 135–155.

Cripps, R. A., Lee, B. B., Wing, P., Weerts, E., Mackay, J. and Brown, D. (2011). A global map for traumatic spinal cord injury epidemiology: towards a living data repository for injury prevention. *Spinal Cord*, *49*(4), 493–501.

Davis, G.M. and Shepherd, R.J. (1988). Cardiorespiratory fitness in highly active versus inactive paraplegics. *Medicine and Science in Sports and Exercise*, *20*, 463-468.

DeGroot, S., Post, M.W., Postma, K., Sluis, T.A. and van der Woude, L.H. (2010). Prospective analysis of body mass index during and up to 5 years after discharge from inpatient spinal cord injury rehabilitation. *Journal of Rehabilitation Medicine*, *42*, 922-928.

De Oliveira, R. F., Oudejans, R.R.D. and Beek, P.J. (2008). Gaze behavior in basketball shooting: further evidence for online visual control. *Research quarterly for exercise and sport*, *79*(3), 399-404.

Ditor, D. S., Latimer, A. E., Ginis, K. A., Arbour, K. P., McCartney, N. and Hicks, A. L. (2003). Maintenance of exercise participation in individuals with spinal cord injury: effects on quality of life, stress and pain. *Spinal* Cord, *41*, 446-450.

Dopsaj, M., Ilić, V., Đorđević-Nikić, M.,Vuković, M., Eminović, F., Macura, M. and Ilić, D., (2015). Descriptive model and gender dimorphism of body structure of phisically active students of Belgrade university: Pilot study. *The Antropologist*, *19*(1), 239-248.

Dopsaj, M., Ivanović, J., Blagojević, M., Koropanovski, N., Vučković, G., Janković, R., Marinković, B., Atanasov, D. and Miljuš, D. (2009a). Basic and specific characteristics of the hand grip explosive force and time parameters in different strength traine population. *Brazilian Journal of Biomotricity*, *3*(2), 177-193.

Dopsaj, M., Kljajić, D., Eminović, F., Đorđević Nikić, M. and Ilić, V. (2013). Bioimpedance body structure reliability measured in different stature position. *Technics Technologies Education Management*, *8*(3), 1448-1455.

Dopsaj, M., Kljajić, D., Eminović, F., Koropanovski, N., Dimitrijević, R. and Stojković, I. (2011). Model indicators of muscle force characteristics in young and healthy persons while performing motor task- hand grip: pilot research. *Special Education and Rehabilitation*, 10(1), 15-36.

Dopsaj, M., Nešić, G. and Ćopić, N. (2010). The multicentroid position of the anthropomorphological profile of female volleyball players at different competitive levels. *Facta universitatis - series: Physical Education and Sport, 8*(1), 47-57.

Dopsaj, M., Nešić, G., Koropanovski, N. and Simikić, M. (2009b). The anthropo-morphological profile of female police students and differently trained athletes: A multicetroid model. *NBPJournal of Criminalistics and Law, 14*(1),145-160.

Dopsaj, M., Vučković, G., Milojković, B., Subošić, D., Eminović, F. and Kekovic, D. (2012). Hand grip scaling in defining risk factors when using authorized physical force. *Facta universitatis - series: Physical Education and Sport, 10*(3), 169-181.

Dorsett, P., Geraghty, T. (2008). Health-related outcomes of people with spinal cord injury - a 10 year longitudinal study. *Spinal Cord, 46*, 386-391.

Dowling, S., McConkey, R., Hass, D., Menke, S., Eminović, F.,Wilski, M., Nadolska, A., Kogut, I., Goncharenko, E., Pochstein, F., Bethge, M., Viranyi, A., Regenyi, E., Felegyhazi, J. and Pasztor, S., (2010). *Unified gives us a chance- Anevaluation of Special Olympics Youth Unified Sports® Programme in Europe/Eurasia,* Belfast: University of Ulster, Special Olympics, (pp. 96). On line: http://www.science.ulster.ac.uk/unifiedsportsunder 'Unified Gives Us a Chance' - Unified Sport - Final Report Sept 2010.pdf.

Duff, J., Evans, M. J. and Kennedy, P. (2004). Goal planning: a retrospective audit of rehabilitation process and outcome. *Clinical Rehabilitation, 18*, 275–286.

D'Hondt, F. and Everaert, K. (2011). Urinary trac infection in patient with spinal cord injuries. *Current Infectious Disease Reports, 13*, 544-551.

Durán, F. S., Lugo, L., Ramirez, L. and Eusse, E. (2001). Effects of an exercise program on the rehabilitation of patients with spinal cord injury. *Archives of Physical Medicine and Rehabilitation, 82,* 1349-1354.

Elfström, M. L., Kreuter, M., Persson, L. O. and Sullivan, M. (2005). General and condition-specific measures of coping strategies in persons with spinal cord lesion. *Psychology, Health and Medicine, 10*, 231-242.

Eminović, F. (2014). *Motor learning and exercise adaptations for athletes with intelectual disabilities.* In: D. Hassan, et al., (eds.). Sport, coaching and intellectual disability, (pp 195-210). London: Routledge.

Eminović, F. and Arsić, S., (2014). Corelation between executive and motor function in patients after a stroke. In: K. Bennett (Ed.). Executive Functioning Role in Early Learning Processes, Impairments in Neurological Disorders and Impact of Cognitive Behavior Therapy (CTB), (pp. 323-358). NewYork: Nova Publishers.

Eminović, F., Čanović, D. and Nikić, R. (2011b). Physical education 1 - Physical education of children with disabilities - scientific monographs. Belgrade: Faculty for Special Education and Rehabilitation.

Eminović, F. and Dimoski, S., (2015). *Handbook of hearing disorders research,* In. C. H. Atkinson (Ed.). Conduct disorders in children and youth with hearing impairment, (pp. 131-155). NewYork: Nova Publishers.

Eminović, F., Kljajić, D., Koropanovski, N., Dimitrijević, R., Dimoski, S. and Dopsaj, M. (2011a). Sex dimorphism of hand grip endurance in healthy and young persons. *Acta Kinesiologica, 5*(2), 53-57.

Figoni, S.F. (2002). Spinal cord injury. In: Durstine, J.L. (Ed.). *ACSM's exercise management for persons with chronic diseases and disabilities*. Champaign, IL: Human Kinetics.

Frankel, H. L., Hancock, D. O., Hyslop, G., Melzak, J., Michaelis, L.S., Ungar, G. H., Vernon, J.D. and Walsh, J.J. (1969). The value of postural reduction in the initial management of closed injuries of the spine with paraplegia and tetraplegia. *Paraplegia*, *7*(3), 179–192.

Frey, G. C., McCubbin, J. A., Dunn, J. M. and Mazzeo, R. (1997). Plasma catecholamin and lactate relationship during graded exercise in men with spinal cord injury. *Medicine and Science in Sports and Exercise*, *29*, 451–456.

Garshick, E., Kelley, A., Cohen, S.A., Garrison, A., Tun, C.G., Gagnon, D. and Brown, R. (2005). A prospective assessment of mortality in chronic spinal cord injury. *Spinal Cord*, 43, 408-416.

Gassaway, J., Dijkers, M., Rider, C., Edens, K., Cahow, C. and Joyce, J. (2011). Therapeutic recreation treatment time during inpatient rehabilitation. *Journal of Spinal Cord Medicine*, *34*(2), 176-185.

Geyh, S., Ballert, C., Sinnott, A., Charlifue, S., Catz, A., D'Andrea Greve J. M. and Post M.W.M. (2013). Quality of life after spinal cord injury: a comparison across six countries. *Spinal Cord*, *51*, 322–326.

Haisma, J. A., Bussmann, J.B., Stam, H.J., Sluis, T.A., Bergen, M.P., Dallmeijer, A.J., de Groot, S. and van der Woude, L.H. (2006). Changes in physical capacity during and after inpatient rehabilitation in subjects with a spinal cord injury. *Archives of Physical Medicine and Rehabilitation*, *87,* 741–48.

Hammond, F. M., Gassaway, J., Abeyta, N., Freeman, E.S. and Primack, D. (2011). Social work and case management treatment time during inpatient spinal cord injury rehabilitation. *The Journal of Spinal Cord Medicine*, *34*(2), 216-226.

Heath, G. W. and Fentem, P. H. (1997). Physical activity among persons with disabilities: a public health perspective. *Exercise Sport Science Reviews*, *25*, 195–234.

Hicks, A. L. and Martin Ginis, K. A. (2008). Treadmill training after SCI: it's not just about the walking. *Journal of Rehabilitation Research and Development*, *45*, 241–248.

Hicks, A. L., Martin, K.A., Ditor, D.S., Latimer, A.E., Craven, C., Bugaresti, J. and McCartney, N. (2003). Long-term exercise training in persons with spinal cord injury: effects on strength, arm ergometry performance and psychological well-being. *Spinal Cord*, *41*, 34–43.

Hicks, A. L., Martin Ginis, K. A., Pelletier, C., Ditor, D.S., Foulon, B. and Wolfe, D. (2011). The effects of exercise training on physical capacity, strength, body composition and functional performance among adults with spinal cord injury: A systematic review. *Spinal Cord*, *49,* 1103–1127.

Hjeltnes, N. and Janssen, T. (1990). Physical endurance capacity, functional status, and medical complications in spinal cord injured subjects with long standing lesions. *Paraplegia*, *28,* 428-432.

Huonker, M., Schmid, A., Sorichter, S., Schmidt Trucksab, A., Mrosek, P. and Keul, J. (1998). Cardiovascular differences between sedentary and wheelchair – trained subjects with paraplegia. *Medicine and Science in Sports and Exercise*, *30,* 609–613.

Hutzler, Y., Vanlandewijck, Y. and Vlierberghe, M. (2000). Anaerobic performance of older female and male wheelchair basketball players on a mobile wheelchair ergometer. *Adapted Physical Activity Quarterly*, *17*, 465-478.

Imai, K., Kadowaki, T., Aizawa, Y. (2004). Standardized indices of mortality among persons with spinal cord injury: accelerated aging process. *Industrial Health*, *42*, 213-218.

Ivanović, J., Koropanovski, N., Vučković, G., Janković, R., Miljuš, D., Marinković, B., Atanasov, B., Blagojević, M. and Dopsaj, M. (2009). Functional dimorphism and characteristics considering maximal hand grip force in top level athletes in the Republic of Serbia. *Gazzetta Medica Italiana Archivio per le Scienze Mediche, 168*(5), 297-310.

Jacobs, P. L. and Nash, M. S. (2004). Exercise recommendations for individuals with spinal cord injury. *Sports Medicine, 34,* 727-751.

Jacobs, P. L., Nash, M.S., Klose, J., Guest, R.S., Needham Shropshire, B.M. and Green, B. (1997). Evaluation of a training program for persons with SCI paraplegia using the Parastep - 1 ambulation system: part 2. Effects on physiological responses to peak arm ergometry. *Archives of Physical Medicine and Rehabilitation, 78,* 794-798.

Janssen, T. W., van Oers, C. A., Rozendaal, E.P., Willemsen, E.M., Hollander, A. P. and van der Woude, L.H. (1996). Changes in physical strain and physical capacity in men with spinal cord injuries. *Medicine and Science in Sports and Exercise, 28,* 551-559.

Jensen, M. P., Truitt, A. R., Schomer, K.G., Yorkston, K.M., Baylor, C. and Molton, I.R. (2013). Frequency and age effects of secondary health conditions in individuals with spinal cord injury: a scoping review. *Spinal Cord, 51,* 882–892.

Jones, M. L., Harness, E., Denison, P., Tefertiller, C. and Evans, N. (2012). Activity-based therapies in spinal cord injury: clinical focus and empirical evidence in three independent programs. *Topics in Spinal Cord Injury Rehabilitation, 18*(1), 34–42.

Jovanović, L., Kovačević, R., Ereš, S. and Kljajić, D. (2013). *Basics of kinesiotherapy.* Belgrade: Atosprint.

Jović, S. (2011). *Medical rehabilitation of people with physical disabilities.* Belgrade: Clinic for Rehabilitation "Dr M. Zotović."

Kasum, G., Lazarević, Lj., Jakovljević, S. and Bačanac, Lj. (2011). Personality of Male Wheelchair basketball players and nonathletes persons with disability. *Facta Universitatis, 9*(4), 407 – 415.

Kawanishi, C.Y. and Greguol, M. (2013). Physical activity, quality of life, and functional autonomy of adults with spinal cord injuries. *Adapted Physical Activity Quarterly, 30,* 317-337.

Kenney, W. L., Wilmore, J., Costill, D. (2011). *Physiology of sport and exercise with web study Guide-5th Edition.* Champaign: Human Kinetics.

Kirshblum, S., Burns, S., Biering Sorensen, F., Donovan, W., Graves, D., Jha., A., Johansen, M., Jones, L., Krassioukov, A., Mulcahey, M.J., Schmidt Read, M. and Waring, W. (2011). International standards for neurological classification of spinal cord injury (Revised 2011). *The Journal of Spinal Cord Medicine, 34*(6), 535-546.

Kljajić, D., Dopsaj, M., Eminović, F. and Kasum, G. (2013). Sport in rehabilitation of persons with impairments. Zdravstvena zaštita, *3,* 58-66.

Kljajić, D., Eminović, F., Trgovčević, S., Dimitrijević, R. and Dopsaj, M. (2012). Functional relationship between dominant and non-dominant hand in motor task – hand grip strength endurance. *Special Education and Rehabilitation, 11*(1), 67-85.

Krassioukov, A., Eng, J.J., Claxton, G., Sakakibara, B.M., Shum, S. (2010). Neurogenic bowel management after spinal cord injury: a systematic review of the evidence. *Spinal Cord, 48*(10), 718-33.

Krause, J. S., Kjorsvig, J. M. (1992). Mortality after spinal cord injury: a four year prospective study. *Archives of Physical Medicine and Rehabilitation, 73,* 558-563.

Kukolj, M. (2006). *Antropomotorics.* Belgrade: Faculty of Sport and Physical Education.

Larson, C. A., Tezak, W. D., Malley, M. S. and Thornton, W. (2010). Assessment of postural muscle strength in sitting: reliability of measures obtained with hand-held dynamometry in individuals with spinal cord injury. *Journal of Neurologic Physical Therapy*, *34,* 24-31.

Marciello, M. A., Herbison, G. J., Ditunno, J. F.Jr., Marino, R.J. and Cohen, M.E. (1995). Wrist strength measured by myometry as an indicator of functional independence. *Journal of Neurotrauma*, *12*(1), 99–106.

Martin Ginis, K. A., Latimer, A. E., Arbour Nicitopoulos, K.P., Buchholz, A., Bray, S.R., Craven, B.C., Hayes, K.C., Hicks, A.L., McColl, M.A., Potter, P. J., Smith, K. and Wolfe, D.L. (2010). Leisure-time physical activity in a population-based sample of people with spinal cord injury. Part I: Demographic and injury-related correlates. *Archives of Physical Medicine and Rehabilitation*, *91,* 722–728.

Martin Ginis, K. A., Latimer, A. E., McKecknie, K., Ditor, D.S., McCartney, N., Hicks, A.L., Bugaresti, J. and Craven, B. (2003). Using exercise to enhance subjective well-being among people with spinal cord injury: The mediating influences of stress and pain. *Rehabilitation Psychology*, *48,* 157–164.

McGrath, J.R., Marks, J.A., Davis, A.M. (1995). Towards interdisciplinary rehabilitation: Further developments at Rivermead Rehabilitation Centre. *Clinical Rehabilitation*, *9,* 320–326.

McVeigh, S.A., Hitzig, S.L. and Craven, B.C. (2009). Influence of sport participation on community integration and quality of life: A comparison between sport participants and non-sport participants with spinal cord injury. *Journal of Spinal Cord Medicine*, *32*(2), 115–124.

Menez, L., Dantas, P. and Filh, JF. (2009). Rhythmic gymnastics on different levels of qualification. *Medicine and Science in Sports and Exercise*, *41*(5), 310.

Milićević, S., Bukumirić, Z., Karadžov Nikolić, A., Babović, R. and Janković S. (2012a). Demographic characteristics and functional outcomes in patients with traumatic and nontraumatic spinal cord injuries. *Vojnosanitetski pregled*, *69*(12), 1061-1066.

Milićević, S., Bukumirić, Z., Karadžov Nikolić, A., Sekulić, A., Stevanović, S. and Janković, S. (2012c). Secondary complications and associated injuries in traumatic and non traumatic spinal cord injury patients. *Serbian Journal of Experimental and Clinical Research*, *13*(1), 15-18.

Muraki, S., Tsunawake, N., Hiramatsu, S. and Yamasaki, M. (2000б). The effect of frequency and mode of sports activity on the psychological status in tetraplegics and paraplegics. *Spinal Cord*, *38,* 309–314.

Muraki, S., Tsunawake, N., Tahara, Y., Hiramatsu, S. and Yamasaki, M. (2000a). Multivariate analysis of factors influencing physical work capacity in wheelchair-dependent paraplegics with spinal cord injury. *European Journal of Applied Physiology*, *81,* 28-32.

Myslinski, M. J. (2005). Evidence-based exercise prescription for individuals with spinal cord injury. *Journal of Neurological Physical Therapy*, *29*(2), 104-106.

Nash, M. S. (2005). Exercise as a health-promoting activity following spinal cord injury. *Journal of Neurological Physical Therapy*, 29: 87-106.

Nash, M. S., Jacobs, P.L., Mendez, A.J. and Goldberg, R.B. (2001). Circuit resistance training improves the atherogenic lipid profiles of persons with chronic paraplegia. *Journal of Spinal Cord Medicine*, *24,* 2–9.

Nash, M.S., Mendez, A.J. (2009). Nonfasting lipemia and inflammation as cardiovascular disease risks after SCI. *Topics in Spinal Cord Injury Rehabilitation*, *14*(3), 15–31.

National Spinal Cord Injury Statistical Centar, Birmingham, Alabama, USA. (2013). Available at: www.nscisc.uab.edu (accessed June 2013).

New, P. W., Cripps, R.A., Bonne Lee, B. (2014). Global maps of non-traumatic spinal cord injury epidemiology: towards a living data repository. *Spinal Cord*, 52: 97–109.

Noreau, L., Shephard, R.J. (1995). Spinal cord injury, exercise and quality of life. *Sports Medicine*, *20*, 226–250.

Official website of the Paralympic Movement (2015). Available at: www.paralympic.org (accessed June 2015)

Oja, P., Tuxworth, B. (1995). *Eurofit for adults: Assessment of health-related fitness.* Tampere, Finland: Council of Europe, Committee for the Development of Sport.

Omorou, Y. A., Erpelding, M. L., Escalon, H. and Vuillemin, A. (2013). Contribution of taking part in sport to the association between physical activity and quality of life. *Quality of Life Research*, *22*, 2021–2029.

Orbell, S., Johnston, M., Rowley, D., Davey, P. and Espley, A. (2001). Self-efficacy and goal importance in the prediction of physical disability in people following hospitalisation: a prospective study. *British Journal of Health Psychology*, *6*, 25–40.

Osterthun, R., Post, M.W., van Asbeck, F.W. (2009). Characteristics, length of stay and functional outcome of patients with spinal cord injury in Dutch and Flemish rehabilitation centres. *Spinal Cord*, *47*(4), 339-344.

Otašević, J., Kljajić, D. (2013). *People with disabilities and their rights in sport. Legal Life, thematic issue of "Rights and dignity,"* Belgrade Association of Serbia, tom 1, *9*, 633-645.

Price, M.J., Campbell, I.G. (1999). Thermoregulatory responses of spinal cord injured and able-bodied athletes to prolonged upper body exercise and recovery. *Spinal Cord*, *37*, 772–779.

Rahimi, R., Arshadi, P., Behpur, N., Sadeghi Boroujerdi, S. and Rahimi, M. (2006). Evaluation of plyometrics, weight training and their combination on angular velocity. *Facta Universitatis*, *4*(1), 1-8.

Ravenek, K.E., Ravenek, M.J., Hitzig, S.L. and Wolfe, D.L. (2012). Assessing quality of life in relation to physical activity participation in persons with spinal cord injury: A systematic review. *Disability and Health Journal*, *5*, 213-223.

Rogan, M., Rogan, M. (2010). Britain and the Olympic Games: Past, Present, Legacy. United Kindom: Matador.

Sawka, M.N., Glaser, R.M., Laubach, L.L., Al-Samkari, O. and Suryaprasad, A.G. (1981). Wheelchair exercise performance of the young, middle-aged, and elderly. *Journal of Applied Physiology*, *50*, 824-828.

Sibilio, M. and Aiello, P. (2010). Some basic elements for a possible classification of motor activities. *Acta Kinesiologica*, *4*(2), 13 - 16.

Sie, I.H., Waters, R.L., Adkins, R.H. and Gellman, H. (1992). Upper extremity pain in the postrehabilitation spinal cord injured patient. *Archives of Physical Medicine and Rehabilitation*, *73*(1), 44-48.

Silva, M.C.R., Oliveira, R.J. and Gandolfo Conceicao, M.I. (2005). Effects of swimming on the functional independence of patients with spinal cord injury. *Revista Brasileira de Medicina do Esporte*, *11*(4), 237-241.

Silva, A.C., Neder, J.A., Chiurciu, M.V., Pasqualin, D.C., da Silva, R.C.Q., Fernandez, A.C., Lauro, F.A.A., de Mello, M.T., Tufik, S. (1998). Effect of aerobic training on ventilatory muscle endurance of spinal cord injured men. *Spinal Cord*, *36*, 240-245.

Sisto, C.A., Dyson Hudson, T. (2007). Dynamometry testing in spinal cord injury. *Journal of Rehabilitation Research and Development, 44*(1), 123–136.

Spinal Cord Injury Facts and Figures at a Glance. *Publication of the National Spinal Cord Injury Statistical Center, Birmingham, Alabama.* (2013). Available at: www.nscisc.uab.edu (accccessed April 2013).

Strauss, D., DeVivo, M. J., Shavelle, R. (2000). Long-term mortality risk after spinal cord injury. *Journal of Insurance Medicine, 32,* 11-16.

Sutbeyaz, S.T., Koseoglu, B.F. and Gokkaya, N.K.O. (2005). The combined effects of controlled breathing techniques and ventilatory and upper extremity muscle exercise on cardiopulmonary responses in patients with spinal cord injury. *International Journal of Rehabilitation Research, 28,* 273–276.

Tasiemski, T, Brewer, B.V. (2011). Athletic identity, sport participation, and psychological adjustment in people with spinal cord injury. *Adapted Physical Activity Quarterly, 28,* 233-250.

Tasiemski, T., Kennedy, P., Gardner, B. and Taylor, N. (2005). The association of sports and physical recreation with life satisfaction in a community sample of people with spinal cord injuries. *NeuroRehabilitation, 20*(4), 253–265.

Taylor-Schroeder, S., LaBarbera, J., McDowell, S., Zanca, J.M., Natale, A., Mumma, S., Gassaway, J. and Backus, D. (2011). Physical therapy treatment time during inpatient spinal cord injury rehabilitation. *The Journal of Spinal Cord Medicine, 34*(2), 149-161.

The International Spinal Cord Society. SCI Global Mapping (2013). Available at: http://iscos.org.uk/sci-global-mapping. (accessed May 2013).

Tomasone, J.R., Wesch, N.N., Martin Ginis, K.A. and Noreau, L. (2013). Spinal cord injury, physical activity, and quality of life: a systematic review. *Kinesiology Review, 2,* 113-129.

Tordi, N., Dugue, B., Klupzinski, D., Rasseneur, L., Rouillon, J.D. and Lonsdorfer, J. (2001). Interval training program on a wheelchair ergometer for paraplegic subjects. *Spinal Cord, 39,* 532-537.

Trgovčević S, Kljajić D, Nedović G. (2011). Social integration as a determinant of the quality of life for people with traumatic paraplegia. *Godišnjak političkih nauka, 5*(6), 493-506.

Trgovcević, S., Milićević, M., Nedović, G., Jovanić, G. (2014). Health condition and quality of life in persons with spinal cord injury. *Iranian Journal of Public Health, 43*(9), 1229-1238.

Uzunković, K., Odović, G., Eminovic, F., Nedović, G., (2011). Suitability of sport facilities for persons with disabilities. In: G., Ćirović (Ed.). Sports Facilities-Standardizations and Trends – SPOFA 11. Belgrade: University of Belgrade Faculty of Sport and Physical Education. pp. 43–57.

Van den Berg Emons, R.J., Bussmann, J.B., Haisma, J.A., Sluis, T.A., van der Woude, L.H., Bergen, M.P. et al., (2008). A prospective study on physical activity levels after spinal cord injury during inpatient rehabilitation and the year after discharge. *Archives of Physical Medicine and Rehabilitation, 89,* 2094–2101.

Van Langeveld, S. A, Post, M. W., van Asbeck, F. W., ter Horst, P., Leenders, J., Postma, K., Rijken, H. and Lindeman, E. (2011). Contents of physical therapy, occupational therapy, and sports therapy sessions for patients with a spinal cord injury in three Dutch rehabilitation centres. *Disability and Rehabilitation, 33*(5), 412-422.

Verhaagen, J., McDonald, J. III (2012). Handbook of Clinical Neurology Series: Spinal Cord Injury. Elsevier.

Vissers, M., van den Berg Emons, R., Sluis, T., Bergen, M., Stam, H. and Bussmann, H. (2008). Barriers to and facilitators of everyday physical activity in persons with a spinal cord injury after discharge from the rehabilitation centre. *Journal of Rehabilitation Medicine, 40,* 461-467.

Zaciorsky, V. M. (1975). Physical properties athletes. Belgrade: Partizan NIP.

Waring, W. P., Biering Sorensen F., Burns, S., Donovan, W., Graves, D. Jha. A., Jones, L., Kirshblum, S., Marino, R., Mulcahe, M. J., Reeves, R., Scelza, W., Schmidt Read, M. and Stein, A. (2010). 2009 Review and revisions of the international standards for the neurological classification of spinal cord injury. *Journal of Spinal Cord Medicine, 33*(4), 346-352.

Washburn, R., Hedrick, B. N. (1997). Descriptive epidemiology of physical activity in university graduates with locomotor disabilities. *International Journal of Rehabilitation Research, 20,* 275-287.

World Health Organization. *Global Burden of Disease.* (2011). Available at: www.who.int/topics/global_burden_of_disease/en/ (accessed July 2013).

World Health Organization. *International Classification of Functioning, Disability and Health (ICF)* (2001). Avalible at: http://www.who.int/classifications/icf/en/ (accessed July 2013).

World Health Organization. *World report on disability.* (2011). Available at: www.who.int/disabilities/world_report/2011/en/index.html (accessed July 2013).

Wu, S., Williams, T. (2001). Factors influencing sport participation among athletes with spinal cord injury. *Medicine and Science in Sports and Exercise, 33,* 177–182.

Wyndaele, M., Wyndaele, J. J. (2006). Incidence, prevalence and epidemiology of spinal cord injury: what learns a worldwide literature survey? *Spinal Cord, 44*(9), 523-529.

In: Physical Activity Effects on the Anthropological Status ...   ISBN: 978-1-63484-782-7
Editors: Fadilj Eminović and Milivoj Dopsaj   © 2016 Nova Science Publishers, Inc.

Chapter 8

DESIGNING UNIVERSAL AND ADAPTED LEARNING ENVIRONMENTS FOR INCLUSIVE PHYSICAL EDUCATION AND SPORT PRACTICE

Yeshayahu Hutzler[*]

Academic College at Wingate Institute, Netanya Israel and the Israel Sport Center
for the Disabled, Ramat-Gan, Israel

ABSTRACT

The purpose of this chapter is to describe the theoretical frameworks supporting inclusive physical education and sport. The inclusion of students and athletes with disability is understood in this respect as a human right according to the United Nations' Convention on Rights of Persons with Disability (CRPD). Several theoretical frameworks are presented in this chapter, namely the International Classification of Function and Disability (ICF), Adaptation Theory including Ecological Task Analysis, Universal Design and Universal Design for Learning. These theoretical perspectives are interwoven into a practical concept of providing universal practices for students with and without disabilities as well as individually adapted practices as needed relating to (a) the selection of the task and specific task criteria, (b) the activity and participation environment, (c) the equipment used, (d) the rules of participation, (e) the instructional modalities and (f) the motivational strategies.

Keywords: adaptation, activity, disability, human rights

INTRODUCTION

The United Nations Convention on Rights of Persons with Disability (CRPD) was adopted in 2006 (UN 2006) and has been ratified by over 151 States Parties to date. This is the most influential document recognizing and influencing legislation regarding the rights of

---

[*] E-mail: Shayke.hutzler@gmail.com.

persons with disability worldwide. This convention expands on the right for persons with disabilities to participate in sport, recreation, and leisure, and on the right of children with disabilities to participate in physical education, play, and sport within their community, as well as in unique frameworks, adapted to their needs. While States Parties of the CRPD acknowledge the right to participation of persons with disabilities on an equal basis with their peers without disabilities, restrictions to this participation continue to be the rule rather than the exception in most countries. Persons with disabilities of all ages still experience many barriers in intrapersonal, interpersonal, organizational, and community domains, which impact their participation in physical activity (Vasudevan et al. 2015).

Inclusion vs. Restriction of Physical Activity Opportunities for Persons with Disability

Based on content analysis of focus group sessions conducted in ten regions across the United States in 2001 and 2002, ten themes were identified: (1) barriers and facilitators related to the built and natural environment; (2) economic issues; (3) emotional and psychological barriers; (4) equipment barriers; (5) barriers related to the use and interpretation of guidelines, codes, regulations, and laws; (6) information-related barriers; (7) professional knowledge, education, and training issues; (8) perceptions and attitudes of persons who are not disabled, including professionals; (9) policies and procedures both at the facility and community level; and (10) availability of resources (Rimmer et al. 2004). However, many barrier studies address the lack of motivation or interest as individual barriers (e.g., Buffart et al. 2009). Thus, it appears that in addition to establishing a barrier-free physical environment, the motivational perspectives of physical activity need be explored in persons with disability, and programs need be developed to increase the physical activity opportunities of persons with disabilities across the age span.

Inclusion vs. Restriction in Physical Education

While most scholar agree that integration entails placing students with disabilities together with their peers without a disability at unaltered mainstream educational settings, there is little consensus among education professionals, scholars, and policy makers regarding the process of "inclusion" (Smith and Thomas 2005). While many stakeholders describe inclusion as designing adaptations and providing supports to students with disabilities in order to suit their abilities and enable their participation in educational settings (e.g., Barton 1993), others more radically demand that school culture be addressed and adapted so as to enable students with disability to be fully included (Corbett and Slee 2000). Typical physical activity modalities in this regard include physical education, recess and excursions.

In contrast to classroom teachers, physical education (PE) teachers are often challenged with negotiating large open spaces and using a variety of equipment pieces in dynamic sessions engaging significant numbers of students. Such situations often encounter safety concerns in addition to having to deal with the variability in learning capacity (Morley et al. 2005). In addition, physical educators are engaged in the challenge of developing life-long health-oriented physical activity behavior (Lee et al. 2007). Under such circumstances, including students with disabilities in a general PE setting is often perceived as a challenging and even threatening task for physical educators. For example, Fejgin et al. (2005) found that among 363 Israeli PE teachers, burnout significantly correlated with the number of students with "behavior problems" included in their classes, as well as with lack of social support. In addition, it was found in this study that in contrast to students with learning and behavior problems, where the majority of teachers reported them to be included to a great or very great extent, the majority of the PE teachers reported that children with sensory or motor impairments were not at all included or only included to some extent. One major reason for PE teachers' relationship between lack of social support and burnout could be their perception of the inappropriate amount of training, knowledge, and skill needed in coping with students with disability within an inclusive setting. Indeed, a significant number of studies, mostly from the United States, have emphasized that PE teachers are not competent enough to provide an educational curriculum that complies with the inclusion principle (e.g., Ammah and Hodge 2006; Hardin 2005; Hodge 1998; Hodge et al. 2009; Kowalski and Rizzo 1996; LaMaster et al. 1998; Lienert et al. 2001). The very recent establishment of the *UNICEF Physical Activity and Sport Task Force (2015) intends to promote mechanisms for cooperation and collaboration to enhance policies and programs that promote the right for children with disabilities to inclusive physical activity, PE, sport, recreation, and play in line with the CRPD* (Physical Activity and Sport Task Force 2015). In this line, Blauwet and Lezzoni (2014) describe a post-2015 development agenda and development goals, including policy recommendations and indicators for achieving inclusion targets by 2030, such as the number of recreational facilities accessible to everyone, including children and adults with disabilities.

Adaptation in Physical Activity

Adaptation can be described as a mode of coping with competition or environmental conditions on an evolutionary time scale (Darwin 1859). Adaptation was first used in the 1950s, in the context of designing physical activity opportunities for students with disabilities (Sherrill 2004). Following the foundation of the International Federation of Adapted Physical Activity (IFAPA) in the mid-1970s by Simard, De-Potter, and their associates (Reid, in press), adaptation became the key attribute of the professional and scholarly discussion on how to provide and facilitate physical activity participation in persons with disability, including children, and an international scholarly journal, the *Adapted Physical Activity Quarterly*, was established in 1984. According to Sherrill (2004), the first systematic attempt to define adapted physical activity in English occurred at the 7th International Symposium on Adapted Physical Activity (ISAPA), held by the IFAPA in Berlin in June 1989. The resulting definition was "Adapted physical activity refers to movement, physical activity, and sports in which special emphasis is placed on the interests and capabilities of individual with limiting conditions, such as the disabled, health impaired, or aged" (Doll-Tepper et al. 1990, p. v.). This definition, which refers to the service delivery/empowerment aspect of adapted physical activity (APA), clearly applies – in addition to those with disabilities – to very young or marginalized populations such as those with cultural-limiting conditions (for example: the requirement for orthodox Moslem or Jewish females to wear long-sleeved clothing. Thus, the adaptation framework was conceptualized into a theory (Sherrill 1995; 2004) suggesting a philosophy, concepts, and strategies applicable not only to physical activity adaptations required for performing under disability conditions, but also to age, gender, and other heterogeneity-related adaptation principles. This conceptual framework was soon transformed into practical models, such as the Australian TREE model referring to adapting a Teaching/coaching style; Rules and regulations; Equipment; and Environments, while including participants with a disability (Australian Sport Commission, n. d.), or the FAMME model, referring to a Functional Approach for Modifying Movement Experiences (Kasser and Lytle 2005).

The ecological system view of person and environment, and a task dynamically evolving out of the interaction between these systems, was suggested within the APA scholarly theory development already by the early 1990s.

Now we realize that it is unjust to assess only the individual with a disability. We must assess his or her environment, or ecosystem, and identify the attitudinal, aspirational, and architectural barriers and affordances that interact to impact the learning and practice of physical activity (Sherrill 1995; p. 34).

More recently, the *adaptation theory* has been defined "as a generic frame of knowledge for enhancing human potential that is practiced when the participant is required to act under limiting conditions" (Hutzler 2007, p. 291).

This principle of the individual acting under limiting environmental and personal conditions is inherent within the more global perspective of planning and programming rehabilitation services, entitled the International Classification of Function and Disability (ICF) (WHO 2001). This is a taxonomy, providing criteria for classification, assessment, and intervention in health and disability. According to the ICF there are three major domains of potential challenges to the interactions of an individual with his or her environment:

1. Impairment of the affected body structures (e.g., lungs, joints, limbs, brain) and functions (e.g., respiration, range of movement, muscular strength, motor control, decision making);
2. Limitation in activities required for daily living, vocational engagement, and leisure time; and
3. Restriction of participation in socially and culturally appropriate activities (WHO 2001).

These challenges to structures and functions, activities and participation are related to the specific health condition (type and degree of disability), as well as to contextual variables based on individual pre-disposition and environmental physical and social factors that could be perceived as facilitators (enablers) or barriers (limiters).

In accordance with this model, and with the underlying principle of person-environment-task interaction, the Systematic Ecological Modification Approach (SEMA) has been developed and presented (Hutzler 2007; Hutzler and Sherrill 2007). This approach to analyzing and designing APA service needs and interventions includes the principal elements that follow.

Task Objective Analysis

The first element of the SEMA is derived from the Ecological Task Analysis (ETA) model of Davis and Burton (1991), and refers to identifying the task that is evolving within the ecological frame of reference. Tasks are expressed as anticipated functional outcomes in respect to the relationship of an individual with his or her environment (Reed 1988). In terms of the ICF a task could be an *activity* outcome, such as throwing, dribbling, or catching a ball, or swimming a breast stroke. A task may also be a *participation* outcome, such as the degree of participation in a soccer game, a class excursion, or a swimming competition.

Task accomplishment under limiting conditions has further been associated with the Judgment and Decision Making Model (JDM), and applied to the teacher-student/coach-athlete interactions when facing functional, activity, and participation limitations (Hutzler and Bar-Eli 2013). It has been suggested that in addition to these barriers, challenging the performance, decision bias, or heuristics related to participants with disability may further affect the teachers' or coaches' ability to enable the tasks' goals. For example, at first glance, most teachers would deny the participation of a child with a physical disability such as cerebral palsy, which requires mobility aids for locomotion, in an excursion where the student must engage in hiking in uneven and non-paved trails.

Most basketball coaches would disallow the participation of an individual sitting in a wheelchair, and most soccer coaches would deny the participation of an individual using crutches for mobility. The reasons for these restrictive intentions may be due to safety concerns, task mastery difficulty, or social interaction difficulty perceptions, which may be biased by heuristics – principles which reduce the complex person-environment interaction to simplistic patterns of decision making and action (Tversky and Kahneman 1974).

Quality Indicators

Each task can be recognized by means of quality indicators, addressing qualitative (typically process-oriented) or quantitative (typically outcome-oriented) indicators. Examples for qualitative outcomes are the accomplishment of all criteria expected within a task, performed at a high skill level.

The Test of Gross Motor Development (TGMD: Ulrich 2000) is an example for this type of assessment, and is widely used for assessing typically developing children and for establishing deviations from the normative performance level, mostly due to intellectual, emotional or coordinative disorders. Quantitative assessment of performance quality is characterized by the ancient and still recognized measures of physical activity "Citius, Altius, Fortius" (Latin for "Faster, Higher, Stronger"; Hay 1993). It should be acknowledged that the quality criteria recommended for non-disabled persons may not always apply to those with disabilities, for whom the personal–environment interactions often require a different set of biomechanical or social constraints. Obviously, the quantitative criteria should be compared with reference to age, gender, and functional impairment.

Limitation and Enablement Criteria

The second element describes the limits within the person-environment framework, including (a) limitations manifested as deficits in the individual functional abilities of the various body systems of the individual, e.g., cognitive, emotional, perceptual, motor control, muscular strength, or range of motion, and (b) environmental limitations such as height of the net for a wheelchair user playing volleyball, size of the soccer court for a person with cerebral palsy, size and color of objects for a person with a visual disorder. However, it is also important to address enablement criteria, which are those available personal or environmental factors that might support a task mastery. For example, peer students who are able and willing to assist their classmate with disability during a game, a race, or an excursion can be considered a resource.

Performance Errors

Most practical textbooks typically follow problem and error descriptions for enhancing instructional cues and feedback practices (e.g., Krause et al. 2008). Identifying errors in performance processes and outcomes is the way most teachers perceive and describe the inability of a student to cope with task criteria, and the very popular Test of Gross Motor Development (2nd edition; Ulrich 2000) evaluates the degree of correctly performed quality criteria of fundamental motor tasks. However, teachers and instructors may be biased by the patterns common in persons without a disability (Hutzler and Bar-Eli 2013), and errors should be addressed within an individual rather than a generic task analysis. The teacher or the coach may be unaware of the individual and environmental constraints leading to the performance patterns observed, and thus his or her instructional strategies may be inappropriate, or even contraindicated. For example, passing a ball in volleyball to a teammate usually requires having a steady platform. If a participant fails to pass a ball in a dynamic position, he or she will usually be instructed to pass the ball from a static position, that is, while standing still. For individuals with a condition such as cerebral palsy, standing still would provide an increased barrier, as planter flexed feet and internal rotated hips limit keeping balance on the base of support. In such a case it would often be more useful to walk or run in order to achieve dynamic balance for supporting the passing action.

Adaptation Recommendations

Actual adaptations for PE (e.g., Davis 2011; Lieberman and Houston-Wilson 2009; van Lent 2006) or for sport training curricula (Winnick 2011) must be the result of a critical analysis of the relations between environmental and individual criteria. This manipulation should be used to pursue beneficial pattern shifts during the acquisition of movement skills or within a social participation event, in spite of the limiting conditions. Adaptation should be suggested by practitioners and discussed with participants within the following domains of the person-environment interaction.

1. *The task.* As demonstrated earlier in this chapter, each performance task has specific criteria which can be modified, either by using a different skill (e.g., wheeling a wheelchair instead of running for moving fast from one place to another), or by changing specific technical criteria such as extending an arm sideways during a long jump performed by an athlete with a leg amputation, thus correcting for the asymmetric inertia;
2. *The environmental conditions.* These variables include, for example, court size, treadmill speed, or ski slope, which can often be manipulated while teaching at the beginner stages in order to facilitate mastery in spite of poor skill.

3. *The equipment used.* Utilizing and modifying equipment is a basic principle in sport events, and the history of sports includes a variety of examples for modifications performed in order to improve performance, such as increasing the size of the racket in tennis, using a variety of running gear for different events, the evolution and regulation of swimming suits, etc. The individually tailored adaptation of sport equipment is a major asset for mastering and improving performance. The utilization of personally suited and technically specific ball weights in Boccia (a ball-throwing game for accuracy in persons with severe disability) is one example. The adaptation of wheelchairs, which 50 years ago had a one size-one design fit for all purposes and persons is another example. The wheelchiar has evolved into a scientifically- and empirically-evidenced practice of selecting custom made designs for specific sport requirements and individual anthropometric and physiological criteria. The interaction of arm size and power with wheel and hand rim sizes is an example for the variety of options available for performance optimization.

4. *The game rules.* Sport game and competition rules have evolved throughout the years as a framework for developing individual and socially-challenging sport activities. Persons with disabilities may be limited by some rules, and therefore changing rules may compensate for their limitations and allow more enabling conditions, thus supporting affirmative action. One example is the two bounces rule in wheelchair tennis. This rule increases the time available for the wheelchair athlete to perform a stroke, and compensates him or her for being hindered in the lateral movement (a wheelchair can't be propelled laterally) and for the dual task nature of the wheelchair-assisted arm and hand stroke, which needs to be synchronized with the propulsion movements performed simultaneously by the same muscle groups.

5. *The instruction modalities.* Most teachers and coaches use verbal instruction, utilizing the command style (Shimon 2011). Modifying the instruction style to other, less authoritarian styles may be beneficial for individuals with attention deficits. Modifying verbal instructions to manual guidance is recommended in cases of students with intellectual disability or visual impairment, who are unable to comprehend or visualize the visual cues, but may be sensitive to somatosensory cues (Block 2015; Lieberman and Houston-Wilson 2009; Sherrill 2004).

Figure 1 depicts a summary model of the systematic ecological modification approach, incorporating (a) task objectives as functional outcomes of the individual-environment relationship, also characterized as the activity or participation categories of ICF; (b) task qualitative and quantitative criteria, typically described as skills or behaviors; (c) limitation (barriers) and enablers (facilitators), depicting personal and environmental contextual factors in ICF terminology; (d) performance errors, for which adaptation is required; and finally (e) a list of adaptation domains, by which performance limitation or participation restriction may be encountered and obviated.

Universal design (UD) is a concept and practice introduced in the late 1990s by the architect R. L. Mace, a senior research associate, research professor, and program director at the Center for Universal Design at the University of North Carolina (Nasar and Evans-Cowley 2007; Story et al. 1998). The concept is intuitive and simple, and is defined as designing all products, buildings, and exterior spaces to be usable by all people to the greatest extent possible (Mace et al. 1991).

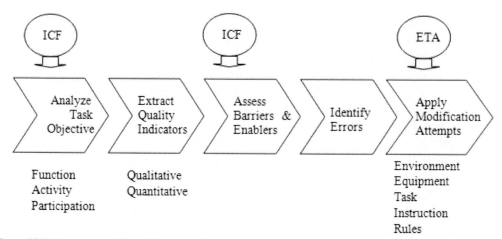

Notes: ICF=International Classification of Function and Disability; ETA=Ecological Task Analysis.
Adapted from Hutzler 2007.

Figure 1. Systematic Ecological Modification Approach with Theoretical Foundations.

In other words, UD should accommodate everyone: young, old, male, female, able and disabled. UD evolved following the changing demography of persons with disability and their longer life expectancy in the late 20th century, increasing their number in the population to between 10-15% (McNeil 1997). UD follows seven design principles (Connell et al. 1997), as listed below.

1. Equitable use. The design is useful and marketable to people with diverse abilities.
2. Flexibility in use. The design accommodates a wide range of individual preferences and abilities.
3. Simple and intuitive use. Use of the design is easy to understand, regardless of the user's experience, knowledge, language skills, or current concentration level.
4. Perceptible information. The design communicates necessary information effectively to the user, regardless of ambient conditions or the user's sensory abilities.
5. Error tolerance. The design minimizes hazards and the adverse consequences of accidental or unintended actions.
6. Low physical effort. The design can be used efficiently and comfortably and with a minimum of fatigue.
7. Size and space for approach and use. Appropriate size and space is provided for approach, reach, manipulation, and use regardless of user's body size, posture, or mobility.

These principles are expected to facilitate accessibility of persons with disabilities to various life events, and therefore increase their participation. However, even though they promote a priori, fixed universally-designed features, the original UD scholars accept that "designers may include adaptable elements ... when needed for a specific user" (Mace et al. 1991, p. 156). A similar situation may appear in the physical activity domain. Even when the universally-accepted use of a wheelchair for mobility enables persons with lower limb mobility impairments to play basketball, tennis, or rugby, some of them still need strapping for keeping them stablilized, and this requires individually-adapted regulations. Therefore, the concept supported in this chapter is that universal design in physical activity needs to include UD elements, which should include a variety of task options, environmental conditions, and equipment solutions, with the addition of individually adapted and tailored solutions, specifically in regard to instructional and motivational strategies and rule modifications.

Universal Design for Learning

During the past decade UD has had a significant impact, and has progressively migrated into education, where the concept of universal design for learning (UDL) was conceived (Ba et al. 1999; Hehir 2009). UDL promoters suggest that "the challenge is not to adapt curricula for students with special needs, but to create an apriori inclusive, affording and enabling environment for all" (Cargiulo and Metcalf 2013). According to UDL followers, three learning frameworks should be considered, namely *recognition, strategy* and *affective networks*, addressing the *what, how,* and *why* of learning, respectively. The adaptation theory principles addressing these UD and UDL foundations include: (a) the representation of the adapted task criteria, environment, rules, and equipment needed to accomplish it (the *what* of learning), (b) the instructional modifications enabling the comprehension and expression of learning and performing the requested task (the *how* of learning), and (c) the motivational strategies used to enhance the engagement of potential participants, necessary for initiating and maintaining participation (the *why* of learning). These motivational strategies and practices may be relevant not only to participants with a disability, but also to peers without disability who are exposed to the opportunities that are opened up by including those with a disability. A summarizing structural frame of reference related to adaptation, as well as to UD and UDL assets, is represented in Figure 2.

The implementation of UD and UDL concepts in physical education and in sports is still in a very early stage, and has not yet achieved a wide base. However, due to the McFadden case (see Lakowski 2011), a trend in this direction started about 10 years ago. Tatyana McFadden, a female high school super athlete with a disability, who won medals for the US in the 2004 Paralympic Summer Games, was not allowed to race and score points for her school. She sued her school and the state athletic association to be included in her high school track team, and although she lost the case, today many school districts in the US enable high-school and university students with a disability to compete on equal status as those without a disability, utilizing an adapted scoring system.

Increasingly, UDL has also been included in US national policy, such as the US Higher Education Opportunity Act of 2008.

Recently, a number of authors in the US (Lieberman et al. 2008; Sherlock-Shangraw 2013) have proposed to incorporate the UDL approach into physical education and sport practice.

Specifically, it has been demonstrated how sport coaches may utilize (a) multiple means of representing the tasks addressed during practice, (b) multiple means of action and expression while engaging in sport tasks, and (c) multiple means of (enhancing) engagement. While in the US a significant development has been observed over the years, in many other countries there is hardly any notion of UD or UDL, and even adaptation has not yet been established and evidenced.

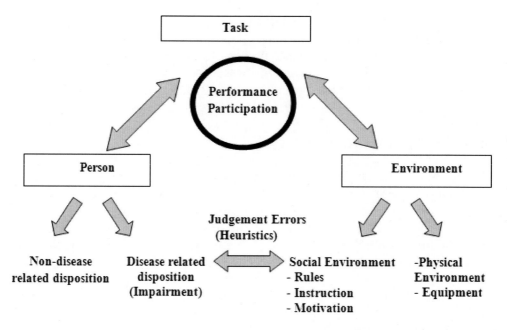

Figure 2. Structural frame of reference related to adaptation, as well as to UD and UDL related assets.

CONCLUSION

This chapter described the evolution of the concepts of adaptation, UD, and UDL in relation to physical activity and sports. It has exposed how these terms merge into a network of concepts, allowing for the development of effective learning and for practicing strategies to ensure the participation of students and athletes with disabilities within a variety of specialized and inclusive frameworks, as recommended within the CRPD.

For this reason, and in order to facilitate the participation of individuals with unique limitations not foreseen within the universal design of sport systems, it is warranted that PE teachers, sport instructors, and coaches learn the principles of task, environment, equipment, and rule adaptations, as well as the various modalities of instructional modifications and motivational strategies, as a core knowledge base required to facilitate participation of persons with disabilities in PE and sports.

REFERENCES

Ammah, J. O., and Hodge, S. R. (2006). Secondary physical education teachers' beliefs and practices in teaching students with severe disabilities: A descriptive analysis. *The High School Journal,* 89(2), 40-54. doi:10.1353/hsj.2005.0019.

Australian Sport Commission (n. d.) Using the DEP activity cards. Australian Sport Commission: Disability Education Program. Online: http://www.ausport.gov.au/__data/assets/ pdf_file /0012/448698/DEP_Activity_cards.pdf.

Bar, L., Galluzzo, J., and Sinfit, S. D. (1999). The accessible school: Universal design for educational settings. Berkeley, CA: MIG Communications.

Barton, L. (1993). Disability, empowerment and physical education. In J. Evans (Eds.), Equality, education and physical education (pp. 43-54). London, UK: The Falmer Press.

Blauwet, C., and and Lezzoni, L. (2014). Thematic paper: Disability inclusive physical activity and sport in the post 2015 development agenda. Physical Medicine and Rehabilitation, 6, S4-S10. Posted online http://www.gpcwd.org/uploads/2/6/0/9/ 26097656/gpcwd_thematic _paper_on_physical_activity.pdf.

Block, M. E. (Ed.) (2000). A teacher's guide to adapted physical education (4th Ed.). Baltimore, MD: Paul H. Brookes.

Buffart, L. M., Westendorp, T., van den Berg-Emons, R., Stam, H. J., and Roebroeck, M. E. (2009). Perceived barriers and facilitators of physical activity in young adults with childhood-onset physical disabilities. Journal of Rehabilitation Medicine, 41, 881-885.

Cargiulo, R. M., and Metcalf, D. (2013). Teaching in todays' inclusive classrooms: A universal design for learning approach (2nd Ed.). Belmont, CA: Wadsworth.

Connell, B. R., Jones, M., Mace, J., Mueller, J., Mullick, A., Ostroff, E., and Vanderheiden, G. (1997). The seven principles of Universal Design. NC State University, The Center for Universal Design. Online: http://www.ncsu.edu/project/design-projects/sites/cud/content/ principles/principles.html.

Corbett, J., and Slee, R. (2000). An international conversation on inclusive education. In F. Armstrong, D. Armstrong, and L. Barton (Eds.), Inclusive education: Policy contexts and comparative perspectives (pp. 133-146). London, UK: David Fulton.

Darwin, C. (1859). On the origin of species. London, UK: John Murray.

Davis, R. (2011). Teaching disability sport: A guide for physical educators (2nd Ed). Champaign, IL: Human Kinetics.

Davis, W. E., and Burton, A. W. (1991). Ecological task analysis: translating movement behavior theory into practice. Adapted Physical Activity Quarterly, 8, 154-177.

Doll-Tepper, G., Dahms, C., Doll, B., and von Selzam, H. (Eds.). (1990). Adapted physical activity: An interdisciplinary approach. Proceedings of the 7th ISAPA, Berlin, June 1989. Berlin: Springer-Verlag.

Fejgin, N., Talmor, R., and Erlich, I. (2005). Inclusion and burnout in physical education. European Physical Education Review, 11(1), 29-50.

Hardin, B. (2005). Physical education teachers' reflections on preparation for inclusion. The Physical Educator, 62(1): 44-56.

Hay, J. G. (1993). Citius, altius, longius (faster, higher, longer): the biomechanics of jumping for distance. Journal of Biomechanics, 23(Suppl. 1), 7-21.

Hehir, T. (2009). Policy foundation of universal design for learning. In D. T. Gordon, J. W. Gravel, and L. A. Schifter (Eds.), A policy reader in universal design for learning (pp. 35-45). Cambridge, MA: Harvard Education Press.

Hodge, S. (1998). Prospective physical education teachers' attitudes toward teaching students with disabilities. The Physical Educator, 55(2), 68-77.

Hodge, S. R., Sato, T., Samalot-Rivera, A., Hersman, B. L., LaMaster, K., Casebolt, K., and Ammah, J. O. A. (2009). Teachers' beliefs on inclusion and teaching students with disabilities. Journal of Multicultural Learning and Teaching, 4(2), 38-58.

Hutzler, Y. (2007). A systematic ecological modification approach to skill acquisition in adapted physical activity. In W. E., Davis and J. Broadhead (Eds.), Ecological perspectives on movement (pp. 179-195). Champaign, IL: Human Kinetics.

Hutzler, Y., and Bar-Eli, M. (2013). How to cope with bias while adapting for inclusion in physical education and sports: A judgment and decision making perspective. *Quest,* 65(1), 57-71.

Hutzler, Y., and Sherrill, C. (2007). Defining adapted physical activity: International perspectives. *Adapted Physical Activity Quarterly*, 24(1), 1-20.

Kasser, S. L., and Lytle, R. K. (2005). A Functional Approach for Modifying Movement Experiences (FAMME) in Inclusive Physical Activity: a lifetime of opportunities. Champaign, IL: Human Kinetics.

Kowalski, E. M., and Rizzo, T. L. (1996). Factors influencing preservice student attitudes toward individuals with disabilities. *Adapted Physical Activity Quarterly*, 13, 180-196.

Krause, J., Meyer, J., and Meyer, D. (2008). Basketball skills and drills (3nd Ed.). Champaign, IL: Human Kinetics.

Lakowski, T. (2011). Advancing equity for students with disabilities in school sports. *Journal of Intercollegiate Sport, 4,* 95-100.

LaMaster, K., Gall, K., Kinchin, G., and Siedentop, D. (1998). Inclusion practices of effective elementary specialists. *Adapted Physical Activity Quarterly, 15,* 64-81.

Lee, S. M., Burgeson, C. R., Fulton, J. E., and Spain, C. G. (2007). Physical education and physical activity: Results from the School Health Policies and Programs Study 2006. *The Journal of School Health*, 77, 435-463.

Lieberman, L., Lytle, R., and Clarcq, J. (2008). Getting it right from the start: Employing the universal design for learning approach to your curriculum. *Journal of Physical Education, Recreation and Dance*, 79(2), 32-39.

Lieberman, L. J., and Houston-Wilson, C. (2009). Strategies for inclusion: A handbook for physical educators (2nd Ed). Champaign, IL: Human Kinetics.

Lienert, C., Sherrill, C., and Myers, B. (2001). Physical educators' concerns about integrating children with disabilities: A cross-cultural comparison. *Adapted Physical Activity Quarterly, 18,* 1-17.

Mace, R. L., Hardie, E. J., and Place, J. P. (1991). Accessible environments: Toward universal design. In W. E. Preiser, J. C. Vischer, and E. T. White (Eds.), Design intervention: Toward a more humane architecture (pp. 155-176). New York, NY: Van Nostrand Reinhold.

McNeil, J. M. (1997). Americans with disabilities: 1994-95. US Bureau of the Census Current Population Reports, P70-61. Washington, DC: US Government Printing Office.

Morley, D., Bailey, R., Tan, J., and Cooke, B. (2005). Inclusive physical education: Teachers' views of including pupils with special educational needs and/or dis-abilities in physical education. *European Physical Education Review,* 11(1), 84-107.

Nasar, J., and Evans-Cowley, J. (2007). Universal design and visitability: From accessibility to zoning. Columbus, OH: The John Glenn School of Public Affairs.

Physical Activity and Sport Task Force, 2015. http://www.gpcwd.org/physical-activity-and-sport.html.

Reed, E. S. (1988). Applying the theory of action systems to the study of motor skills. In O. G. Meijer and K. Roth (Eds.), Complex movement behaviour: The motor-action controversy (pp. 45-86). Amsterdam, The Netherlands: Elsevier.

Reid, G. (in press). IFAPA: Historical perspectives. Palaestra.

Rimmer J. H., Riley, B., Wang, E., Rauworth, A., and Jurkowski, J. (2004). Physical activity participation among persons with disabilities: barriers and facilitators. *American Journal of Preventive Medicine,* 26(5), 419-425.

Sherlock-Shangraw, R. (2013). Creating inclusive youth sport environments with the universal design for learning. *Journal of Physical Education, Recreation and Dance,* 84(2), 40-46.

Sherrill, C. (1995). Adaptation theory: The essence of our profession and discipline. In I. Morisbak and P. E. Jørgensen. (Eds.) Quality of life through adapted physical activity and sport – a lifespan concept. Proceedings of 10th ISAPA, 1995 (pp 32- 44). Oslo and Beitostølen, Norway: ISAPA Organizers.

Sherrill, C. (2004). Young people with disability in physical education/physical activity/sport in and out of schools: Technical report for the World Health Organization. International Council of Sport Science and Physical Education. Online: http://www.icsspe.org/ sites/default/files/YOUNGPEOPLE.pdf.

Shimon, J. M. (2011). Introduction to teaching physical education: Principles and strategies. Champaign, IL: Human Kinetics.

Smith, A., and Thomas, N. (2005). Inclusion, special educational needs, disability and physical education. In K. Green and K. Hardman (Eds.), Physical education: Essential issues (pp. 220-237). London, UK: Sage.

Story, M., Mace, R., and Mueller, J. (1998). Designing for people of all ages and abilities. Raleigh, NC: Center for Universal Design, NC State University.

Tversky, A., and Kahneman, D. (1974). Judgment under uncertainty: Heuristics and biases. *Science,* 185(4147),1124-1131.

Ulrich, D. A. (2000). Test of Gross Motor Development (TGMD-2) (2nd ed.). Austin, TX: ProdEd.

United Nations (2006). Convention on the rights of persons with disabilities. New York: NY, United Nations.

van Lent, M. (2006). (Ed.). Count me in: A guide to inclusive physical activity, sport and leisure for children with a disability. Leuven, Belgium: Acco.

Vasudevan, V., Rimmer, J. H., and Kviz, F. (2015). Development of the barriers to physical activity questionnaire for people with mobility impairments. *Disability and Health Journal,* May 14. pii: S1936-6574(15)00055-2. doi: 10.1016/j.dhjo.2015.04.007. [Epub ahead of print].

Winnick, J. (2011). Adapted physical education and sport (5th Ed.). Champaign, IL: Human Kinetics.

World Health Organization [WHO] (2001). International classification of functioning, disability and health (ICF). Geneva, Switzerland: Author [On-line]. Available: http://www3.who.int/icf/icftemplate.cfm.

In: Physical Activity Effects on the Anthropological Status ...   ISBN: 978-1-63484-782-7
Editors: Fadilj Eminović and Milivoj Dopsaj   © 2016 Nova Science Publishers, Inc.

Chapter 9

RECREATIONAL ACTIVITIES IN INTEGRATED SETTINGS FOR PEOPLE WITH DISABILITIES

Keith Storey[*]*, PhD, BCBA-D*
Graduate School of Education,
Touro University, Vallejo, CA, US

ABSTRACT

Both recreation and integration are important for people with disabilities. Unfortunately, many individuals with disabilities receive only segregated recreational services.

This segregation in recreational settings may also increase segregation in other areas of their lives such as in employment, residential, and community settings. Desirable "best practices" recreational services for people with disabilities has changed from specialized and segregated services to providing services in inclusive settings with appropriate supports. Individuals may need a variety of appropriate supports such as systematic instruction, natural supports, and social skills training to be successfully integrated socially and be able to have the skills to competently participate in the recreational setting.

The empirical research base indicates that services and supports in integrated recreational settings with appropriate supports is the best way of achieving meaningful quality of life outcomes for persons with disabilities. This chapter covers the three basic approaches for the inclusion of people with disabilities in community recreation: a) including the integration of existing generic programs, b) reverse mainstreaming, and c) zero exclusion.

Keywords: integration, inclusion, instruction, supports

---

[*] E-mail: keith.storey@tu.edu.

INTRODUCTION

What Is Integration in Recreational Settings?

Integration has been elusive to define and measure. No single definition of integration enjoys consensus and a comprehensive definition has been elusive. Ford and Davern (1989) pointed out that integration is a complex social phenomenon while Mank and Buckley (1989) described integration as "in its simplest and most elegant form as a degree of community presence and participation for persons with disabilities that is no different from that enjoyed by persons without a disability label" (p. 320). Thus, in recreational settings it involves individuals with disabilities participating in recreational activities in their communities in which people without disabilities participate and are the majority of people in that setting. This chapter is based on the premise that all humans desire some sort of social life and that important social life often occurs in recreational settings. One only has to look at past research to see that positive relationships with others are associated with less stress (House 1981), better health (House 1981), and a higher quality of life (Hughes et al. 1995; Schalock 2000). In the disability field, four different components of integration have generally been considered (Mank and Buckley 1989; Storey 1993). These are physical integration, social integration, relationships, and social networks.

Physical Integration

Physical integration is a necessary first step for other types of integration. Physical proximity is a basic assumption for integration. Wehman (1988) defines physically integrated settings as situations where non-disabled workers or members of the public at large predominate. Without physical integration there cannot be social integration, relationships, and social networks. But mere physical presence may not necessarily lead to other forms of integration. For example, a person with a disability may attend a dance class at a health club (physical integration) but not interact with anyone which would be a physically integrated setting but a socially segregated situation. Amado (1993) points out that it is important not to assume that a person who is physically integrated into a community setting is automatically socially integrated into the community. As noted above, the act of participating in an activity does not indicate that someone is a member of that community. If social integration and social relationships are to be attainable it is important to analyze not only at relationships within a specific setting (such as the health club), but also the diverse relationships possible within one's broader community. By supporting the person's exploration of interests through community connections, we can support opportunities to create a wider array of relationships. Table 1 provides tips for promoting friendship and inclusion.

Social Integration

Social integration has been defined as regular access to interactions with individuals without a disability and regular use of normal community resources (Will 1984). Therefore, for social integration to occur, interactions between the person with a disability and non-disabled individuals are a necessary condition. Social interactions have been found to predict likability and friendship patterns (Gresham 1982), are often conceptualized as forms of conversation and communication (Certo and Kohl 1984), and competent social interactions elevate social perceptions of persons with disabilities (Gaylord-Ross and Peck 1985).

Table 1. Tips for promoting friendship and inclusion

1.	Shift the focus from activities to relationships. Going to a recreational activity (e.g., music, bowling) does not mean that a person will necessarily meet someone and form a friendship
2.	"It never hurts to ask."
3.	Focus on gifts, strengths, and contributions.
4.	"One person, one environment." "Even when a small number of people with disabilities, 2 or 3 for example, participates in a larger group, subtle "us" and "them" divisions can arise....it's also easier for people without disabilities to have the opportunity to get to know and befriend one person, rather than a whole group."
5.	"First impressions" are normal reactions, and people can be helped to get past them. Education can help.
6.	Sometimes coaching is necessary.
7.	It takes work.
8.	You have to prioritize.

Adapted from Amado, A., 2004.

Relationships

Social relationships are often defined in connection to social support and may be analyzed in terms of quantity, structure, and function (House and Kahn 1985).

"Relationships depend on social interactions that are ongoing and usually involve reciprocal participation in activities" (Mank and Buckley 1989, p. 320). It has been theorized that social interaction progresses in stages (Shelden and Storey 2014; Trower 1979).

Relationships and friendships move from formality to intimacy, at each stage exchanging quite different information, making different inferences, and filtering potential friends before allowing deeper levels of intimacy to develop (Stainback and Stainback 1987).

Social Networks

Social networks have been difficult to define but generally refer to the people identified as socially important to a person (Barrera 1986). Mank and Buckley (1989) refer to social networks as involving "repeated contact with a number of people who identify the relationships that exist within the group as 'socially important'" (p. 320).

Social contact patterns and social supports are directly related to social networks and are often conceptualized under the term "social life" (Kennedy et al. 1990).

Social networks generally have been assessed by measuring the size, structure, functions, and adequacy of the network (Barrera 1986; Heitzmann and Kaplan 1988). Self-fulfillment and satisfaction with one's quality of life have been highly associated with a stable social network (Haring 1991; McKinney et al. 1982).

Personal Choice in Recreational Settings

Personal choice for persons with disabilities in recreational settings is a critical issue (Dattilo 2012). Each individual will have their own needs and desires. Some people will want to have a large social network and have frequent interactions across a variety of recreational settings. Others may be satisfied with a few acquaintances and spending much of their time in a single recreational setting. It is important that an individual have opportunities for choice of recreational options and that these be meaningful choices and also that they be taught choice-making skills (Agran et al. 2010). It is often necessary for an individual to experience a recreational setting to know if they actually like it or not. For example you may be asked if you like to play soccer or eat in a restaurant but until you do so you are not making an informed choice. And if your choice is between going to a Special Olympics event on a Saturday afternoon or doing nothing that is not a true choice.

It is extremely critical that there are appropriate supports for the individual to be successful in the recreational setting. Without appropriate supports informed choices become meaningless. For example, an individual with an intellectual disability who is joining a health club may need to learn how to take the bus to and from the facility, orientation to the facility, instruction on how to use the equipment, teaching of skills necessary for participating in a yoga group, and social skills instruction for learning how to appropriately interact with staff and other participants in the various settings.

What Does It Mean to Be Physically and Socially Integrated in a Recreational Setting?

Dattilo (2012) notes that "inclusion is good" as it promotes valuing of differences, promotes positive attitudes toward disability, can reduce stigma and stereotypes, can reduce discrimination and segregation, and promote quality of life outcomes. The problem facing service providers is not whether integration is important, but how to best achieve successful integration in recreational settings.

Persons with disabilities often have an abundance of leisure time due to unemployment or underemployment, lack of appropriate community and social networks, and/or the lack of skills to utilize their free time creatively or constructively. In other words, individuals with disabilities may have limited engagement in appropriate recreational activities unless systematic instruction and appropriate supports are provided (Storey and Miner 2011). Yet for many of us it is our recreational pursuits that offer us the richest opportunities to develop social relationships and to enhance our quality of life. When we engage in recreational activities, we typically have opportunities to meet people with interests similar to our own, hence giving us better odds on a relationship "clicking."

What constitutes appropriate and "state-of-the art" recreational services for people with disabilities has changed dramatically over the past 40 years from specialized and segregated services to providing services in inclusive settings with appropriate supports (Anderson 2012; Mactavish and Schleien 2000; Modell and Valdez 2002, Schilling and Coles 1997; Schleien 1993; Schleien et al. 1990). However, segregated recreational services still predominate and segregated activities are often seen as the norm for individuals with a disability, especially those with more significant disabilities (Dattilo 2002). In contrast to these segregated services, an increasing research base indicates that services and supports in typical recreational settings may be the best way of achieving meaningful quality of life outcomes for persons with disabilities (Anderson and Heyne 2012; Dattilo and McKenney 2011; Kuntsler et al. 2013; Miller et al. 2009).

What does it mean to be physically and socially segregated in a recreational setting?

In some ways it is easier to say what integration is not, in other words, what are segregated recreational programs? These segregated programs serve only people with disabilities or at best provide short term physical and social integration. These programs are perhaps best exemplified by the Special Olympics (Hourcade 1989; Wolfensberger 1995). Storey (2008a; 2008b) has provided a critique of these segregated programs and advocated that they lack meaningful outcomes and should be done away with and replaced with integrated recreational programs. There are a variety of reasons why this segregation in recreational settings occurs such as inadequate funding, lack of integrated services, lack of individual skills, and lack of appropriate supports.

Providing Support in Recreational Settings

For some individuals, the primary issue keeping them from achieving their recreational goals might not be their own skill level, but rather more basic support needs. Recreational professionals can work toward success by addressing an individual's need for additional supports.

Natural supports. The overarching purpose behind developing natural supports is to develop an individualized system of supports for a person that is effective without being overly intrusive. A common way of viewing natural supports is to consider drawing support from people within the setting other than staff members paid to provide support. In a recreational setting, an individual might draw support from coworkers, neighbors, family, friends, and acquaintances formed in community settings. These individuals might provide support by providing transportation, assisting with communication, providing advocacy, serving as a mentor, directly teaching skills, and/or introducing the person to new people.

Reciprocity. Once initiated, relationships in a recreational setting take work and time to develop and sustain. Reciprocity tends to be critical to sustaining relationships. In other words, both parties in a relationship need to feel they are benefiting from the relationship. For individuals with disabilities, there may be unique barriers to sustaining relationships and demonstrating reciprocity, brought on by a lack of accessibility, inadequate transportation, or rigid program rules. Newton, Olson, and Horner (1995) distinguished between tangible and interpreted reciprocity in discussing relationships between individuals with and without cognitive disabilities. Tangible reciprocity refers to a sense that one is seeing an equitable exchange of items or materials in a relationship. For instance, we typically expect that we will receive holiday gifts from individuals to whom we give holiday gifts. Interpreted reciprocity refers to a sense that one is getting emotional benefit from a relationship, such as a sense of support or mutual enjoyment. Newton et al. found that community members who had relationships with adults with intellectual disabilities often found tangible reciprocity (e.g., exchanging cards and gifts) to be missing from their relationships, while interpreted reciprocity (e.g., complete acceptance, satisfaction from an interaction) was present and appreciated. Mutual effort and need also were identified as important to sustaining these relationships.

Recreational support staff may need to remind and assist an individual to send a birthday card or text to say hello, or assist a person in identifying activities that would be of common interest and initiating the planning for that activity. Of course, the level of support needed to sustain a relationship depends on the individuals involved. One person may need assistance in composing an appropriate message and texting it. Another person might need social skills instruction on how to greet team members appropriately when first joining a team. As with all recreational services, the nature and intensity of support depends on the individual's needs and preferences.

Contextual Interventions

Contextual interventions are those strategies that involve manipulating or accessing additional opportunities to interact. More simply, contextual interventions are focused on creating more or better opportunities for social interactions and subsequent social relationships to develop. Contextual interventions can be used in initial support for an individual at a recreational activity. In that activity it might be possible to create opportunities for interaction by having the person with a disability bring coffee for others or suggesting a rearrangement of where people are situated in an exercise group so that that the participant with a disability is situated around some friends who can model what is happening and provide encouragement to the individual.

Creating Opportunities

Newton et al. (1995) interviewed fourteen community members (ten ex-staff, three volunteers and one friend of staff), each of who had a social relationships with a person with a disability. Relationships formed from different origins. Some ex-staff reported that they just "clicked" with the individual when they were on staff. Others reported that the relationship began when they assisted the individual through difficult times or that they had filled the role of a "missing" family person. Based upon these findings, Newton et al. recommend that rather than attempting to match individuals with disabilities and other community members, staff would be more helpful in assisting the person to meet as many new people as possible and eventually a relationship will "click."

Recreational staff can assist people with disabilities by supporting multiple and diverse opportunities to meet people and assisting them in exploring the community and identifying places and opportunities of recreational interest.

Amado (1993) suggests looking for places where there are opportunities for relationships to develop. Potential arises from opportunities to see the same people over time, or being a "regular," and having a basis for exchange. She also suggests accessing environments where other community members engage in personal business, leisure and recreation, hobbies, continuing education and personal development, clubs and organizations, and volunteer opportunities.

Overview of Integrated Recreational Services

Schleien and associates (1995) have outlined key tenets regarding recreational programming. These are:

1. people have a right to recreation that is personally satisfying;
2. the essence of recreation is freedom: freedom to choose between a variety recreational opportunities and experiences;
3. the recreational experience differs between individuals; therefore, supports should be designed to address various needs, interests, and abilities.

There are currently three basic approaches for the inclusion of people with disabilities in community recreation, including the integration of existing generic programs, reverse mainstreaming, and zero exclusion.

Integration of Existing Generic Programs

In this approach the individual chooses an already existing traditional, age-appropriate recreation program. An integration specialists or other professional identifies and ameliorates discrepancies between skill requirements of the program and the individual's capabilities. People with disabilities have been successfully integrated into non-competitive recreational activities (Cooper and Browder 1997; Hamre-Nietupski et al. 1992; Schleien and Larson 1986).

In addition, including those with more severe disabilities, are often quite capable of competing successfully in competitive sports with non-disabled participants (Bernabe and Block 1994; Devine et al. 1998; Roper and Silver 1989).

The advantages of integration of existing generic programs include:

1. Participation of people with disabilities reflects the natural proportion to peers without disabilities;
2. The program activities are age-appropriate and of high interest;
3. Opportunities exist for extended natural peer interactions.

The disadvantages of integration of existing generic programs include:

1. Only a small number of participants with disabilities can be served at one time;
2. Too much attention is often directed toward participants with disabilities;

3. Participants with disabilities are not always welcome;
4. The generic recreation staff may not be trained to work with and provide appropriate supports for people with disabilities.

Reverse Mainstreaming

In this approach, programs designed for people with disabilities are modified to attract peers without disabilities.

The advantages of reverse mainstreaming include:

1. A large number of participants with disabilities can be served at one time;
2. The program is designed to meet the needs of participants with disabilities;
3. The program staff members are trained to work with and provide supports for people with disabilities;
4. People without disabilities are welcome to join the program.

The disadvantages of reverse mainstreaming include:

1. Natural proportions do not exist;
2. Recreation skills taught may not generalize to other settings;
3. A segregated model of services is perpetuated;
4. Opportunities for extended peer interactions do not exist;
5. Individuals without disabilities may be reluctant to join the recreational program.

Zero Exclusion

In this approach, therapeutic recreation specialists and generic recreation program leaders collaborate to design programs meeting the needs of all participants, with or without disabilities.

The advantages of zero exclusion include:

1. The recreation needs of all individuals can be met;
2. The cooperation between therapeutic recreation staff members and generic recreation staff members is promoted;
3. Participants with disabilities and their nondisabled peers have equal status;
4. No one is excluded from the group.

The disadvantages of zero inclusion include:

1. The initial start-up costs may be high;
2. Parents and people with disabilities who prefer segregated programs may fear that those programs will be eliminated (Schleien et al. 1993).

Best Practices Recommendations for Providing Integrated Recreational Services

Increasing Access to Environments and Activities

Increasing the number of environments and variety of activities that an individual participates in may be an initial critical consideration in providing supports. For example, some individuals with disabilities have limited exposure to their communities, only traveling between school or adult program and home five days per week. Visiting and trying a variety of recreational opportunities may increase the person's understanding of what is available and what they may be interested in. Teaching a recreation skill can also increase access as the person would then have the skills to participate in activities in a specific setting. For example, teaching circuit training on weight lifting machines at the local health club would add another place in which the individual goes during the week as well as increase opportunities for choosing other activities such as dressing or purchasing a soft drink.

Environmental Analysis Inventory

Schleien and Ray (1988) have recommended the use of an Environmental Analysis Inventory for recreational activities. The Environmental Analysis Inventory serves multiple purposes. First, it provides a step-by-step procedure to integrate people into community-based recreational activities. Second, it offers an individualized approach to facilitating community participation. Third, it provides information to support providers (e.g., how to plan and prepare for a recreational activity). Fourth, it assists in identifying basic skills and other information for participation in the targeted activity.

In addition to facilitating more efficient recreational skills training and supports, an Environmental Analysis Inventory can also assist in identifying critical and useful recreational skills for the activity, as well as environmental demands and the "culture" of the particular activity (Brown et al. 1979). That information can then be used to assist an individual in initiating interactions and developing relationships within the setting. This top down approach includes identifying current and future environments, the critical activities, and skills required. Figure 1 provides an example of an ecological inventory for going to a movie.

Once the priority environments are identified (in this example the movie theater), the recreational support person conducts an analysis using the ecological inventory process. The steps of the ecological inventory are:

Step 1: Identify the curriculum domain.
Step 2: Identify and survey the environment that the person will be recreating in.
Step 3: Breakdown the major environment into sub-environments.
Step 4: Identify relevant activities.
Step 5: Identify skills required in each activity setting.

Completing the ecological inventory involves observing and analyzing an environment in which the individual currently participates or will participate at a later time.

Ecological Inventory
Domain: Recreation/Leisure
Name: Magnus

Figure 1. Ecological inventory form.

Major Environment Going to Movie							
Sub-environment Ticket Window		Sub-environment Snack Bar		Sub-environment Restroom		Sub-environment Main Area of Theater	
Activity #1	Activity #2	Activity #1	Activity #2	Activity #1	Activity #2	Activity #1	Activity #2
Purchasing ticket	Giving ticket to ticket taker and entering	Selecting snacks	Paying for snacks	Using restroom	Washing hands Skills Turn water on Put hands under water	Locating seat	Watching movie
Skills	Skills	Skills	Skills	Skills	Put soap on hands Rub hands together Rinse hands Turn water off Get paper towel Dry hands Throw away towel	Skills	Skills

Next, the various sub-environments are identified. For example, if a learner wishes to increase recreational skills by going to a movie, the ecological inventory is conducted at the movie theater where the person will be going (see Figure 1). The domain is recreation, the environment is the movie theater, and the sub-environments would include ticket window, snack bar, restroom, and main theater area. Activities, such as purchasing tickets at the ticket window, selecting and purchasing snacks at the snack bar, using the restroom, and locating seat and watching the movie are identified within the sub-environments. These activities may be broken down into individual skills required or task analyzed for instruction (in this example the hand washing task analysis is presented).

Accommodations and Modifications in Recreational Settings

Making changes or modifications to instruction and supports can be a key component of recreational services. It is not always necessary that the individual do the recreational activity in exactly the same way as others or to the same criterion. The terms accommodations and modifications are often used interchangeably, but they represent two different changes. Accommodations provide different ways for individuals to take in (access) information or to display their knowledge or skill in the recreational setting. These changes don't alter or lower the standards or expectations for a task. Accommodations do not substantially change the instructional level, the content, or the performance criteria for the individual. Using a chair in a yoga class would represent an accommodation in a recreational setting.

Modifications are changes in the delivery, content, or completion level of tasks. They result in changing or lowering expectations and create a different standard for some individuals. Modifications do change the expected performance level for an individual. Having a person hit off of a batting tee in a softball game (when other players are not) is an example of a modification.

Use of Systematic Instruction Strategies for Teaching Specific Skills

Participation and integration in recreational settings are all based upon individuals having the skills necessary to be competent in specific situations (e.g., playing on a sports team, participating in workout group, eating at a restaurant, etc.). For many individuals, such competence is not acquired incidentally. In other words, the emphasis of instruction must be to develop competence to function successfully in recreational settings. Systematic instruction provides evidence-based methods to teach those skills (Storey and Miner 2011).

What Is the Best Way to Break Down a Task for Instruction?

For instructional purposes, a task analysis is the key to building instruction. A task analysis is a process of breaking a task or activity into its required component responses, and listing these responses in an appropriate sequence (Bellamy et al. 1979). In other words, it is a complete description of each and every behavior needed to accomplish a specific activity.

The purpose of task analysis is to facilitate instruction by focusing the instructor's attention on the specific demands of a task/activity and by providing a method for gathering data during instruction about the acquisition of the task/activity by the learner. The teaching of complex tasks proceeds most efficiently if people learn simpler component responses and chain them together ultimately to perform the complex target behavior (Cuvo 1978).

Construction of a task analysis before instruction begins meets three instruction needs: a) it increases the likelihood that the instructor has a thorough understanding of the task/activity; b) the task analysis provides the basis for a system for data collection; and c) the identification of discriminative stimuli from which to direct instructional strategies. In developing a task analysis it is important to consider the following points:

1. The specific objective for the task/activity should be identified and recorded;
2. The person who will be doing the instruction should perform the task/activity several times before constructing the task analysis (this is important because there is often more than one method of completing a task/activity, such as putting on a coat);
3. The person who will be doing the instruction should analyze the task and construct the task analysis;

4. The task/activity should be broken down into response units small enough to instruct the learner successfully. For some learners bigger "chunks" are fine as response units (or steps) of the task analysis (such as enter the health club, go to the locker room, change into workout clothes, go to weight room, etc) while other learners might need more detailed response units (such as enter door to health club, get out identification card, put card into scanner, enter through gate, walk to locker room, etc.);

5. The steps in the task/activity should be sequenced in the exact order in which they will be performed;

6. Mandatory steps in the task analysis should be identified (certain steps in the task analysis which are considered essential). These are steps which if not performed or are performed incorrectly, the terminal outcome is not achieved successfully;

7. The discriminative stimulus for each step should be identified (Cuvo 1978; Gold 1976; Mank and Horner 1988; Powell et al. 1991). This identification of the discriminative stimulus that the learner needs to respond to is extremely important as the point of instruction is for the learner to respond appropriately to relevant stimuli in the environment.

How Are Learner Errors Analyzed?

As mentioned previously, data must be kept in order to know if the learner has mastered the activity to criterion levels.

Steps on a task analysis that are repeatedly incorrect must be examined in order to make appropriate modifications to instruction. The primarily three types of errors are 1) initiation errors, 2) discrimination errors, and 3) response errors.

For example while learning to go to a movie, if the learner makes a mistake in paying for the ticket, this step could then be broken down in greater detail to teach the correct response.

What Is the Difference between Cues and Corrections?

Cues and corrections are two different things. A cue refers to information provided to a learner before a behavior is performed. A correction refers to supplementary or corrective information to communicate to a learner that a response already performed is incorrect or that a different response is needed.

Cues

Cues (also known as prompts) are an added antecedent stimulus which increases the probability of a correct response. Antecedent means that the cue is provided before the behavior is to occur.

The reasoning for the use of cues is that they occur before the behavior should happen and thus increase the likelihood of a correct response so that that response can be reinforced and thus increase the likelihood that in the future the behavior will occur in response to the natural cue (the ticket taker at the theater asks for the ticket) without the instructor cue ("when you see the ticket taker hand them your ticket"). The purpose of cues is to assist the learner in performing behaviors (skills) in response to naturally occurring discriminative stimuli.

The learner is thus: a) alerted to important discriminative stimuli that provide information about behaviors to emit and b) be able to respond appropriately. As Steere and Pancsofar (1995) have written "The cue is the clue to do something new." There are different types of cues which may be used to provide information to learners and they may be used in different ways.

Verbal Cues

These are statements or questions provided by an instructor that draw the learner's attention to the discriminative stimuli. Verbal cues may state specifically what the individual should do such as "Hand your ticket to the ticket taker."

Verbal cues may also be nonspecific questions (i.e., indirect verbal cues) that alert the learner that something should be noticed such as "What do you do with your ticket to enter the theater?" Specific verbal cues provide more information than nonspecific verbal cues.

Modeling

With modeling the instructor does the step to show the learner how to perform that step of the task analysis. For example, the instructor could hand their ticket to the ticket taker.

Gestures

These are movements made by the instructor to draw attention to discriminative stimuli. Pointing, motioning, or shadowing movements are examples. For example, the instructor could point to the ticket and then to the ticket taker.

Physical Guidance

This involves physical contact between the instructor and the learner and it may involve full physical prompting (hand over hand) to direct the learner's movements, or just a light touch. For example, the instructor could take the learner's hand that is holding their ticket and help them hand the ticket to the ticket taker.

Correction Procedures

The basic assumption should be that errors are a result of incorrect or inadequate instruction, not inherent to the learner because of a disability label. Errors are not random. Few learners perform with unpredictable error patterns. The two most common errors are due to prior history (where the person has learned an inappropriate response to a discriminative stimulus) and incomplete instruction (Horner et al. 1984).

Errors are of equal, if not greater, importance for instructors to attend to in order to deliver quality and effective instruction (Horner 1984). And it is important to collect data that documents error patterns. When a learner makes an error, the instructor should stop the learner immediately. It is important to interrupt the learner as soon as an error is initiated or observed and interrupt in a non-punitive manner. You do not want the learner to continue on the task after an error because they are learning incorrect performance. Second, recreate the situation in which the error occurred. Third, have the learner to repeat the step using enough assistance to assure success. Be sure to deliver praise for the correct response. Finally, repeat the step again using less assistance. There are three types of errors that a learner may make: initiation errors, discrimination errors, and response errors.

Initiation Errors

An initiation error is when the learner fails to initiate a behavior in response to the discriminative stimulus in the environment. For example, when entering the theater after purchasing a ticket the learner stops and stands there and fails to initiate the next step of handing the ticket to the ticket taker. Respond to initiation errors by:

1. isolating the preceding two steps of the task analysis and the step on which the initiation error was made;
2. identify cues for instruction to ensure correct responding on that step of the task analysis;
3. pair cue and task stimuli;
4. fade the cue after correct responding;
5. immediately reinforce self-initiation of the correct step;
6. fade reinforcement.

Discrimination Errors

These are errors where the learner responds to the wrong discriminative stimulus in the environment. For example, handing one's ticket to another customer rather than the ticket taker would be a discrimination error. Respond to discrimination errors by:

1. highlighting the relevant dimension of stimulus that the learner should respond do;
2. presenting examples with very similar stimuli;
3. increasing the intensity and frequency of reinforce for correct responses;
4. fade reinforcement.

Response Errors

These are errors where the learner makes an incorrect response. For example, the learner hands money to the ticket taker instead of their ticket. Respond to response errors by:

1.   identifying cues to ensure correct responding;
2.   presenting examples in cumulative sequence;
3.   increasing intensity and frequency of reinforcer.

Social Skills Instruction

Combs and Slaby (1977) define social skill as "the ability to interact with others in a given social context in specific ways that are socially acceptable or valued and at the same time personally beneficial, mutually beneficial, or beneficial primarily to others. In other words, social skills involve the person interacting appropriately with others from the perspective of the other people. Gresham, Sugai, and Horner (2001) have identified five dimensions of social skills: a) peer relational skills (getting along with others), b) self-management skills (controlling one's own behavior), c) academic skills (social behaviors related to academics such as listening to the teacher), d) compliance skills (following directions), and e) assertion skills (using skills learned with others) (pp. 333-334).

We often underestimate just how much social behavior can affect persons' success in integrated recreational settings. Individuals with disabilities must interact appropriately with others in addition to performing specific recreational activities. Attending a movie, participating in an exercise group, eating at a restaurant are recreational activities that all involve the need for appropriate social interactions. For example, at a restaurant one most greet the hostess, request a table, greet and give order to the waitress, and pay the cashier. Deficits in any of these interactions can negatively impact the quality of service, or of even being able to receive any service at all.

Preparing a plan to teach social skills should involve having instructional goals and objectives, a planned direct instructional sequence, an opportunity for the individual to demonstrate the behavior and a systematic assessment process to determine whether the skill has been learned or if the person needs more instruction (Sugai and Lewis 1996). The use of the new social skill should be periodically monitored over weeks and months to see if the individual is still using the social skills successfully. Positive reinforcement should always be provided at these monitoring times to strengthen the skill use.

Published Social Skill Curricula

Examining the numerous published social skills curricula can serve as a starting point to teach commonly desired social behaviors. A list of available programs to consider is provided in Table 2. For selecting the most appropriate program, it is important to review the program content targeted and what methods are used to teach the social skills.

Multimedia and Video Modeling

Multimedia (virtual environments, simulations, videos, pictures, and other multimedia) can be very effective strategies for teaching recreational skills (Sigafoos et al. 2007). Video peer modeling (VPM) and video self-modeling (VSM) use visual instruction to teach recreational skills. VSM involves the target person observing her or himself on video performing a skill to be learned, while VPM involves the target person observing a friend or other person on video performing the skill to learn. An advantage to video modeling is that it eliminates support provider prompting, allowing the individual to completely focus on the model being presented. Convenience is another factor for using this tool. Support providers are able to manipulate the camera, zooming in and out, editing as necessary and the results can be viewed repeatedly by the individual.

Another advantage is that it is easy to see the antecedent-behavior-consequence relationship in a. These situations can be manipulated so that the person can see both appropriate and inappropriate demonstrations of the recreational skill so that they can make the appropriate discrimination. For example, an individual could be videoed in a mock practice session on how to interact socially with others in a cooking class (such as asking for an item, excusing oneself when accidently bumping into another student in the class, how to ask the instructor for help). A person in the mock situation could make an error in the first recording. A second recording can show the person correcting the error and performing the skills correctly. The individual can then compare the correct behavior to the incorrect behavior. Facial expression, body language, voice tone, and emotions can all be seen and evaluated as use as role models using VSM (Prater 2007).

Table 2. Selection of published programs for social skills instruction

The ACCEPTS Program (Walker et al), Middle School to High School ages http://www.proedinc.com/customer/productView.aspx?ID=625andSearchWord=ACCEPTS%20PROGRAM
ACHIEVE Stop and Think Social Skills Program, (Knoff) Pre K through 8th grade, http://projectachieve.us/stop-think/stop-and-think.html
The EQUIP Program (Gibbs, Potter and Goldstein), adolescents, 12 – 17 yrs, http://www.researchpress.com/scripts
I Can Problem Solve programs (Shure) Grades K though 6th, http://www.researchpress.com/product/item/4628/
PATHS curriculum (Kusche and Greenburg), PreK through 6th grade, http://www.channing-bete.com/prevention
The PREPARE program (Goldstein) Middle School and High School Students http://www.researchpress.com/product/item/5063/
Skillstreaming Program (Goldstein and McGinnis) Pre K through12[th] grade, http://www.skillstreaming.com/
Teaching Social Competence to Youth and Adults with Developmental Disabilities (D.A. Jackson, N.F. Jackson and Bennett) Adolescents and Adults, http://www.proedinc.com/customer/productView.aspx?ID=1428

CONCLUSION

The shift from segregated to integrated recreational services has been important for improving the quality of life for people with disabilities. The question is now not if integrated services are better than segregated but how to provide appropriate skill building and supports so that each individual is successfully integrated into community recreational settings of their choosing. Storey (1993) has noted that integration is a *means* (i.e., a set of methods to make behaviors and activities happen), an *outcome* (i.e., the result of having done given things to get individuals more completely involved in the usual fabric of the "normal" recreational world), and it is a *social policy* objective (i.e., we use it as a means to accomplish particular lifestyle outcomes, and those outcomes and means are intertwined).

REFERENCES

Agran, M., Storey, K., and Krupp, M. (2010). Choosing and choice making are not the same: Asking "what do you want for lunch?" is not self-determination. *Journal of Vocational Rehabilitation, 33*(2), 77-88.

Amado, A. N. (1993). Friendships and community connections between people with and without developmental disabilities. Baltimore: Paul H. Brookes.

Amado, A. (2004). Lessons learned about promoting friendships. *TASH Connections, 30*(½), 8-12.

Anderson, L. (2012). Why leisure matters: Facilitating full inclusion. *Social Advocacy and Systems Change Journal, 3*(1), 1-13.

Anderson, L., and Heyne, L. (2012). Therapeutic recreation practice: A strengths approach. State College, PA: Venture Publishing, Inc.

Barrera, M. (1986). Distinctions between social support concepts, measures, and models. *American Journal of Community Psychology, 14*, 413-445.

Bernabe, E. A., and Block, M. E. (1994). Modifying rules of a regular girls softball league to facilitate the inclusion of a child with severe disabilities. *Journal of the Association for Persons with Severe Handicaps, 19*, 24-31.

Brown, L., Branston-McLean, M. B., Hamre-Nietupski, S., Pumpian, I., Certo, N., and Gruewald, L. (1979). A strategy for developing age appropriate and functional curricular content for severely handicapped adolescents. *Journal of Special Education, 13*, 81-90.

Certo, N., and Kohl, F. L. (1984). A strategy for developing interpersonal interaction instructional content for severely handicapped students. In: N. Certo, N. Haring, and R. York (Eds.), *Public school integration of severely handicapped students: Rational issues and progressive alternatives (pp. 221-244).* Baltimore, MD: Paul H. Brookes.

Combs, M. L. and Slaby, D. A. (1977). Social skills training with children. In B. B. Lahey and A. E. Kazdin (Eds.), *Advances in clinical child psychology (Vol. 1) (pp. 161-201).* New York: Plenum Press.

Cooper, K. J., and Browder, D. M. (1997). The use of a personal trainer to enhance participation of older adults with severe disabilities in community water exercise classes. *Journal of Behavioral Education, 7*, 421-434.

Dattilo, J. (2002*). Leisure education program planning: A systematic approach (2nd Ed.).* State College, PA: Venture.

Dattilo, J. (2012). *Inclusive leisure services (3rd Ed.).* State College, PA: Venture.

Dattilo, J., and McKenney, A. (2011). *Facilitation techniques in therapeutic recreation (2nd Ed.).* State College, PA: Venture.

Devine, M. A., McGovern, J. N., and Hermann, P. (1998). Inclusion in youth sports. *Journal of Park and Recreation Administration, 17,* 56-72.

Ford, A., and Davern, L. (1989). Moving forward with school integration: Strategies for involving students with severe handicaps in the life of the school. In: R. Gaylord-Ross (Ed.), *Integration strategies for students with handicaps (pp. 11-31).* Baltimore, MD: Paul H. Brookes.

Gaylord-Ross, R., and Peck, C. A. (1985). Integration efforts with severely mentally retarded populations. In: D. Bricker and J. Filler (Eds.), *Severe mental retardation: From theory to practice (pp. 185-207).* Reston, VA: Council for Exceptional Children.

Gresham, F. M. (1982). Social interactions as predictors of children's likability and friendship patterns: A multiple regression analysis. *Journal of Behavioral Assessment, 4,* 39-54.

Gresham, F. M., Sugai, G., and Horner, R. H. (2001). Interpreting outcomes of social skills training for students with high-incidence disabilities. *Exceptional Children, 67,* 331-344.

Hamre-Nietupski, S., Krajewski, L., Riehle, R., Sensor, K., Nietupski, J., Moravec, J., McDonald, J., and Cantine-Stull, P. (1992). Enhancing integration during the summer: Combined educational and community recreation options for students with severe disabilities. *Education and Training in Mental Retardation, 27,* 68-74.

Heitzmann, C. A., and Kaplan, R. M. (1988). Assessment of methods for measuring social support. *Health Psychology, 7,* 75-109.

Hourcade, J. J. (1989). Special Olympics: A review and critical analysis. *Therapeutic Recreation Journal, 23,* 58-65.

House, J. S. (1981). *Work stress and social support.* Redding, MA: Addison-Wesley.

House, J. S., and Kahn, R. L. (1985). Measures and concepts of social support. In S. Cohen and S. L. Syme (Eds.), *Social support and health (pp. 83-108).* Orlando, FL: Academic Press.

Hughes, C., Hwang, B., Kim, J., Eisenman, L. T., and Killian, D. J. (1995). Quality of life in applied research: A review and analysis of empirical measures. *American Journal on Mental Retardation, 99,* 623-641.

Kennedy, C. H., Horner, R. H., and Newton, J. S. (1989). Social contacts of adults with severe disabilities living in the community: A descriptive analysis of relationship patterns. *Journal of The Association for Persons with Severe Handicaps, 14, 190*-196.

Kuntsler, R., Thompson, A., and Croke, E. (2013). Inclusive recreation for transition-age youth: Promoting self-sufficiency, community inclusion, and experiential learning. *Therapeutic Recreation Journal, 47*(2), 122-136.

Mactavish, J. B., and Schleien, S. J. (2000). Exploring family recreation activities in families that include children with Developmental Disabilities. *Therapeutic Recreation Journal, 34,* 132-153.

Mank, D. M., and Buckley, J. (1989). Strategies for integrating employment environments. In: W. Kiernan and R. Schalock (Eds.), *Economics, industry, and disability: A look ahead (pp. 319-335).* Baltimore, MD: Paul H. Brookes.

Miller, K. D., Schleien, S. J., and Lausier, J. (2009). Search for best practices in inclusive recreation: Programmatic findings. *Therapeutic Recreation Journal, 43*(1), 27-41.

Modell, S. J., and Valdez, L. A. (2002). Beyond bowling: Transition planning for students with disabilities. *Teaching Exceptional Children, 34,* 46-52.

Newton, J. S., Olson, D., and Horner, R. H. (1995). Factors contributing to the stability of social relationships between individuals with mental retardation and other community members. *Mental Retardation, 33,* 383-393.

Prater, M. A. (2007). *Teaching strategies for students with mild to moderate disabilities (pp. 452-453).* Upper Saddle River, NJ: Pearson.

Roper, P. A., and Silver, C. (1989). Regular track competition for athletes with mental retardation. *Palaestra, 5,* 14-16, 42-43, 58-59.

Schalock, R. L. (2000). Three decades of quality of life. *Focus on Autism and Other Developmental Disabilities, 15,* 116-127.

Schilling, M. L., and Coles, R. (1997). From exclusion to inclusion: A historical glimpse at the past and reflection of the future. *The Journal of Physical Education, Recreation and Dance, 68,* 42-45.

Schleien, S. J. (1993). Access and inclusion in community leisure services. *Park and Recreation, 28,* 66-72.

Schleien, S. J., Heyne, L. A., Rynders, J. E., and McAvoy, L. H. (1990). Equity and excellence: Serving all children in community recreation and leisure services in a community setting. *Journal of Physical Education, Recreation, and Dance, 61,* 45-48.

Schleien, S. J., and Larson, A. (1986). Adult leisure education for the independent use of a community recreation center. *Journal of the Association for Persons with Severe Handicaps, 11,* 39-44.

Schleien, S., Meyer, L., Heyne, L., and Brandt, B. (1995). *Lifelong leisure skills and lifestyles for persons with developmental disabilities.* Baltimore, MD: Paul Brookes.

Schleien, S., and Ray, M. T. (1988). *Community recreation and persons with disabilities: Strategies for integration.* Baltimore: Paul H. Brookes Publishing Co.

Shelden, D. L., and Storey, K. (2014). Social life. In K. Storey and D. Hunter, (Eds.). *The road ahead: Transition to adult life for persons with disabilities (3rd Ed.) (pp. 233-254).* Washington, DC: IOS Press.

Sigafoos, J., O'Reilly, M., and de la Cruz, B. (2007). *How to use video modeling and video prompting.* Austin, TX: Pro-Ed.

Stainback, W., and Stainback, S. (1987). Facilitating friendships. *Education and Training in Mental Retardation, 22, 18-25.*

Storey, K. (1993). A proposal for assessing integration. *Education and Training in Mental Retardation, 28(4),* 279-287.

Storey, K. (2008a). The more things change, the more they are the same: Continuing concerns with the Special Olympics. *Research and Practice for Persons with Severe Disabilities, 33(3),* 134-142.

Storey, K. (2008b). A response to Hughes and McDonald's and MacLean's commentaries: Yes things have changed, and they are still the same! *Research and Practice for Persons with Severe Disabilities, 33(3),* 150-151.

Storey, K., and Miner, C. (2011). *Systematic instruction of functional skills for students and adults with disabilities.* Springfield, IL: Charles C. Thomas Publisher, Inc.

Sugai, G., and Lewis, T. J. (1996). Preferred and promising practices for social skills instruction. *Focus On Exceptional Children, 29(4),* 11-27.

Trower, P. (1979). Fundamentals of interpersonal behavior: A social-psychological perspective. In: A. S. Bellack and M. Hersen (Eds.), *Research and practice in social skills training (pp. 3-40).* New York: Plenum Press.

Wehman, P. (1988). Supported employment: Toward zero exclusion of persons with severe disabilities. In P. Wehman and M. S. Moon (Eds.), *Vocational rehabilitation and supported employment (pp. 3-16).* Baltimore, MD: Paul H. Brookes.

Will, M. (1984). *Supported employment for adults with severe disabilities: An OSERS program initiative.* Washington, DC: Office of Special Education and Rehabilitative Services.

Wolfensberger, W. (1995). Of "normalization" lifestyles, the Special Olympics, deinstituionalization, mainstreaming, integration, and cabbages and kings. *Mental Retardation, 33,* 128-131.

In: Physical Activity Effects on the Anthropological Status ...   ISBN: 978-1-63484-782-7
Editors: Fadilj Eminović and Milivoj Dopsaj   © 2016 Nova Science Publishers, Inc.

Chapter 10

EFFECT OF SPECIAL OLYMPICS PROGRAM ON CROSS-COUNTRY SKIERS: ASPECTS OF HEALTH RELATED VARIABLES

*Hana Válková**

Faculty of Sport Studies, Masaryk University, Brno, Czech Republic

ABSTRACT

Focused attention on the healthy lifestyle of individuals with intellectual disability has been realised thanks to the Special Olympics Healthy Athlete Program, particularly "Health Promotion and FUNFitness." A comparison of healthy behaviour and fitness variables will provide an important background to this study, not only for involvement in so-called Low Level and Intermediate Level events in individual sports, but also for training and for education in healthy living and therapy for people with mental disabilities. Involvement in sports at a competitive level is relevant to SO philosophy, with participation in competitions depending on the level of ability for which a coach is responsibility. Being that cross-country skiing is very popular in Czech Republic, this article has thus been oriented towards this sport. The aim of the study was: 1. to collect data related to the health and fitness variables of Special Olympians competing as cross-country skiers; 2. to compare this data with the real results of cross-country skiing competition according to the gender and the level of event. 3. To formulate recommendations for participants. A cohort of Czech Special Olympians (39 male, 15 female) were included in the research and analysis. These were cross-country skiers of an average age of 39.79 years, all of them in the spectrum of a moderate level of intellectual disability, with 3 years' experience in cross-country training and competition. The data was collected over one week during the Czech National Winter Games. *Data collection*: a) a verbal survey oriented towards healthy lifestyles; b) assessment of fitness variables regarding Special Olympics Healthy Athlete Manual in clusters of cardiovascular fitness, Body Mass Index, strength of legs, strength of abdominal muscles, strength of hands; c) results of cross-country race at Low Level and Intermedium Level. Descriptive statistics and logical data analysis was used in statistical analysis. The results showed that all the variables determined were lower compared to the general population in this age group,

---

* Corresponding author: Hana Válková. Email: valkova@fsps.muni.cz.

especially in terms of Heart Rate variables. The BMI was comparable to the average of the general population, especially in Intermediate competitors. There were no dramatic differences between gender groups, but significant differences were found between ability levels in all aspects of variables. This fact can be considered as providing a positive selection for adequate competitive level (responsibility of coaches) but probably the lack of training, being that some of variables important for cross-country mastering (balance, hand strength, cardiovascular fitness) marked higher abilities, which is then the challenge for their involvement in a higher level of competition events. Even the age cohort (25-45 years) and level of intellectual disability (moderate) was similar to the wide, heterogeneous spectrum of fitness variables that were found. We can conclude that the individual strategy concerning the healthy or non-healthy life style of people with intellectual disability is similar to that of the general population. In spite of the fact that the physical fitness variables of SO athletes is lower comparing with general population, several athletes presented an optimal level of fitness. Irrespective of some adverse results, a lot of athletes can participate in sports thanks to the Special Olympics which can help to address issues concerning the healthy behavior and lifestyle of people with intellectual disabilities.

Keywords: mental disability, healthy athlete program, fitness variables, low level events, intermediate level events

INTRODUCTION

Physical Activities of Persons with Intellectual Disability

Focus on the importance of physical activities for the health of people with intellectual disabilities (formerly termed - mental disability, or mental retardation) started in the 1970s. Due to the progressive ideas of pioneering authors, the topic has survived up to today (Broadhead & Church, 1984; Faith, 1972; Roswal et al., 1984). The first research projects usually paid more attention to the description of motor abilities and motor skills development in designing cross-sectional studies (Cratty, 1972; Pitetti et al., 1989; Rarick et al., 1970; Rintala & Palsio 1994; Vermeer, 1990; Vermeer & Davis, 1995; Winnick & Short, 1985).

In spite of the focus on motor ability development, early findings have shown the benefit of either general physical activities, games or sports training for the psycho-social advancement of people with mental disabilities. This is the reason why research projects have spread from only addressing fitness variable to targeting active life style variables. The most important topic is therefore involvement in daily physical activities, health status and the obesity of individuals with intellectual disability. Here we can make a comparison of the findings of Vargas-Cuesta et al. (2010) regarding the benefits of physical activities between two groups of older adults with intellectual disability, participating in different levels of sport practice (low intensity - high intensity).

In this study, they confirmed fitness a personal prosperity due to higher frequency of physical activity. Similar findings have been oriented towards school PE lessons and leisure activities during an individual's life-span, supporting the idea of the importance of physical activity in leisure time (Dixon-Ibarra et al., 2013; Faison-Hodge & Poretta, 2004; Rimmer et al., 2004; Sit et al., 2008). Physical activities have also been indicated in terms of improving physical, social and general life competence as the basis for community inclusion (Ninot et al., 2000; Temple & Walkley, 2003).

A cohesive monograph, edited by Taggart and Cousins (2014), has since given a picture of typical health problems sub-jointed with intellectual disability, such as perception impairment, diabetes, epilepsy, cancer, obesity, cardiovascular diseases and nutrition problems. Health promotion requires a community and, in the context of leisure time, the significance of physical activities and sports have been underlined (Nankervis et al., 2014).

Physical Activities in the Framework of Special Olympics

"The mission of Special Olympics is to provide year-round sports training and athletic competitions in variety of Olympic-type sports for children and adults with intellectual disabilities, giving them continuing opportunities to develop physical fitness, demonstrate courage, experience joy and participate in a sharing of gifts, skills and friendship with their families, other Special Olympics athletes and the community." (Special Olympics, 2010, p. 14)

The Special Olympics (SO) philosophy is based on the principle of relativity which means that all Special Olympians can participate in appropriate groups according to their abilities, skills and limits, with respect to the training effect. Seeing that the SO program has become the expanding intervention sports program the effect of SO participation has been analysed according to various aspects: the influence on separation or community integration, healthy lifestyle, social competence, independence and self-awareness (Coreen et al., 2009; Dykens & Cohen, 1996; Dykens et al., 1999; Hourcade, 1989; Orelove et al., 1982; Özer et al., 2012; Roswal et al., 2003; Válková et al., 1999; Wilhite & Kleiber, 1992).

The motives for participation and the influence on the life of SO athletes and their families in community were assessed because the SO program was recognised as constituting an unique physical activity in leisure time (Goodwin et al., 2006; Shapiro, 2003; Wolfensberger, 1995). Descriptions of the participants with intellectual disability in Special Olympics and improvements in sports and complementary programs have also been included in Special Olympics International anniversary reports (Special Olympics, 2005, 2007). The prevalence of the authors has confirmed the presence of less female participants in SO programmes than males (Coreen et al., 2009; Eichstaedt & Lavay, 1992; Faith, 1972; Foley et al., 2013; Rimmer et al., 2004; Taggart et al., 2012; Temple and Walkley, 2003; Winnick & Short, 1985).

Issue of Obesity and Overweight

Obesity and overweight are frequent topic in all population groups including those addressing both physically active and sedentary people (Dixon-Ibarra and Dugala, 2013), as well as including persons with intellectual disability. This issue is presented from various points of view in addressing age, gender, type and intensity of disability and the type of living environment (Emerson, 2005; Onyewadume, 2006; Lahtinen et al., 2007; Sohler et al., 2009;

Temple et al., 2006; Temple et al., 2010; Winter et al., 2011). The findings of these researchers confirm a higher Body Mass Index (BMI) of females and growing trends according to age in both females and males (Faison-Hodge & Poretta, 2004; Foley et al., 2013; Gába et al., 2012; Harris et al., 2003; Shepard, 1990). These results have been found in different corners and environment of the world: Northern England (Emerson, 2005); Africa (Onyewadume, 2002); Finland (Lahtinen et al., 2007); New Zealand (Stedman & Leland, 2010) and the Czech Republic (Bartková, 2014; Gába et al., 2012; Válková, 1998).

The assessment of the BMI of Special Olympic athletes has drawn the attention of several authors claiming that the connection between physical activity and obesity seemed to be antagonistic. Yet opposing findings have also been revealed (Harris et al., 2003; Onyewadume, 2006; Special Olympics, 2011). An investigation of nearly 11,000 Special Olympians from 145 nationalities who have participated in different sports within World Summer SO Games in 2003 reported that 30% of athletes were obese and 27% overweight (Special Olympics, 2005). Similar findings were repeated several years later (Special Olympics, 2011). BMI trends amongst adult US Special Olympians in the 2005-2010 period were then processed and presented in a cohesive review provided by Foley, Lloyd and Temple (2013). General trends were also confirmed of some BMI indexes, particularly for young adults showing underweight and nutrition problems.

Exercise and Training Effect on Cardiovascular Fitness

Historically, the issue of physical activities and the sport training effect on both BMI and cardiovascular fitness in the context of persons with intellectual disabilities have been interesting up to the present day (Dixon-Ibarra et al., 2013; Wright & Cowden, 1986). The connection between the variables of Special Olympians has been investigated by several research teams (Pitetti et al., 1997; Rintala et al., 1992; Stanish & Draheim, 2007). The effects of training and health related fitness have also been covered by Chynias, Reid and Hoover (1998) and Draheim, Williams and McCubbin (2003).

The tendency towards a low level of heart rate has generally been recognised in relation to 'SO physical activities,' but the type of sport has not been defined particularly. It is logical that different sports need different cardiovascular fitness (compare gymnastics, softball through, unified football, cross-country skiing). Two groups of trained runners with and without intellectual disability were compared by Frey et al. (1999), while Cluphf and associates (2001) have monitored the influence of intensive dance activity on cardiovascular fitness. A Special Olympics swimming training program effect on cardiovascular endurance and conceptions of self has also been investigated by Chrysagis et al. (2009).

Assessment of cardiovascular endurance seems to be crucial issue that has warranted endless investigation since the last century and up to the present day. There is the necessity in this matter to anticipate the problem of age, somatotype, task understanding and the long-term motivation of people with intellectual disability which can negatively impact upon their real endurance ability. Therefore, specialists in aerobic fitness and endurance testing have searched for appropriate tests, such as the 12 minute run, shuttle run, one mile walk or two km walk, the laboratory treadmill walk or run, and modification of the classical step-test (Lejčarová, 2012; Lotan et al., 2004; Pitetti et al., 1997; Rintala et al., 1992; Rintala et al.,

1997; Shepard, 1990; Válková, 1998). In summary, the step-test appeared to be the most available and accessible means for screening cardiovascular endurance and its modification was included in the Special Olympics Healthy Athlete Test Battery.

Motor Abilities and Fitness Assessment

The importance of motor abilities in relation to the quality of life, mobility and the wellbeing of persons with intellectual disability has been a very frequent topic in the pioneering period of research, as well as in recent society and social studies (Broadhead & Church, 1984; Cratty, 1972; Eichstaedt & Lavay, 1992; Faith, 1972; Lahtinen et al., 2007; Lotan et al., 2004; Pitetti et al., 1989; Rintala & Palsio, 1994; Winnick & Short, 1985). The origin of instruments used for this purpose, including for Special Olympian testing, came from the AAHPER, UNIFIT, EUROFIT systems (Měkota & Kovář, 1995; Pitetti et al., 2010; Reid et al., 1985; Shepard, 1990).

The availability of cohesive test battery for the testing of individuals with intellectual disability (Eurofit Special) has validated the findings of Skowronski et al. (2009). Only mild modifications have been recommended, excepting the measurement of endurance. The basic problem, which it has been necessary to anticipate, has been communication and motivation. The results of testing are mostly cross-sectional, which have served as documents detailing the level of abilities possible to compare with the norms of general population or to presented differences according to age cohort, gender or Special Olympians versus non-Special Olympians (Dixon-Ibarra et al., 2013; Foley et al., 2013; Lahtinen et al., 2007; Onyewadume, 2002). Experimental studies oriented towards fitness and lasting longer than three weeks are rare (Cluphf et al., 2001; Frey et al., 1999; Lotan et al., 2004; Válková, 2011).

Skills in basketball, volleyball or table tennis have been experimentally proven to be parallel with fitness assessment (Downs & Wood, 1996; Shapiro and Dummer, 1998; Van Biesen et al., 2010; Vargas-Cuesta et al., 2010).

Special Olympics Healthy Athlete Program

The study presented here is based on the principles of the Special Olympics Healthy Athlete (SO HA) Assessment.

The Healthy Athlete Program is one of the complementary programmes but still proves very popular.

The key objectives of Special Olympics Healthy Athletes are to:

- Improve access to care at event-based and other health screening clinics;
- Make appropriate referrals for follow-up to community health professionals;
- Train health care professionals and students on the needs of people with intellectual disabilities;
- Collect, analyse and disseminate data on the health needs of people with intellectual disabilities; and

- Advocate for improved health policies and programs for people with intellectual disabilities.

The seven Healthy Athletes Disciplines are (the year of start):

- Special Olympics – Lions Clubs International Opening Eyes® (1991)
- Special Olympics Special Smiles® (1992)
- Special Olympics FUNfitness (1999)
- Special Olympics Healthy Hearing (2000)
- Special Olympics Health Promotion (2001)
- Special Olympics Fit Feet (2003)
- Special Olympics MedFest® (2007)

(www.specialolympics.org/health programs, the year of beginning of the program in bracket)

The screening of Special Olympians within the SO Healthy Athlete programme is included in the spectrum of complementary programs, during all of the SO World or Regional Summer and Winter Games. Educated clinical directors, medical staff and physiotherapists with trained volunteers then provide the screening. This programme is sponsored by many stakeholders, including medical companies. This is the reason why athletes can receive, if necessary, new glasses, tooth braches, soaps, catalogues of healthy meals and reports for home medical care, including vouchers for hearing aids. The national Special Olympics programmes provide the opportunity to participate and develop HA programmes in their home environment. Czech SO jointly ran this program in 2000. Since that first time, the HA program has been realised within national games or tournaments once or twice per year, especially FUNFitness and Health Promotion. The programme has, for a long time, been financially supported by the SOI and the EU.

The content of the HA FUNfitness test battery was developed according to the know-how of AAHPHER, and later for EUROFIT tests, with mild modification available for persons with intellectual disabilities e.g., "partial sit-up" (www.specialolympics.org/health programs). It includes the Time-Stand Test, the Partial Sit-UP-Test, the Single Leg Balance Test on the Right – Left leg, the Hand Grip Test of Right – Left hand, the Body Mass Index and the Heart Rate Index (www.specialolympics.org/health programmes).

The Fitness Test Battery (in the Czech SO arrangement) has been realised as a 'fitness decathlon' in order to ensure that the athletes are strongly motivated. Successful results, as well as the level of fitness improvement, are awarded with special HA ribbons. Athletes look foreword to results from FUNFitness screening because athletes, parents and coaches receive results after a comparison with their last achievements and assessment of the training effects, as well as for healthy behavior recommendations.

Within the University Affiliated Program, which is another very important SO complementary program, the Czech SO has developed a teaching pack for teaching HA skills. University student volunteers have the chance to access field practice and elaborate on their bachelor or master theses. Gába et al. (2012) have assessed the anthropological status of SO athletes according to the age cohort. Of the athletes who have passed their training at least twice per week 12% of them were found in the category 'obesity.' A trend of growing obesity has proved linear with a higher age.

Franek (2009) has compared the FUNFitness Battery results for three subgroups of participants in the Czech Athletic National Tournament: simple intellectual disability, Down syndrome and cerebral palsy. In comparing the subgroup with Down syndrome and with simple intellectual disability, significant differences were found in terms of flexibility (better results in Down syndrome group) and items of strength (worse for those with Down syndrome). The results of the participants in the subgroup with cerebral palsy were not homogeneous. These results should influence the choice of an appropriate sport and event.

Graciasová (2010) has assessed cross-country skiers in statistical balance on one leg with opened eyes through special laser technique. The athletes were able to pass quite complicated laboratory tests successfully. The balance test results were unexpectedly good even in very limited participants. Thus athletes and coaches should be pushed to train for more demanding events. The FUNFitness Battery results for cross-country skiers showed the best, average and the worst performances in competition (Bártková, 2014; Ševčíková, 2014). Winners showed better cardiovascular fitness than skiers with a worse performance but a lower than recommended norm for general population. Other fitness results created the typical cluster important for success in cross-country skiing: strength of hands and legs, abdominal muscle strength and balance.

The goal for the future of Czech SO is to describe a profile of health-related variables of athletes, according to the typical sports or events, being that the different sports can be influenced by different clusters of fitness variables and abilities. Thus, the training effect should be formulated and completed with a recommendation for healthy life style improvement.

Cross-Country Skiing within Special Olympics

Cross-country skiing is a winter sport in which participants propel themselves across snow-covered terrain using skies and poles (Rees, 2007). Recently the sport has been offered as one of 4 Special Olympics snow sports, along with alpine skiing, snow-boarding and snow-shoeing. Federation Internationale de Ski (FIS) Rules are applied with mild modifications (Special Olympics, 2010).

The competition events are divided into comparable categories according to the SO philosophy of providing opportunities according to age, gender and ability – so giving everyone a reasonable chance to win. The Low Level events are: 50 m and 100 m distance; Intermediate Level – 500 m, 1 km and 2, 3 or 5 km; and Advanced Level – 5 km, 7.5 km and 10 km. Athletes can combine races event within their level. A race of 3 km is exceptional as athlete can combine their races either in Intermediate Level or in Advanced Level. It is necessary to pass Low Level events with a diagonal step (more demanding for balance), while Intermediate Level events can be passed with a free technique, and athletes on the Advance Level events have to select and register either classical or skating style.

Low Level events are managed on a flat terrain, while Intermediate and Advanced races respect a plasticity of terrain: flat parts, curves, up and down parts, and the steepness of slope which demands fitness, skills and decision making, as well as motivation. It is necessary to underline the demanding training required. Some races are conducted using interval starts with one or two athletes starting intervals every 30 seconds, while others start with a simple pistol shot per maximum 8 athletes in one race (www.specialolympics.org/sports/crosscountry/). Cross-country skiing has been included in the SO program since the first Winter SO Games in 1977, Colorado, US (DePaw & Gavron, 2005, p. 101).

These developments to the traditional Winter Olympic Games structure have happened due to its popularity in a lot of countries. Cross-country skiing is a very common, frequent and accessible (not expensive) sports activity in countries with natural geographical and weather conditions; for instance, snow the during winter season. The CZ SO programme has developed cross-country since it was established in 1990. Movement, games and physical activities in the winter countryside have included cross-country skiing, while training can help athletes accommodate variants of cold, chill and frost, as well as a different profile of terrain, and the accommodation of ski equipment and social environment. These conditions create a strong cohesive composition of effective training for future health related fitness.

Ensuring effective training is the responsibility of educated coaches in several domains: intellectual disability, communication and social behavior, fitness loading, and cross-country skiing skills and technologies. Coaches have the opportunity to use textbooks or internal syllabuses of sports federations oriented towards fitness and the skills of the general population of different age (from preschoolers – beginners up to adult age and advanced competitors). However, the manuals for practical training of individuals with intellectual disabilities are rare, with the exception of the SO coaches manual (Special Olympics, 2010) and Canadian Long Term Athletes Development in cross-country (Rees, 2007, 2009).

DePaw and Gavron (2005) have presented the history and structure of SO management, competitions within the Special Olympics, including cross-country skiing. Text books in the original Czech language are very general in terms of syllabus design; only s survey of competitive events is presented, with the accent on mono-skiing and blind skiing, with no interest in skiing for athletes with intellectual disability. Moreover, general brief information is repeated several times (Jesina, 2007; Jesina, Janecka et al., 2008). The explanation of cross-country competition structure, rules and basic principles of training effects within CZ SO program has been formulated by Válková (2013).

INTENTION

Experimental studies have focused on cross-country skiing, while the training effect of the fitness of Special Olympians remains a rare topic (Válková, 2011, 2013). In accordance to the needs of the CZ SO program, the evidence-based investigations have been arranged, oriented towards the training influence on the personal fitness of cross-country skiers. Besides a description of health related fitness variables, the main intention of the project has been a comparison of fitness profiles with the level of each race. The continuum of follow-up steps was: a) to collect the data of fitness variables; b) to compare the data with real results in cross-country competition races and with gender; c) to summarise the training effect on personal fitness and to formulate recommendations for SO skiers.

The current goal is the definition of an adequate profile of skiers with different skills and limits, while making an argument for their involvement in the sport and adapted activities and for their improvement of physical fitness and appropriate healthy behavior. In regarding to the local field conditions, a limited number of real participants (but within specialisation) had to be accepted hence the first pilot study should be considered as progressive.

Basic questions concerning the project intention are as follows:

1. What are the average values of fitness variables for cross-country skiers?
2. What are the differences in fitness test performance when comparing recommendations for a general adult population?
3. Can we find some gender differences? If yes, which?
4. What is the role the of fitness variables from the aspect of lower and intermediate competitive events?
5. Is it possible to define the root cluster of fitness variables connected with a Lower or Intermediate Level of events?
6. Is it possible (on the bases of fitness variables achievements) to deduce the training effect on the anthropological and fitness status of adult Special Olympians competing as cross country skiers?

The investigations move across real sports environment with the aim of improving knowledge which can then be used by coaches, parents and volunteers in practice.

METHODS

Participants

The investigation was realised over one week of the Czech National Winter Games in 2015 and across a spectrum of sports: cross-country, downhill, snow-boarding. Only cross-country skiers were assessed. The study involved a cohort of adult Czech Special Olympians (39 male, 15 female) cross-country skiers of 25-45 years age, with all of them in the spectrum of moderate levels of intellectual disability (below 70 points of IQ) without any additional disability.

According to the Special Olympics Rules, participants of the national SO games had to pass minimum one year training. Our selected participants were engaged in several SO sports like track and field, swimming, cycling once or twice per week.

Participants had a former cross-country experience as they participated three times or more in winter SO competition. This means that it may be possible to deduce the effect of cross-country skiing training. The criteria for selection were: a) registration in Special Olympic programme with training in cross-country; b) independent competition in Low Level events (50-100 metres run) or Intermediate Level events (500 m – 1 km – 3 km); c) capability to pass independently Healthy Athlete - Fitness Test Battery (Table 1). A lower number of female participants was the reality because females do not practice sports as frequently as males (Coreen et al., 2009; Eichstaedt & Lavay, 1992; Foley et al., 2013; Rimmer et al., 2004; Taggart et al, 2012; Temple et al., 2003; Winnick and Short, 1985). Only two males and no females competed in the 5 and 10 km events, which was the reason why this category was not involved in this study.

Table 1. Survey of cross-country skiing participants

Gender	50 m cc-ski race	1 km cc-ski race	3 km cc-ski race	Avg. age	Total No of participants
Male	11	20	8	30.79	39
Female	5	8	2	30.78	15
Total No of participants	16	28	10	30.79	54

Table 2. Survey of used Special Olympics Healthy Athlete Tests (FUNFitness)

Abbreviation	Title	Purpose	Explanation	Measured unit
TST	Stand Up	strength of legs	stand up from sitting position on the chair as quick as possible	time for 10 attempts in sec.
PSUT	Partial Sit-Up	strength of abdominal muscles	sit up from laying position, legs on the chair, as quick as possible	number of attempts in 60 sec.
SLBR/SLBL	Single Leg Balance Test	static balance	stand on Right leg stand on Left leg	10 sec. is maximum
HGR/HGL	Hand Grip Test	strength of hands	Dynamometry of Right, Left hand in sitting position	2 attempts for each hand, better result in kg
BMI	Body Mass Index	body composition	height, weight, waist periphery	Processed index
HR QHR	Heart Rate Quiet Heart Rate	cardiovascular fitness	pulse, heart beat	pulse per minute

According http://www.specialolympics.org/healthprograms.

Data Collection and Processing

The data from two domains was collected: a) official final results of competition (50 m – 1 km – 3 km); b) HA FUNFitness Test Battery variables. Basic demographic data (age, level of mental disability, training history, etc.) was extracted from the registration protocol and events protocol.

In spite of the fact that a real HA FUNFitness Test Battery is very complex, selected variables relevant to the purpose of cross-country performance were used. Corresponding former knowledge and training experience for a cross-country performance is influenced by somatic characteristics (BMI), cardiovascular capacity, the dynamic strength of legs, the strength of abdominal muscles, hand-grip strength and balance (Frey et al., 1999; Graciasová, 2010; Rees, 2009; Shephard, 1990; Ševčíková, 2014; Válková, 2013).

As the number of athletes in this study was limited, the data was only processed according to descriptive statistics (average, mean, percent). The differences determined according to the criteria of 'gender' (male-female) and 'events requirements' (50 m – 1 km – 3 km) were processed in a visual comparison of average variables. This approach can be considered as appropriate for the first pilot study.

Research Procedures

The assessment was realised over one week during the Czech National Winter Games in 2015. The registration of athletes in CZ SO was supported by the permission of parents and caregivers for participation in the HA program, with request of anonymity and feedback. Feedback WAs an important part of screening which is relevant with SO rules (Special Olympics, 2007). This means that a complete research program was realised, related to ethical consent. The author knew nearly all of participants personally (their families too) and so we checked their demographic data from official documents.

a) Competition (preliminary and final) was realised in accordance with official time schedule: only one preliminary or final competition per day for each event. Quality of track corresponded with local conditions, but relevant to cross-country regulation of event. Coaches and athletes were pushed to prepare skiing (equipment, waxing) which was checked by officials. A collective start per maximum 8 athletes was used which is a common preference comparing an interval start in CZ SO. This design can provide a higher motivation for athletes, including competition for medals, ribbons or awards. Digital measurements of results (minutes and seconds) were provided by experienced coaches and officials.

b) Fitness variable assessment (HA FUNFitness Test Battery) was organised every day in the free time of athletes according to their competitions schedule, but in an appropriate time before their competition (not after). The athletes were motivated to achieve their best by being 'awarding' for their achievements with special ribbons. Athletes passed the tests without coaches' support. Ten trained volunteers assessed the athletes' fitness in the following circle: BMI (height – weight - waist), balance (single leg balance test, right – left leg), hands strength (hand grip test right – left hand), strength of legs (time-stand test), strength of abdominal muscles (partial sit-up test), heart rate index (step-test). Heart rate in quiet situation was measured in the morning before breakfast.

The individual results were discussed with coaches.

RESULTS AND COMMENT

Seeing that the Special Olympic Athletes in cross-country skiing are included in regular fitness and skills training for more than one year we can consider the results presented here as the effect of the SO program. These results are then presented relating to basic anthropological variable (BMI) and basic assessed abilities: cardiovascular fitness, strength (upper and lower limbs and abdominal muscles) and static balance (stand on one leg).

Body Mass Index (BMI) and Cardiovascular Fitness

An increasing number of obese and overweight people in the general population is a worldwide problem. Several authors not that the same trends of intellectual disability have been discovered in populations from different geographical, cultural or economy environment (Emerson, 2005; Lahtinen et al., 2007; Lejčarová, 2012; Onyewadume, 2006; Sohler et al., 2009; Stanish & Draheim, 2007; Stedman & Leland, 2010; Temple et al., 2006; Temple et al., 2010). Corresponding to these findings, researchers have also documented the BMI index of Special Olympic athletes with intellectual disability as a part of population (Foley et al., 2013; Harris, et al., 2003; Special Olympics, 2005, 2011). A cohesive survey by Foley´s team (Foley et al., 2013) has presented the trends in BMI of US adults athletes; here, the growing BMI in relation of age cohorts is significantly higher for SO female. In spite of the fact that only 39 males and 15 females have participated in the Czech study, the different Czech sports-culture environment has to be accepted, especially for participants recruited from cross-country skiers. Comparing Foley´s et al.'s review (2013) we can see general findings: the BMI index was comparable with average of general population particularly in group of skiers of an Intermediate Level (1 km, 3 km). There were no dramatic differences between gender groups, but great differences were found between ability levels in all aspects of variables even if on the border of the 'overweight zone.'

Female performed at a higher index than the males, even if all the participants underwent regular training for several years. On the other hand, the effect of regular training seems also to have been documented, as they are only 'on the border' in their adult age. The data banks of the body composition in persons with intellectual disability has not been collected in Czech Republic. Thus we can deduce that the results of the BMI values are not so bad, but that a lot of athletes should change their eating habits (according to the author's experience during their cross-country camps). Some of them eat too much or prefer sweets, while some of them have problems with meals which can be considered a general problem of SO athletes. This should thus be a challenge for parents' care and the coaches' training process.

Despite these adverse results a lot of athletes can do sports thanks to SO, which has started to solve the problems of people with intellectual disability, including physical performance. The differences in BMI amongst participants in different events level are visible; for instance, participants in Low Level events show a higher BMI index – the zone of 'overweight.' The question is, what is primary and what is a secondary problem? Somatic and cognitive limits, including obesity, cannot permit participation in 1 km and longer distances, or the lack of movement influence overweighting. The first idea seems to be valid according to practical experience with SO training and competitions, and this fact can be considered to constitute a positive involvement in adequate sports and competitive level (coaches responsibility), but it can probably also be taken as a marker of lack of training.

The identical explanation that we can formulate about this issue involves the heart rate (Table 3). QHR is very weak in all cases; either we use the norms of World Health Organization for general population or 'soft' recommendation of SOI to make comparison. Several values of individuals were extreme (e.g., 1 girl – skier: QHR 102 pulses, the same girl

107 pulses after step-test). Extremely low differences after step-test loading and consequently mild difference between QHR and HR after a 2 minute rest were found. Standard HR during loading in training (and step-test loading) should be about 130-150 pulses per minute for a SO population with intellectual disability. The gaps in comparison to a healthy population were found in resting the heart rate which showed physical performance and sports fitness. The men's heart rate returned to resting value better than the women's return. Female presented worse performance than female and men again, and the level of event also proved very strong determinant. We hence need to underline more intensive physical activity in the future.

Table 3. Results of heart rate indexes and BMI of cross-country skiers

Gender		Male			Female		
event		50 m	1 km	3 km	50 m	1 km	3 km
No		N = 11	N = 20	N = 8	N = 5	N = 8	N = 2
average achievement/min		0:38	10:12	19:26	1:34	11:36	19:04
Mean		x	x	x	x	x	x
QHR (puls/min)		83.2	91.2	87.0	76.0	94.7	91.0
aft S-T (puls/min)		105.8	115.5	103.3	101.6	105.3	101.0
aft 2 min (puls/min)		91.7	99.4	86.4	78.0	100.0	89.0
% difference - QHR		7.5	8.2	0.6	0.0	6.5	- 2.2
BMI		25.2	24.2	24.9	27.5	25.1	24.04
BMI – WHO recommendation	norm	18.5 - 24.9			18.5 - 24.9		
	overweight	25.0 - 29.9			25.0 - 29.9		

Legend: QHR: heart rate in quite situation; aft S-T: after step-test; aft 2 min: after 2 minutes rest; % difference - QHR: difference between QHR and returned heart rate after 2 minutes rest; BMI: body mass index; WHO – World Health Organization.
http://www. netfit.co.uk/fitness/test/resting-heart-rate.htm, Manual FUNfitness Special Olympics (2007, p. 56).

Table 4. Comparison of cross-country skiers QHR with general norms and SOI recommendation

Gender	Criterion of QHR	Norm of QHR age 25-35	Norm of QHR age 36-45
Male	average	71-74	75-81
	under average	75-81	76-82
	week	more than 82	more than 83
	research sample	83-91	
Female	average	73-76	74-78
	under average	77-82	79-84
	week	more than 83	more than 85
	research sample	74-95	
SOI Healthy Athletes recommendation, male + female more than 18	excellent	under 70	
	average	70-90	
	week	more than 90	

http://www.netfit.co.uk/fitness/test/resting-heart-rate.htm, Manual FUNfitness Special Olympics (2007, p. 56).

Selected Fitness Variables

In spite of the fact that the real HA FUNFitness Test Battery is very complex, we selected variables relevant only to the purpose of cross-country performance: somatic characteristics (BMI), cardiovascular capacity, dynamic strength of legs, abdominal muscles strength, hand-grip strength and balance (Graciasová, 2010; Rees, 2009; Ševčíková, 2014).

The findings that the people with intellectual disabilities have lower physical fitness than the non-disabled is documented in a lot of studies (Foley et al., 2013; Lahtinen et al., 2007; Onyewadume, 2006; Pitetti & Yarmer, 2002; Pitetti et al., 2010; Reid et al., 1985; Rintala et al., 1997; Temple, et al., 2006; Válková, 1998, 2011; Van Biesen et al., 2010). In spite of this fact, we can only compare average values of assessed variables gender differences, which were very mild, even in males presented in higher ranking. The specific results in balanced abilities were nearly equal, although hand grip strength was an exception as male values were dramatically different (Table 4). Knowing the athletes, we can then add the men involved in sheltered jobs that use manual work strength (butchers, bricklayers, repairmen) parallel with their training, and women working in cleaning and washing jobs that are not too demanding on hand grip strength. Comparing the norms for the general population (EUROFIT norms), our cross-country skiers presented lower level performance. Thus, compared to the norms of Skowronski (2009) for a population with intellectual disability, our results were in accordance with this recommendation.

Seeing that different events (50 m – 1 km – 3 km) are logically different and demanding on fitness, we analysed selected fitness variables according to the individual events. Running distances of 1 km and 3 km are influenced by cognitive loading, while competitors also have to pass the ski track independently so solving problems the technique required (slope up, slope down, curves, etc.), cardiovascular and breathing problems and fatigue coping, while maintaining intrinsic motivation for a longer time. The average time for 1 km was about 10:12 minutes for males, 11:36 min for female, for 3 km 19:26 min for males and 19:04 min for females (but the results were distorted by the fact that there were only two very well trained girls). In spite of using only descriptive statistics, the average test items was well documented. A lower level event involves a lower level of fitness performance within both male and female gender groups. Strong visible gaps were found between 50 m and 1 km runs, but not so strong between 1 km and 3 km races.

Being that our athletes are involved in SO physical activity program lasting for more than 3 years, we can deduce the training effect is evident when even their average age is more than 30 years (Table 1). From the opposite perspective, balance the ability of even 'lower level' athletes can be considered as good background for their participation in higher levels of events. We need to underline the equal request as in the case of cardiovascular fitness; that is, more time for training, more intensive physical activity and more specialised training in cross-country skiing.

CONCLUSION

The training effect on the fitness of the general population is a well-known fact too assessed in the environment of people with intellectual disability (Dixon-Ibarra, et al., 2013;

Emerson, 2005; Lahtinen, et al., 2007; Lotan, et al., 2004; Onyewadume, 2002; Pitetti, et all., 2002, 2010; Temple, et al., 2006; Válková, 1998, 2014; Vargas-Cuesta, et al., 2010). General facts about the benefit of non-specified physical exercises, motor activities and their influence on health-related fitness variables can be useful for daily physical loading. In terms of sports participation, it is necessary to apply general knowledge to specific sports.

Another issue is the spectrum of acceptance within the domain of 'intellectual disability' which is very broad. Health related variables are influenced both by intellectual background and training. According to both the philosophy and rules of the Special Olympics, participation either in Low Level or Intermediate Level (or high one) events should be in accordance with mental limits: cognitive, emotional and socio-behavioral. In secondary terms, the design of the description of fitness variables within the domain 'event level' can provide a comparison between these categories so assess developmental trends in athletes' improvement.

Table 5. Survey of fitness variables of cross-country skiers comparing the gender

gender	Male N = 39		Female N = 15		Skowr	Skowr
	Mean	SD	Mean	SD	M/F IQ 55-69	M/F IQ 40-54
TST (s)	21.63	± 5.79	20.51	± 5.13		
PSUT (attempts)	20.36	± 6.62	18.91	± 5.92	21.7/16.4 ± 4.9/± 6.0	15.7/11.1 ± 5.7/± 4.9
SLBR (s)	8.69	± 2.18	8.61	± 2.53	6.0/5.9 ± 0.2/± 0.6	5.6/5.4 ± 0.7/± 0.1
SLBL (s)	8.42	± 2.38	8.81	± 2.91		
HGR (kg)	16.70	± 12.71	5.45	± 8.66		
HGL (kg)	16.19	± 11.76	58.30	± 8.92		

Legend: TST (s) - Time-Stand Test in seconds; PSUT (attempts in 60 seconds) – Partial Sit-UP-test; SLBR/SLBL (stand in seconds) - Single Leg Balance Test (Right – Left leg); HGR/HGL (kg) - Hand Grip Test (Right – Left hand; Skowr – norms of Skowronski et al. (2009).

Table 6. Survey of fitness variables of cross-country skiers comparing the events

Gender	Male			Female		
event N	50 m N = 11	1 km N = 20	3 km N = 8	50 m N = 5	1 km N = 8	3 km N = 2
Mean	x	x	x	x	x	x
achievement/min	0:38	10:12	19:26	1:34	11:36	19:04
TST (s)	22.30	21.33	21.12	22.35	20.75	20.50
PSUT (attempts)	18.36	20.36	20.88	17.05	18.91	18.50
SLBR (s)	6.43	10.00	10.00	6.07	8.15	10.00
SLBL (s)	5.78	9.32	10.00	5.42	8.05	10.00
HGR (kg)	14.80	18.45	18.66	5.12	6.45	12.00
HGL (kg)	14.21	18.11	18.23	5.15	5.83	11.50

Legend: TST (s) - Time-Stand Test in seconds; PSUT (attempts in 60 seconds) – Partial Sit-UP-test; SLBR/SLBL (stand in seconds) - Single Leg Balance Test (Right – Left leg); HGR/HGL (kg) - Hand Grip Test (Right – Left hand).

The future goal is then to analyse systematically the cohesive athletes' profiles of SO sports in common with the Czech Special Olympics programme. The aim is therefore to formulate the arguments for their involvement in the available sports levels, both to improve their health-related fitness variables and to include the variables of psycho-social wellbeing.

We are limited to presenting the following achievements of our study:

- the number of participants – 54 (see Table 1),
- the age cohort (age span 25-45 years, average 30.79),
- data processing only with descriptive statistics.

The homogenous variables involve a moderate level of intellectual disability and more than three years participation in SO sports programmes. Despite the limits described, it is possible to conclude:

- involvement of our described participants in SO cross-country skiing program is only one chance to be active in training and competitions in the winter season;
- doing a regular sport in an age range of between 25-45 years can be considered as an unique finding generally compared to an able-bodied population;
- the results of BMI index were on the border of the overweight–obesity zone, both in males and females;
- the results of all the cardiovascular fitness indexes were very weak, again both in male and female, which is a significant warning not only for performances in cross-country skiing, but even for daily activities and general health;
- the fitness variables assessed were lower compared to the results of regular population (Měkota & Kovář, 1995) but adequate compared to recommendation for individuals with intellectual disability (Skowroński, 2009; Special Olympics, 2007, 2011);
- the gender differences with respect to the event level (50 m – 1 km – 3 km distances) were minimal (male results higher than female), except with hand grip strength where males showed a dramatically higher performance than female;
- all fitness variables were relevant to the event level, and were weak in results of 50 m race participants, visible differences between 50 m and 1 km findings;
- all the fitness variables were weak, but for the 50 m run participants it seemed (logically) to be enough for future involvement in higher level events;
- the cluster of crucial variables important for cross-country skiing consisted of BMI, cardiovascular fitness, balance, the strength of abdominal muscles, dynamic strength of legs, hand grip strength which should be accepted as the criterion for the improvement of fitness oriented on success in cross-country skiing;
- the SO philosophy and formulated regulation dealing with events level (Low – Intermediate – Advanced) are valid both for theory and training practice, which is useful for the safety, fitness, skills and psychosocial development of athletes;
- the coaches of cross-country skiers in CZ SO did a good job as they selected and trained athletes at an adequate event level with the respect to their physical and mental abilities and limits. In spite of these findings, more intensive training had to be stressed step by step;

- the effect of cross-country skiing, as well as other interventions, was important for competition and for daily life, including sheltered manual jobs;
- the Special Olympics Healthy Athlete programme is documented as being beneficial for the healthy lifestyle of SO athletes.

ACKNOWLEDGMENTS

The project was supported by a Special Olympics Europe/Eurasia Healthy Athletes Grant – Fitness Innovation Progress, 2015.

REFERENCES

Bártková, K. (2014). Analýza výsledků step-testu a běžeckého lyžování sportovců Speciálních olympiád [Analyses of step-test results of Special Olympics cross-country skiers]. *Diplomová práce bakalářská* [Bachelors theses]. Olomouc: Palacký University, Faculty of Physical Culture.

Broadhead, G., and Church, G. (1984). Influence of test selection on physical education placement of mentally retarded children. *Adapted Physical Activity Quarterly, 2,* 112-118.

Chrysagis, N., Douka, A., Nikopoulos, M., Apostopoulu, F., and Koutsouki, D. (2009). Effects of aquatic program on gross motor function of children with spactic cerebral palsy. *Biology of Exercise,* 5(2), 13-25.

Chynias, A.K., Reid, G., and Hoover, M.H. (1998). Exercise effect on health-related fitness of individuals with an intellectual disability. *Adapted Physical Activity Quarterly,* 15, 119-40.

Cluphf, D., O'Connor, J., and Vanin, S. (2001). Effects of aerobic dance on the cardiovascular endurance of adults with intellectual disabilities. *Adapted Physical Activity Quarterly,* 18, 60-71.

Coreen, M., Harada, C., M., and Siperstein, G. N. (2009). The sport experience of athletes with intellectual disabilities: a national survey of Special Olympics athletes and their families. *Adapted Physical Activity Quarterly,* 26, 68-85.

Cratty, B. (1972). *The Special Olympics: A national opinion survey.* UCLA.

DePaw, K.P., and Gavron, S.J. (2005). *Disability Sport.* Champaign, IL: Human Kinetics, ICL.

Dixon-Ibarra, A., Lee, M., and Dugala, A. (2013). Physical activity and sedentary behavior in older adults with intellectual disabilities: A comparative study. *Adapted Physical Activity Quarterly*, 30(1), 1-19.

Downs, B.S., and Wood, T.M. (1996). Validating a Special Olympics volleyball skills assessment test. *Adapted Physical Activity Quarterly,* 13, 166-179.

Draheim, C.C., Williams, D.P., and McCubbin, J. A. (2003). Cardiovascular disease risk factor differences between Special Olympians and non-Special Olympians. *Adapted Physical Activity Quarterly*, 20, 118-133.

Dykens, E.M., and Cohen, D. (1996). Effects of Special Olympics international on social competence in persons with mental retardation. *Journal of the American Academy of Child and Adolescent Psychiatry,* 35(2), 223-229.

Dykens, E.M., Valkova, H., and Mactavish, J.B. (1999). Psychosocial correlates of participants in Special Olympics International. *Report presented at the Strategic Research Symposium of Special Olympics*, Fearrington House, Pitsboro, NC.

Eichstaedt, C.B., and Lavay, B.W. (1992). *Physical activity for disabled with mental retardation*. Champaign, IL: Human Kinetics.

Emerson, E. (2005). Underweight, obesity and exercise among adults with intellectual disability in supported accommodation in Northern England. *Journal of Intellectual Disability Research*, 49, 134-143.

Faison-Hodge, J. and Poretta, D.L. (2004). Physical activity levels of students with mental retardation and students without disabilities. *Adapted Physical Activity Quarterly*, 21, 139-152.

Faith, F. (1972). *Special Physical Education*. Philadelphia: W.B. Saunders Company.

Foley, J.T., Lloyd, M., and Temple, V.A. (2013). Body mass index trends among adult US Special Olympians, 2005-2010. *Adapted Physical Activity Quarterly*, 30, 373-386.

Franek, J. (2009). Analýza programu FUNFitness u osob s mentální retardací – účastníků Speciální olympiády [Analysis of FUNFitness program for persons with mental retardation - Special Olympics participants]. *Diplomová práce magisterská* [Master diploma theses]. Praha: Faculty of Physical Education and Sports.

Frey, G.C., McCubbin, J.A., Hanningan-Downs, S. Kasser, S.L., and Skaggs, S. O. (1999). Physical fitness of trained runners with and without mental retardation. *Adapted Physical Activity Quarterly,* 16, 126-137.

Gába, A., Přidalová, M., Válková, H., Walkley, J., and Gábová, Z. (2012). Hodnocení tělesného složení u jedinců se středně těžkou mentální retardací [Analysis of the body composition in individuals with moderate mental retardation]. *Česká antropologie* 61(1), 15-20.

Goodwin, D.L., Fitzpatrick, D.A., Thurmeier, R., and Hall, C. (2006). The decision to join Special Olympics: Parents' perspectives. *Adapted Physical Activity Quarterly,* 23, 163-83.

Graciasová, T. (2010). Postural stability of females with an intellectual disability participating in Special Olympics. *Erasmus-Mundus diploma theses*. Olomouc: Palacky University, Faculty of Physical Culture.

Harris, N., Rosenberg, A., Jangda, S., O´Brien, K., and Gallagher, M.L. (2003). Prevalence of obesity in international Special Olympic athletes as determined by body mass index. *Journal of the American Dietetic Association*, 103, 235-237.

Hourcade, J.J. (1989). Special Olympics: a review and critical analysis. *Therapeutic Recreation Journal*, 23, 58-65.

Ješina, O. (2007). *Aplikované pohybové aktivity v zimní přírodě* (Adapted Physical Activity in winter nature). Olomouc: Univerzita Palackého.

Ješina, O., Janečka, Z. (2008). *Aplikované pohybové aktivity v zimní přírodě II* (Adapted Physical Activity in winter nature). Olomouc: Univerzita Palackého.

Lahtinen, U., Rintala, P., and Malin, V. (2007). Physical performance of individuals with intellectual disability: A 30-year follow-up. *Adapted Physical Activity Quarterly*, 24, 125-143.

Lejčarová, A. (2012). Motorická výkonnost osob s intelektovým postižením v závislosti na úrovni jejich intelektových schopností (Motor performance of people with intellectual disabilities, depending on the level of their intellectual abilities) In: P. Tillinger (Ed.) *Sport osob s intelektovým postižením,* 135-148. Praha: Charles University, Carolinum.

Lotan, M., Isakov, E., Kessel, S., and Merrick, J. (2004). Physical Fitness and Functional Ability of Children with Intellectual Disability: Effects of a Short-Term Daily Treadmill Intervention. *The Scientific World Journal*, 4, 449-457. Retrieved 23. 3. 2014 from the World Wide Web: http://www.hindawi.com/journals/tswj/2004/950740/abs/.

Měkota, K., and Kovář, R. (1995). *UNIFITTEST (6-60): tests and norms of motor performance and physical fitness in youth and in adult age.* Olomouc: Palacky University.

Nankervis, K., Cousins, W., Válková, H., and Macintyre, T. (2014). Physical activity, exercise, and sport. In: L. Taggart, W. Cousins (Eds.). *Health Promotion for People with Intellectual and Developmental Disabilities*, 174-183. McGraw Hill: Open University Press.

Ninot, G., Billard, J., Delignieres, D., and Sokolowski, M. (2000). Effects of integrated sports participation on perceived competence for adolescents with mental retardation. *Adapted hysical Activity Quarterly,* 17, 208-221.

Orelove, F.P., Wehman, P., and Wood, J. (1982). An evaluative review of Special Olympics: Implications for community integration. *Education and Training of the Mentally Retarded,* 325-329.

Özer, D., Baran, F., Aktop, A., Nalbant, S., Aglamis, E., and Hutzler, Y. (2012). Effects of a Special Olympics unified sports soccer program on psycho-social attributes of youth with and without intellectual disability. *Research in Developmental Disabilities,* 33, 229-239.

Onyewadume, I.U. (2006). Fitness of black African early adolescents with and without mild mental retardation. *Adapted Physical Activity Quarterly*, 23, 277-292.

Onyewadume, I.U. (2002) Physical fitness profile of Special Olympic-bound athletes: implications for performance success, injury proneness and future preparations. *Research Bi-annual for Movement*, 18(2), 18-36.

Pitetti, K.H. et al. (1989). Fitness and level of adult Special Olympics participants. *Adapted Physical Activity Quarterly*, 6, 354-370.

Pitetti, K.H., Fernhall, B., Stubbs, N., and Stadler, L. Jr. (1997). A step test for evaluating the aerobic fitness of children and adolescents with mental retardation. *Adapted Physical Activity Quarterly*, 9(2), 127-135.

Pitetti, K.H., Jackson, J. A, Stubbs, N.B., Campbell, K.D., and Battar, S.S. (2010). Fitness levels of adult Special Olympic participants. *Adapted Physical Activity Quarterly*, 6(4), 354-370.

Pitetti, K.H., and Yarmer, D.A. (2002). Lower body strength of children and adolescents with and without mild mental retardation: a comparison. *Adapted Physical Activity Quarterly*, 26, 324-333.

Rarick, G. L., Widdop, J. H., and Broadhead, G. D. (1970). The physical fitness and motor competence of educable mentally retarded children. *Exceptional Children*, 36, 509-519.

Rees, D. (2007). Cross-country skiing: Sport for life. Able-bodied LTAD Guide. (http://www.cccski.com/getmedia/13d28c29-2b22-45c8-9caf-0a855583fe08/LTAD-guide-CCC.pdf.aspx).

Rees, D. (2009). Cross-country skiing: Disabled LTAD Guide. http://www.cccski.com/getmedia/0c392394-4715-4874-9534-58416fe99fe1/CCC-AWAD-Fin2small.pdf.aspx.

Reid, G., Montgomery, D.L., and Seidl, C. (1985). Performance of mentally retarded adults on the Canadian standardized test of fitness. *Canadian Journal of Public Health*, 76, 187-190.

Rimmer, J.H., Riley, B., Wang, E., Rauworth, A., and Jurkowski, J. (2004). Physical activity participation among persons with disability. *American Journal of Preventive Medicine,* 26, 419-425.

Rintala, P., Dunn, J. M., McCubbin, J. A., and Guinn, C. (1992). Validity of a cardiorespiratory fitness test for men with mental retardation. *Medicine and Science in Sports and Exercise,* 24, 941-945.

Rintala, P., McCubin, J.A., Downs, S.B., and Fox, S.D. (1997). Cross-validation of the 1-mile walking test for men with mental retardation. *Medicine and Science in Sports and Exercise,* 29, 133-137.

Rintala, P., and Palsio, N. (1994). Effects of physical education programs on children with learning disabilities. In: K. Yabe et al. (Eds.) *Adapted Physical Activity: Health and Fitness.* Tokyo: Springer Verlag.

Roswal, G.M., Roswal, P.M., and Dunleavy, A.O. (1984). Normative health related fitness data in Special Olympians. In: C. Sherrill (Ed.), *Sport and Disabled Athletes.* Champaign, IL: Human Kinetics Publishers.

Roswal, G.M., Damentko, M.B., Smith, G.W., Braycich, M.J., and Krogulec, M. (2003). Sport for individuals with mental disabilities in Asia, Eurasia, and Europe. *Palaestra,* 19 (4), 20-24.

Shapiro, D.R., and Dummer, G.M. (1998). Perceived and actual basketball competence of adolescent males with mental retardation. *Adapted Physical Activity Quarterly,* 15, 179-190.

Shapiro, D. R. (2003). Participation motives of Special Olympics athletes. *Adapted Physical Activity Quarterly,* 20, 150-165.

Shepard, R.J. (1990). *Fitness in Special population.* Champaign, IL: Human Kinetics, Inc.

Sit, C.H.P., McKenzie, T.L., Lian, J.M.G., and McManus, A. (2008). Activity levels during physical education and recess in two special schools for children with mild intellectual disabilities. *Adapted Physical Activity Quarterly,* 25, 247-259.

Skowronski, W., Horvat, M., Nocera, J., Roswal, G., and Croce, R. (2009). Eurofit Special: European fitness battery score variation among individuals with intellectual disabilities. *Adapted Physical Activity Quarterly,* 26, 54-67.

Sohler, N., Lubetkin, E., Levy, J., Soghomonian, C., and Rimmerman, A. (2009). Factors associated with obesity and coronary heart disease in people with intellectual disabilities. *Social Work in Health Care,* 48, 76-89.

Special Olympics (2005). Changing attitudes, changing the world: the health and health care of people with intellectual disabilities. In: *(SOI) Turning research knowledge into action.*

Special Olympics (2007). *Healthy choices, healthy athletes: health promotion guide for Clinical Directors.* Washington DC: Special Olympics.

Special Olympics (2010). *Special Olympics General Rules.* www.specialolympics.org.

Special Olympics (2011). 2011 Special Olympics reach report. *Adapted Physical Activity Quarterly,* 26, 54-67.

Stanish, H.I., and Draheim, C.C. (2007). Walking activity, body composition, and blood pressure in adults with intellectual disabilities. *Journal of Applied Research in Intellectual Disabilities,* 20(3), 183-190.

Stedman, K.V., and Leland, L.S. (2010). Obesity and intellectual disability in New Zealand. *Journal of Intellectual and Developmental Disability,* 35, 112-115.

Ševčíková, K. (2014). Výsledky programu Zdravý atlet u sportovců s mentálním postižením Speciálních olympiád v běžeckém lyžování [FUNfitness results of athletes with intellectual disability participating in Special Olympics cross-country skiing]. *Bachelor diploma theses.* Olomouc: Faculty of Physical Culture, Palacky University.

Taggart, L., andCousins, W. (2014). *Health Promotion for People with Intellectual and Developmental Disabilities.* London: Open University Press.

Temple, V.A., Frey, G.C., and Stanish, H.I. (2006). Physical activity of adults with mental retardation: review and research needs. *American Journal of Health Promotion,* 21(1), 2-12.

Temple, V.A., Walkley, J.W., and Greenway, K. (2010). Body mass index as an indicator of adoposity among adults with intellectual disability. *Journal of Intellectual and Developmental Disability,* 35, 116-120.

Temple, V.A., and Walkley, J.W. (2003). Physical activity of adults with intellectual disability. *Journal of Intellectual and Developmental Disability,* 28(4), 342-352.

Válková, H. (2011). Changes in perceived health related variables of Special Olympians after two years intervention program. In: J. Labudová and B. Antala (Eds.) *Healthy active life style and physical education.* 192-204. *FIEP book of scientific and professional articles.* Topolčianky: Slovak society for education and sport.

Válková, H. (1998). The development of indices of motor competence and social behavior of participants and non-participants in the Special Olympics movement. *Acta Universitatis Palackianae Olomucensis Gymnica,* 28, 53-59.

Válková, H. (2013). Zimní sporty ve Speciálních olympiádách (Winter sports in the Special Olympics). In: D. Trávníková, V. Pacholík (Eds.). *Aplikované pohybové aktivity,* (pp. 283-298). Brno: Masaryk´ University, Faculty of Sport Studies.

Válková, H., Hansgut, V., and Nováčková, M. (1999). The reflection of Special Olympics sports international programme in inner experience of adolescents with mental retardation. *Acta Universitatis Palackianae Olomucensis Gymnica,* 29, 57-64.

Van Biesen, D.,Verellen, J., Meyer, C., Mactavish, J., Van de Vliet, P., and Vanlandewijck, Y. (2010). The ability of elite table tennis players with intellectual disabilities to adapt their service/return. *Adapted Physical Activity Quarterly,* 27(3), 242-257.

Vargas-Cuesta, A.I., Lourido-Paz, B., and Rodriguez, A. (2011). Physical fitness in adults with intellectual disabilities: Differences between levels of sport practice. *Research in Developmental Disabilities,* 32, 788-794.

Vermeer, A. et al. (1990). *Motor development, adapted physical activity and mental retardation.* Basel: Karger.

Vermeer, A., and Davis, W. E. (Eds.). (1995). *Physical and motor development in mental retardation.* Bassel: Karger.

Wilhite, B., and Kleiber, D.A. (1992). The effects of Special Olympics participation on community integration. *Therapeutic Recreation Journal,* 4, 9-20.

Winnick, J.P., and Short, F. (1985). *Physical fitness testing of the disabled.* Champaign, IL: Human Kinetics.

Winter, C.F., Bastiaanse, L.P., Hilgenkamp, T.L.M., Evenhuis, H.M., and Echteld, M.A. (2011). Overwight and obesity in older people with intellectual disability. *Research in Developmental Disabilities,* 33, 398-405.

Wolfensberger, W. (1995). Of "normalization," lifestyles, the Special Olympics, deinstitutionalization, mainstreaming, integration, and cabbages and kings. *Mental retardation*, 33, 128-131.

Wright, J., and Cowden, J.E. (1986). Changes in self concept and cardiovascular endurance of mentally retarded youth in Special Olympics swim training program. *Adapted Physical Activity Quarterly*, 3, 177-183.

In: Physical Activity Effects on the Anthropological Status ...   ISBN: 978-1-63484-782-7
Editors: Fadilj Eminović and Milivoj Dopsaj   © 2016 Nova Science Publishers, Inc.

Chapter 11

EFFECTS OF DIFFERENT PHYSICAL EXERCISE LEVELS ON THE BODY STRUCTURE IN ADULTS OF BOTH GENDER

Milivoj Dopsaj[1],, Marina Đorđević-Nikić[1] and Miloš Maksimović[2]*

[1]University of Belgrade, Faculty of Sport and Physical Education,
Belgrade, Serbia
[2]University of Belgrade, Faculty of Medicine, Belgrade, Serbia

ABSTRACT

Physical inactivity is one of the key health risk factors, directly related to both the increase in prevalence of noncommunicable diseases and to the reduction in work ability and functional capacity in the general population. Another result of reduced physical activity is noticeable in the emerging pandemic of obesity. The main aim of this study was to define relations between physical activity and/or exercise, and characteristics of body composition in working-age population of both genders living in Belgrade, the capital city of Serbia. The sample included 4489 apparently healthy Serbian males (N = 3065) and females (N = 1424) aged 18 to 69.9 years. The total sample was divided into four groups with respect to the frequency of physical activity or exercise: Group 1 – Sedentary, with subjects who performed ≤ 1 exercise/physical activity sessions/week; Group 2 – Casual, with subjects who performed 2-3 exercise/physical activity sessions/week; Group 3 – Committed, with subjects who performed 4-5 exercise/physical activity sessions/week; and, Group 4 – Steady, with subjects who performed ≥ 6 exercise/physical activity sessions/week). Body composition was measured via multisegmental bioelectrical impedance analysis using InBody 720 Tetrapolar 8-Point Tactile Electrode System. The research study used eight variables to describe the body composition of the sample: body height (BH), body mass (BM); body mass index (BMI); fat free mass (FFM); body fat mass (BFM); percent of body fat (PBF); fat free mass index (FFMI); and, body fat mass index (BFMI). MANOVA, ANOVA and t-test were

---

* Corresponding Author, Email: milivoj@eunet.rs.

used to establish the differences among groups, while linear regression analysis was used to define the trends of change. The results obtained suggest that an increase in physical activity and exercise had positive effects on body structure. The results showed a greater impact of physical activity/exercise on the change in body composition in men than in women, with the average change trend in all variables in men higher by 27.04%, ranging between 5.35% in FFM to 59.07% in BM. Finally, the results may indicate that the minimal frequency of physical activity/exercise should be at least four times per week in both men and women, with the duration of between 274 and 307 min of exercise/physical activity per week, i.e., between 60 and 67 min of exercise/physical activity per session.

Keywords: physical activity, physical exercise, bioimpedance, adults, body composition

INTRODUCTION

It is well known that deviations from normal values for weight, body composition, adiposity or percent of body fat are associated with health risk (WHO, 2000; Adams et al., 2006). One of the key factors of the growing prevalence of noncommunicable diseases in the late 20th century resulted from a dramatic increase in overweight and obesity in the population of both developed and developing countries (Kolata, 1985; Caban et al., 2005; Boričić et al., 2013). As early as 1985, it was established that 60% of US black women between ages 45-55 were obese, relative to 30% of similar US white women and 26% of the entire US population (Kolata, 1985). The data for the period 2009-2010 showed that the prevalence of obesity in U.S. children and adolescents aged 2-19 years was 18.6% and 15.0% for boys and girls, respectively, as well as 35.63% and 36.50% for the adult men and women, respectively (Ogden et al., 2012); at the same time, higher obesity prevalence rates peaked in motor vehicle operators, i.e., 31.7% and 31.0% in men and women, respectively (Caban et al., 2005).

On the molecular level, it is maintained that obesity is caused by a multidimensional problem with three underlying mechanisms: feeding control, control of energy efficiency and adipogenesis (Palou et al., 2000). In practice, this means that the changes in the lifestyle patterns towards sedentary behavior (driving a car, sitting at home and at work, television viewing, surfing the Internet, or playing video games) that replaced more active pursuits result in a sustained positive energy balance. In turn, this leads to an increase in the prevalence of overweight and obesity, cardiovascular or metabolic disease risk factors, in children and adults of both genders (Kolata, 1985; De Lorenco et al., 2011; Ogden et al., 2012; Boričić et al., 2013; Đorđević-Nikić et al., 2013). The results of studies published in leading scientific journals worldwide document that during the last fifty years there has been a significant trend towards an increase in the prevalence of overweight and obesity both among children (Moreno et al., 2005; Ogden et al., 2012) and adults (Eiben et al., 2005; Ogden et al., 2012); this has occurred worldwide (Moreno et al., 2005; Ogden et al., 2012; Ahmed et al., 2012); this has been recognized as a global health phenomenon (Lewis et al., 2000; Wang et al., 2002), which significantly reduces the quality of life (Hopman et al., 2007).

In Canada between 1981 and 1996, the prevalence of obesity in children more than doubled over that period, from 5% to 13.5% for boys and 11.8% for girls (Tremblay and Willms, 2000). The prevalence of obesity increased in the U.S. starting in the 1980s, and for the period 1985-1986 to 1995-1996, each race-sex group experienced significant secular weight gains ranging from 0.96 kg/year in African-American women to 0.55 kg/year in white women

(Lewis et al., 2000). Generally, evidence suggests that obesity prevalence continued to increase in the young and in men, while some researchers found that it may have reached a plateau in women. Some results showed that at least 32% of adults in the U.S were obese, but extreme obesity (BMI ≥ 40 kg•m^{-2}) was higher in women than in men, with 6.9% vs 2.8%, respectively (WHO, 2000). Recent results for U.S. obesity rates showed a significant increase over the period between 1986 and 2002, irrespective of race and gender, with the average yearly change from 0.61% (±0.04) from 1986 to 1995, to 0.95% (±0.11) from 1997 to 2002 (Caban et al., 2005).

Generally, obese and overweight children had the greatest risk of becoming obese or overweight young adults. Their weight history shows that 40.0% of males and 48.6% of females who were obese at the age of 18 had already been obese at the age of 7 (Starc and Strel, 2011). With respect to Serbia, recent results indicate that the overall prevalence of overweight and obesity in schoolchildren aged 6–14 years was at 39.0% (31.7% overweight and 7.3% obese). This was slightly lower in boys, at 38.3% (31.5% overweight and 6.8% obese) than in girls, at 40.4% (32.2% overweight and 8.2% obese) (Ostojić et al., 2011). The most recent published study was designed to assess the prevalence of overweight and obesity in urban schoolchildren in Serbia, coming from schools located in the capital city of Belgrade. From the sample of 14% of Belgrade elementary school population aged 9-15 years, there was 24.2% prevalence in the total sample, 19.2% of which accounted for overweight, and 5.0% for obese schoolchildren.

Monitoring changes in the body composition across different age groups is of paramount importance not only for epidemiological and scientific reasons, but also for the control of the status in a particular population.

Biologically, in relation to the macro level, the human body is composed of four main measurable components: water, fat, mineral, and protein (Đorđević-Nikić et al., 2013). For the sake of research and clinical work, certain morphological indices can also be defined in order to determine the ratio between particular components, or even segmentary ratios of the same components, which would complement the information on the basic elements of the body structure (Dopsaj et al., 2015).

According to the indicators issued by the Institute of Public Health, the adult population in Serbia is among the world's top-ranked regarding the rates of morbidity and mortality from heart and blood vessel diseases, metabolic and malignant diseases and others (Boričić et al., 2013). On the other hand, physical activity and exercise have been recognized as significant predictors considering the prevention of various noncommunicable diseases (Hopman et al., 2007), and have therefore been included among the desirable routine and behavioral patterns of the modern age. The documented effectiveness of an exercise regime regarding the body composition across all age groups can prove highly significant in preventive as well as curative treatments.

Therefore, the main aim of this study was to define the relations between physical activity and exercise, and the characteristics of the body composition in the working-age population of both genders living in Belgrade, the capital city of Serbia.

METHODS

Participants

Subjects and Study Design

The research was realized as a non-experimental, cross-sectional study. The total sample included 4489 apparently healthy Serbian men and women aged 18 to 69.9 years, who mostly lived in central Serbia and the Belgrade area. The descriptive characteristics of the male sample (N = 3065) were: Age = 33.5±9.2 yrs; Length of working life = 14.0±9.1 yrs; Body height = 181.8 ± 6.7 cm; Body mass = 86.3±13.7 kg; and, Body mass index = 26.08 ± 3.64 kg • m^{-2}. The descriptive characteristics of the female sample (N = 1424) were: Age = 33.3±11.2 yrs; Length of working life = 13.6 ± 10.0 yrs; Body height = 167.9±6.6 cm; Body mass = 65.8 ± 13.0 kg; and, Body mass index = 23.37±4.57 kg • m^{-2}. All respondents were volunteers fully informed about the aim of the study. The study excluded any respondents who actively competed in any sports, as well as any subjects with a medical diagnosis of motor skill or metabolic disorder. Respondents who participated in the study were recruited using combined techniques of personal and public information.

All respondents were divided into four groups according to the frequency of physical activity/exercise (Carrick-Ranson et al., 2014), as follows:

- Group 1 – Sedentary: subjects who performed ≤1 exercise/physical activity sessions/week (males, N = 408, 0.2 ± 0.4 exercise/physical activity sessions/week, 11 ± 22 min/week of exercise/physical activity, and 11 ± 22 min of exercise/physical activity per session; females, N = 219, 0.1±0.3 exercise/physical activity sessions/week, 4 ± 14 min/week of exercise/physical activity, and 4 ± 14 min of exercise/physical activity per session);
- Group 2 – Casual: subjects who performed 2-3 exercise/physical activity sessions/week (males, N = 875, 2.5±0.5 exercise/physical activity sessions/week, 137 ± 60 min/week of exercise/physical activity, and 54±18 min of exercise/physical activity per session; females, N = 247, 2.6 ± 0.5 exercise/physical activity sessions/week, 153 ± 61 min/week of exercise/physical activity, and 59 ± 21 min of exercise/physical activity per session);
- Group 3 – Committed: subjects who performed 4-5 exercise/physical activity sessions/week (males, N = 1019, 4.6±0.5exercise/physical activity sessions/week, 274 ± 94 min/week of exercise/physical activity, and 60 ± 18 min of exercise/physical activity per session; females, N = 454, 4.5±0.5 exercise/physical activity sessions/week, 307 ± 162 min/week of exercise/physical activity, and 67 ± 30 min of exercise/physical activity per session); and,
- Group 4 – Steady: subjects who performed ≥6 exercise/physical activity sessions/week (males, N = 763, 7.8 ± 1.9 exercise/physical activity session/week, 604 ± 274 min/week of exercise/physical activity, and 77 ± 28 min of exercise/physical activity per session; females, N = 504, 7.2 ± 1.4 exercise/physical activity sessions/week, 501 ± 212 min/week of exercise/physical activity, and 69 ± 26 min of exercise/physical activity per session).

All data about exercise (jogging, running, Pilates, gym, tennis, basketball, football, swimming) and physical activity sessions (walking, hiking, and cycling) were obtained using a standardized questionnaire (Djordjevic-Nikic and Dopsaj, 2013).

The study was realized in accordance with the guidelines for physicians conducting biomedical research involving human subjects set out in the Declaration of Helsinki (http://www.cirp.org/library/ethics/helsinki/). It was approved by the Ethics Committee of the Faculty of Sport and Physical Education, University of Belgrade.

Body Composition Measuring

Multisegmental bioelectrical impedance method was applied in all body composition measuring, using a body composition analyzer (BIA) of the latest generation – InBody 720 Tetrapolar 8-Point Tactile Electrode System (Biospace Co. Ltd., Seoul, Korea), which uses DSM-BIA principle of measuring (Direct Segmental Multi-frequency Bioelectrical Impedance Analysis) (InBody720, 2005; Gába and Přidalová, 2014; Dopsaj et al., 2015). As a technique, BIA has gained acceptance as an accurate method (due to its interclass reliabilities, error of measurement and estimation) for fat-free mass (FFM), body fat (BF), percent of body fat (PBF) etc. in clinical and sports medicine, weight reduction programs, hospitals, nutrition centers, as well as scientific and laboratory research (Sun et al., 2005).

All measurements were performed in the period October 2012–Jun 2015 at Teaching-Research Laboratory (*MIL*) of the Faculty of Sport and Physical Education of University of Belgrade. Standardized testing process was applied (Gába and Přidalová, 2014; Dopsaj et al., 2015). All testing complied with the general medical requirements and the specific measuring equipment procedure (ACSM, 2006; InBody720, 2005): measurements were taken in the morning hours (between 8:00 am and 11:00 am); the evening before the test the respondents did not consume any heavy meals after 8 pm, while on the test day no food or drink was allowed before measurement; 48 hours before the test the respondents were not allowed to undertake any vigorous physical exercise or effort, or to consume alcohol; all respondents were asked to defecate on the day of the test, and to urinate minimum 15 minutes before the test; no measurements were taken from female respondents during the menstrual period; female respondents were measured either in their light sportswear (shorts and a sleeveless/short-sleeved T-shirt) or in underwear; before the test the respondents removed all metal objects (rings, chains, earrings, watches, piercing, underwear bras, hairpins, etc.); no measurements were taken from the respondents with edema, with metal objects in the body, or pregnant women; all respondents were asked to stand for at least 5 min before measurement. In addition, the room temperature during measurement was between 20 and 25 degrees Celsius, in accordance with the manufacturer's recommendations.

Variables

The following eight variables were used in this study to describe the body composition of the research sample (Schutz et al., 2002; Đorđević-Nikić et al., 2013; Gába and Přidalová, 2014; Dopsaj et al., 2015):

- BH, body height, measured according to the international biological standard, in cm;
- BM, body mass, measured with InBody720 analyzer, in kg;
- BMI, body mass index, calculated using the formula: $BMI = BM \ (kg) \ / \ BH \ (m^2)$, in $kg \bullet m^{-2}$;
- FFM, fat free mass, calculated using the formula: $FFM = BM - BFM$ (body fat mass), in kg;
- BFM, body fat mass, measured with InBody720 analyzer, in kg;
- PBF, percent of body fat, calculated using the formula: $PBF = BF/BM$, in %;
- FFMI, fat free mass index, calculated using the formula: $FFMI = FFM \ (kg)/BH \ (m^2)$, in $kg \bullet m^{-2}$;
- BFMI, body fat mass index, calculated using the formula: $BFMI = BFM \ (kg)/BH \ (m^2)$, in $kg \bullet m^{-2}$.

Statistical Methods

Basic descriptive statistical parameters were calculated for all results in order to define parameters of central tendency and dispersion of data measures (Mean ± SD). Multivariate analysis of variance – MANOVA was used to establish the differences between body composition variables relative to gender and exercise/physical activity groups, calculated using the Wilks' Lambda criterion. The difference between individual variables was determined using the Bonferroni criteria test. A linear regression analysis was used to establish the relationship between the criterion (independent) variable (exercise/physical activity groups), and body composition variables were used as predictive (dependent) variables. The level of difference of measurements between individual variables was determined on the probability level of 95%, that is, p value of 0.05 (Hair et al., 1998). The SPSS Statistics 17.0 was used for all statistical analyses.

RESULTS

Table 1 shows the descriptive statistical data for the overall sample of men and women. Table 2 shows MANOVA results for the overall sample of men and women. Table 3 shows descriptive statistical data for the men subsamples divided according to physical exercise levels with between-group differences (ANOVA and Bonferroni criteria t test).

Table 4 shows descriptive statistical data for the women subsamples divided according to physical exercise levels with between-group differences (ANOVA and Bonferroni criteria t test).

Figures 1 to 7 present the results of the obtained linear regression analysis models for the men and women subsamples divided according to physical exercise levels with the model of change trends for the analyzed body constitution variables relative to the groups.

Table 1. Basic descriptive statistics for overall male and female sample

Variables	Male (N = 3065)			Female (N = 1424)			Tests of Between-Subjects Effects		Partial Eta^2
	Mean	SD	cV%	Mean	SD	cV%	F	Sig.	
Age (yrs.)	33.47	9.17	29.78	33.32	11.16	33.71	0.876	0.848	0.000
BH (cm)	181.80	6.70	3.68	167.90	6.61	3.94	295.6	0.000	0.084
BM (kg)	86.28	13.70	16.60	65.78	12.99	13.18	1668.5	0.000	0.324
BMI (kg•m^{-2})	26.08	3.64	14.73	23.37	4.57	4.66	285.2	0.000	0.076
FFM (kg)	70.22	8.42	11.99	46.83	5.76	12.30	1345.1	0.000	0.312
BFM (kg)	16.11	8.82	54.75	18.96	9.83	51.85	309.7	0.000	0.098
PBF (%)	17.96	7.27	40.52	27.04	8.86	9.04	1269.1	0.000	0.267
FFMI (kg•m^{-2})	21.20	1.77	8.33	16.58	1.49	1.49	6340.8	0.000	0.646
BFMI (kg•m^{-2})	1.25	0.81	64.80	6.78	3.61	2.70	93.8	0.000	0.026

Table 2. MANOVA results for overall male and female sample

Multivariate Tests[c]						
Effect		Value	F	p	Partial Eta^2	Observed Power[b]
Gender	Wilks' Lambda	0.184	1396.9[a]	0.000	0.816	1.000
a. Exact statistic; b. Computed using alpha = 0.05; c. Design: Intercept + Gender						

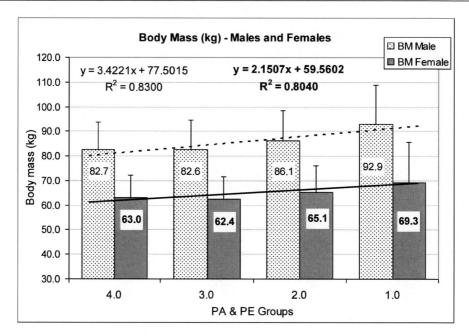

Figure 1. BM change trend model for male and female subsamples divided according to physical exercise levels.

The obtained linear regression model for BM trend change according to physical activity (PA) or physical exercise (PE) groups indicates that reduced exercise frequency resulted in a statistically significant body mass gain in men at the level of F = 242.46, and p = 0.000 with the constant increasing trend of 3.42 kg, while in women BM rose significantly at the level of F = 55.55, and p = 0.000 with the constant increasing trend of 2.15 kg. The difference in BM constant trend change between men and women was 59.05%, i.e., 1.27 kg. In other words, exercise frequency in men was by 59.07% more effective than in women relative to BM change. This means that by changing exercise frequency, men could reduce their BM by as much as 1.27 kg compared to women.

The obtained linear regression model for BMI trend change according to physical activity (PA) or physical exercise (PE) groups indicates that reduced exercise frequency resulted in a statistically significant body mass gain in men at the level of F = 411.30, and p = 0.000 with the constant increasing trend of 1.168 kg•m^{-2}, while in women BMI rose significantly at the level of F = 89.93, and p = 0.000 with the constant increasing trend of 0.957 kg•m^{-2}. The difference in BMI constant trend change between men and women was 22.05%, i.e., 0.211 kg•m^{-2}. In other words, exercise frequency in men was by 22.05% more effective than in women relative to BMI change. This means that by changing exercise frequency, men could reduce their BMI by as much as 0.211 kg•m^{-2} compared to women.

Table 3. Basic descriptive statistics for male subsamples divided according to physical exercise levels with ANOVA and Bonferroni test between group differences

	Descriptives - Males	Mean	SD	cV%	95% Confidence Interval for Mean		Min.	Max.	F	p sig.
					Lower Bound	Upper Bound				
BM (kg)	Sedentary	92.91	15.90	17.11	91.78	94.04	56.10	183.00	98.262	0.000
	2 to 3 exercise/Week	86.07*	12.27	14.25	85.25	86.75	49.90	155.60		
	4 to 5 exercise/Week	82.58#,♣	12.07	14.61	81.87	83.49	56.70	160.80		
	≥6 exercise/Week	82.67♦,¥	10.94	13.23	81.60	83.73	55.90	123.90		
BMI (kg·m⁻²)	Sedentary	28.32	4.27	15.09	28.01	28.62	18.04	52.90	167.15	0.000
	2 to 3 exercise/Week	25.95*	3.11	11.97	25.74	26.13	15.89	47.76		
	4 to 5 exercise/Week	24.89#,♣	3.06	12.29	24.72	25.12	18.19	52.03		
	≥6 exercise/Week	24.78♦,¥	2.68	10.82	24.52	25.04	18.82	36.92		
BFMI (kg·m⁻²)	Sedentary	7.01	3.06	43.72	6.80	7.23	0.64	27.92	369.76	0.000
	2 to 3 exercise/Week	5.03*	2.07	41.16	4.89	5.14	0.62	16.96		
	4 to 5 exercise/Week	3.63#,♣	2.02	55.73	3.51	3.79	0.61	25.11		
	≥6 exercise/Week	3.26♦,¥,£	1.64	50.17	3.10	3.42	0.62	11.19		
PBF (%)	Sedentary	23.93	6.93	28.98	23.44	24.42	3.00	54.33	476.25	0.000
	2 to 3 exercise/Week	18.87*	5.78	30.63	18.48	19.19	2.96	43.98		
	4 to 5 exercise/Week	14.07#,♣	5.73	40.74	13.75	14.52	3.00	48.26		
	≥6 exercise/Week	12.82♦,¥,£	5.14	40.10	12.32	13.32	2.99	32.31		
FFM (kg)	Sedentary	69.99	8.84	12.63	69.36	70.62	43.33	111.34	9.16	0.000
	2 to 3 exercise/Week	69.42	8.00	11.52	68.91	69.89	45.34	102.43		
	4 to 5 exercise/Week	70.60♣	8.39	11.89	70.06	71.18	49.39	110.12		
	≥6 exercise/Week	71.83♦,¥	8.47	11.79	71.01	72.66	45.90	103.75		
BFM (kg)	Sedentary	22.95	10.06	43.84	22.23	23.66	2.00	89.60	440.79	0.000
	2 to 3 exercise/Week	16.64*	6.86	41.25	16.17	17.00	2.00	56.80		
	4 to 5 exercise/Week	11.99#,♣	6.69	55.83	11.62	12.52	1.90	77.60		
	≥6 exercise/Week	10.84♦,¥,£	5.42	50.01	10.31	11.37	2.30	38.60		
FFMI (kg·m⁻²)	Sedentary	21.31	1.89	8.89	21.18	21.45	16.45	28.01	14.91	0.000
	2 to 3 exercise/Week	20.92*	1.62	7.75	20.82	21.02	14.44	26.83		
	4 to 5 exercise/Week	21.27♣	1.76	8.27	21.16	21.40	15.69	28.36		
	≥6 exercise/Week	21.52*	1.78	8.29	21.34	21.69	16.81	27.91		

Post Hoc Test, Bonferroni criteria – Males: * $p > 0.05$, Sedentary vs 2 to 3 exercise/Week; # $p > 0.05$, Sedentary vs 4 to 5 exercise/Week; ♦ $p > 0.05$, Sedentary vs 6 and more exercise/Week; ♣ $p > 0.05$, 2 to 3 exercise/Week vs 4 to 5 exercise/Week; ¥ $p > 0.000$, 2 to 3 exercise/Week vs 6 and more exercise/Week; £ $p > 0.05$, 4 to 5 exercise/Week vs 6 and more exercise/Week;

Table 4. Basic descriptive statistics for female subsamples divided according to physical exercise levels with ANOVA and Bonferroni test between group differences

Descriptives - Females		Mean	SD	cV%	95% Confidence Interval for Mean		Min.	Max.	F	p sig.
					Lower Bound	Upper Bound				
BM (kg)	Sedentary	69.25	16.27	23.49	67.83	70.67	39.40	164.00	22.23	0.000
	2 to 3 exercise/Week	65.10*	11.15	17.14	64.07	66.12	44.10	143.70		
	4 to 5 exercise/Week	62.43#,♣	9.20	14.74	61.28	63.59	45.20	117.40		
	≥6 exercise/Week	62.97♦	9.37	14.88	61.72	64.22	45.30	101.90		
BMI (kg·m⁻²)	Sedentary	24.89	5.75	23.10	24.38	25.39	14.43	56.28	35.27	0.000
	2 to 3 exercise/Week	23.07*	3.85	16.69	22.72	23.43	17.45	48.63		
	4 to 5 exercise/Week	21.97#,♣	3.02	13.75	21.59	22.35	16.57	44.73		
	≥6 exercise/Week	22.06♦,¥	3.02	13.69	21.66	22.46	17.20	36.10		
BFMI (kg·m⁻²)	Sedentary	8.35	4.34	51.98	7.97	8.73	1.96	31.06	66.27	0.000
	2 to 3 exercise/Week	6.53*	2.98	45.64	6.25	6.80	2.28	26.40		
	4 to 5 exercise/Week	5.39#,♣	2.36	43.78	5.09	5.68	1.17	23.47		
	≥6 exercise/Week	5.23♦,¥	2.53	48.37	4.90	5.57	1.83	18.29		
PBF (%)	Sedentary	31.18	9.28	29.76	30.37	31.99	7.42	55.28	87.89	0.000
	2 to 3 exercise/Week	26.91*	7.55	28.06	26.22	27.61	6.95	54.28		
	4 to 5 exercise/Week	23.08#,♣	7.48	32.41	22.14	24.02	5.82	52.47		
	≥6 exercise/Week	22.26♦,¥	7.24	32.52	21.30	23.23	6.23	50.67		
BFM (kg)	Sedentary	23.13	11.91	45.80	22.09	24.17	5.60	90.50	62.91	0.000
	2 to 3 exercise/Week	18.35*	8.14	41.58	17.60	19.10	6.30	78.00		
	4 to 5 exercise/Week	15.23#,♣	6.33	44.34	14.44	16.03	3.50	61.60		
	≥6 exercise/Week	14.81♦,¥	6.78	45.80	13.91	15.72	5.60	51.60		
FFM (kg)	Sedentary	46.15	6.08	13.17	45.62	46.69	31.07	73.48	6.43	0.000
	2 to 3 exercise/Week	46.75	5.23	11.18	46.27	47.24	33.20	65.69		
	4 to 5 exercise/Week	47.20	5.80	12.30	46.47	47.93	35.02	74.49		
	≥6 exercise/Week	48.12♦,¥	5.82	12.09	47.35	48.90	35.33	64.48		
FFMI (kg·m⁻²)	Sedentary	16.55	1.75	10.57	16.39	16.70	12.29	25.22	2.287	0.077
	2 to 3 exercise/Week	16.51	1.35	8.18	16.39	16.64	13.37	22.23		
	4 to 5 exercise/Week	16.56	1.40	8.45	16.39	16.74	12.63	23.56		
	≥6 exercise/Week	16.82	1.19	7.07	16.66	16.98	13.87	19.95		

Post Hoc Test, Bonferroni criteria – Females: * p > 0.05, Sedentary vs 2 to 3 exercise/Week; # p > 0.05, Sedentary vs 4 to 5 exercise/Week; ♦ p > 0.05, Sedentary vs 6 and more exercise/Week; ♣ p > 0.05, 2 to 3 exercise/Week vs 4 to 5 exercise/Week; ¥ p > 0.000, 2 to 3 exercise/Week vs 6 and more exercise/Week; £ p > 0.05, 4 to 5 exercise/Week vs 6 and more exercise/Week;

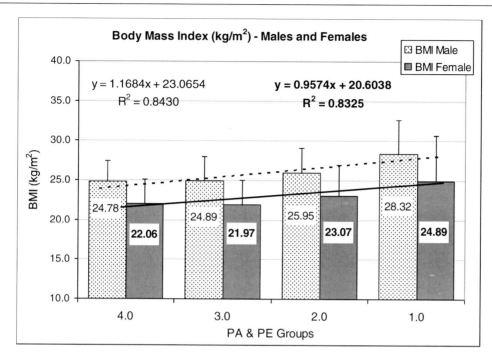

Figure 2. BMI change trend model for male and female subsamples divided according to physical exercise levels.

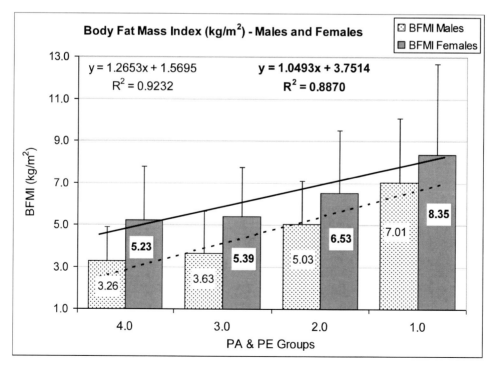

Figure 3. BFMI change trend model for male and female subsamples divided according to physical exercise levels.

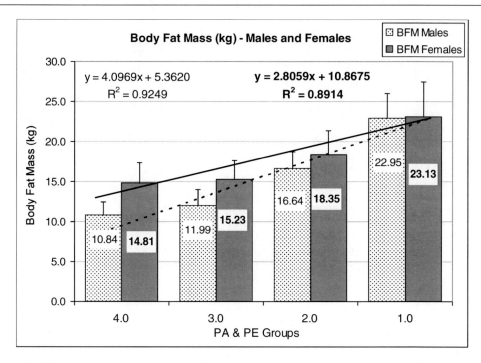

Figure 4. BFM change trend model for male and female subsamples divided according to physical exercise levels.

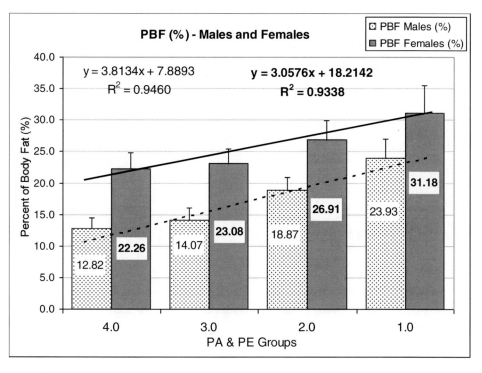

Figure 5. PBF (%) change trend model for male and female subsamples divided according to physical exercise levels.

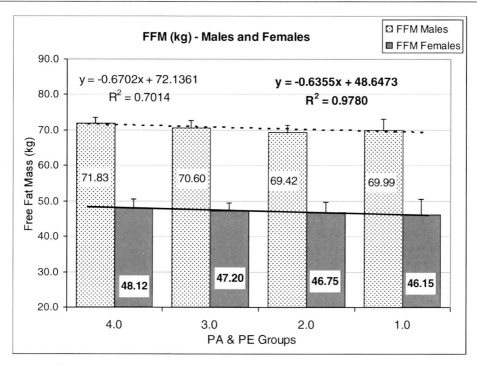

Figure 6. FFM change trend model for male and female subsamples divided according to physical exercise levels.

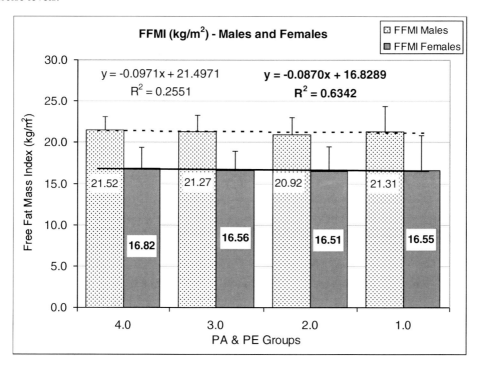

Figure 7. FFMI change trend model for male and female subsamples divided according to physical exercise levels.

The obtained linear regression model for BFMI trend change according to physical activity (PA) or physical exercise (PE) groups indicates that reduced exercise frequency resulted in a statistically significant increase in the body fat mass standardized by the square of body height in men at the level of F = 999.52, and p = 0.000 with the constant increasing trend of 1.265 kg•m^{-2}, while in women BFMI rose significantly at the level of F = 176.67, and p = 0.000 with the constant increasing trend of 1.049 kg•m^{-2}. The difference in BFMI constant trend change between men and women was 20.59%, i.e., 0.216 kg•m^{-2}. In other words, exercise frequency in men was by 20.59% more effective than in women relative to BFMI change. This means that by changing exercise frequency, men could reduce their BFMI by as much as 0.216 kg•m^{-2} compared to women.

The obtained linear regression model for BFM trend change according to physical activity (PA) or physical exercise (PE) groups shows that reduced exercise frequency resulted in a statistically significant increase in overall body fat mass in men at the level of F = 964.11, and p = 0.000 with the constant increasing trend of 4.097 kg, while in women BFM grew significantly at the level of F = 168.87, and p = 0.000 with the constant increasing trend of 2.806 kg. The difference in BFM constant trend change between men and women was 46.01%, i.e., 1.291 kg. In other words, exercise frequency in men was by 46.01% more effective than in women relative to BFM change. This means that by changing exercise frequency, men could reduce their BFM by as much as 1.291 kg compared to women.

The obtained linear regression model for PBF (%) trend change according to physical activity (PA) or physical exercise (PE) groups shows that reduced exercise frequency resulted in a statistically significant increase in percentage of fat mass in men at the level of F = 1326.65, and p = 0.000 with the constant increasing trend of 3.813%, while in women PBF rose significantly at the level of F = 247.51, and p = 0.000 with the constant increasing trend of 3.058%. The difference in PBF constant trend change between men and women was 24.69%, i.e., 0.755 per cent less. In other words, exercise frequency in men was by 24.69% more effective than in women relative to PBF change. This means that by changing exercise frequency, men could reduce their PBF by as much as 0.755 per cent compared to women.

The obtained linear regression model for FFM trend change according to physical activity (PA) or physical exercise (PE) groups indicates that reduced exercise frequency resulted in a statistically significant decrease in fat free body mass in men at the level of F = 16.06, and p = 0.000 with the constant decreasing trend of 0.670 kg, while in women the decrease was also statistically significant at the level of F = 18.96, and p = 0.000 with the constant decreasing trend of 0.636 kg. The difference in FFM constant trend change between men and women was only 5.35%, i.e., 0.034kg. In other words, exercise frequency in men was by 5.35% more effective than in women relative to FFM change. This means that by changing exercise frequency, men could gain 0.034 kg more fat free body mass than women.

The obtained linear regression model for FFMI trend change according to physical activity (PA) or physical exercise (PE) groups demonstrates that reduced exercise frequency resulted in a statistically significant decrease in the overall fat free body mass standardized with respect to body height in men at the level of F = 6.33, and p = 0.012 with the constant decreasing trend of 0.097 kg•m^{-2}. The same trend was also found in women, with the decrease showing a borderline statistical significance of F = 3.88, and p = 0.049 with the constant decreasing trend of 0.087 kg•m^{-2}. The difference in FFMI constant trend change between men and women was 11.49%, i.e., 0.541 kg•m^{-2}. In other words, exercise frequency in men was by

11.49% more effective than in women relative to FFMI change. This means that by changing exercise frequency, men could gain 0.541 kg•m^{-2} more fat free body mass than women.

DISCUSSION

The results for the analyzed variables that describe body composition in a sample of men and women showed statistically significant differences on a general level of Wilks' Lambda value = 0.184, F = 1396.9, p = 0.000 (Table 2). The difference accounted for 81.6% of the total variance of the results, which can be accepted with the reliability of 100%.

Furthermore, the results indicated that there were statistically significant differences in all analyzed variables among the four men subsamples grouped according to the frequency of weekly physical activity/exercise (Table 3). The results suggest that men with different levels of physical activity/exercise had significantly different body compositions. The highest level of difference was found in the variable describing the percentage of body fat (PBF, F = 476.25, p = 0.000, Table 3), whereas the least difference was observed in the variable describing the fat free mass (FFM, F = 9.16, p = 0.000, Table 3).

In women, the results showed that there were statistically significant differences in six analyzed variables among the subsamples grouped according to physical activity/exercise (BM, BMI, BFMI, PBF, BFM and FFM), while one variable did not yield a difference (FFMI, Table 4). As well as in men, the results for women also showed that there was a statistically significant difference in body composition relative to differing levels of physical activity/exercise. The highest level of difference was established in the variable describing the percentage of body fat (PBF, F = 87.89, p = 0.000, Table 4), while the least significant difference was found in the variable describing fat free mass (FFM, F = 6.43, p = 0.000, Table 3). The FFMI variable did not yield a statistically significant difference, which suggests that irrespective of the level of physical activity/exercise, the quantity of fat free mass by height in the analyzed women sample was constant.

Regarding the variable of body mass (BM) in men, no differences were found only between Groups 3 (4 to 5 exercises/week) and 4 (≥6 exercises/week) on a partial level (82.58 vs 82.67, Table 3), while there was a statistically significant difference between other groups (F = 98.262, p = 0,000, Table 3). The structure of statistically significant differences for BMI was exactly the same (Table 3).

The variables that defined the structure of body fat (BFMI, PBF and BFM) showed the following patterns of between-group differences: there was no difference in the given variables between Groups 4 (6 and more exercises/week) and 3 (4 to 5 exercises/week), while both groups yielded statistically significant differences relative to Groups 2 (2 to 3 exercises/week) and 1 (Sedentary); Group 1 (Sedentary) was significantly different from the other three groups (Table 4). These results imply that the frequency of engaging in a physical activity and/or sports higher than 4 sessions a week, with the duration of 274±94 min/week or 60 ± 18 min/individual session, has a statistically significant positive effect on the morphological status in men, with respect to body fat reduction. The average values for BFMI, PBF and BFM for Groups 3 and 4 were on the levels of 3.63 ± 2.02 vs 3.26 ± 1.64 kg•m^{-2}, 14.07 ± 5.73 vs 12.82 ± 5.14% and 11.99 ± 6.69 vs 10.84 ± 5.42 kg, respectively (Table 3).

Considering the variables that predominantly describe the quantity of muscle and bone tissue in the body (FFM and FFMI), it was established that the respondents in Groups 3 and 4 had significantly more such tissue on an absolute level (FFM); however, when the given variables were partialized relative to body height (FFMI), there was nonhomogeneity in the differences (Table 3). The results may suggest that physical activity/exercise not only reduced body fat but also resulted in increasing muscle mass, which is a definitely desirable and well-known effect of such activities (Garrick-Ranson et al., 2014).

The results in the women sample were similar to those in men. For BM, BMI, BFMI and BFM, it was found that Groups 3 (4 to 5 exercises/week) and 4 (4 to 5 exercises/week) showed no difference on a partial level (Table 4), while Groups 1 (Sedentary) and 2 (4 to 5 exercises/week) yielded a statistically significant difference both between-group and relative to the other two groups (Table 4). The highest statistically significant difference between the groups was observed in PBF (F = 6291, p = 0.000), while the lowest one was in FFM (Table 4, F = 6.43, p = 0.000).

The only variable without a statistically significant difference was FFMI (Table 4, F = 2.29, p = 0.077). This means that the amount of fat free body mass in the women sample was the same regardless of the frequency or the volume of physical activity or exercise. Similar to men, the results found in women may indicate that physical activity/exercise generally reduced body fat; however, it did not seem to result in the increase in muscle mass. Besides hormonal and physiological reasons, such specific adaptation to exercise in women may probably be due to the choice of physical activity/exercise, which predominantly involves aerobic activities that do not cause muscular hypertrophy (Blair, 2009; Kjonniksen et al., 2009).

In the men sample, the results for the dependence between the change in the analyzed body constitution variables and different levels of physical activity/exercise showed the following model characteristics:

An increasing trend was established –

- with the reduction in physical activity/exercise relative to the defined group models, BM showed a statistically significant constant increasing trend of 3.42 kg;
- with the reduction in physical activity/exercise relative to the defined group models, BMI showed a statistically significant constant increasing trend of 1.168 kg•m^{-2};
- with the reduction in physical activity/exercise relative to the defined group models, BFMI showed a statistically significant constant increasing trend of 1.265 kg•m^{-2};
- with the reduction in physical activity/exercise relative to the defined group models, BFM showed a statistically significant constant increasing trend of 4.097 kg;
- with the reduction in physical activity/exercise relative to the defined group models, PBF showed a statistically significant constant increasing trend of 3.813%;

A decreasing trend was established –

- with the reduction in physical activity/exercise relative to the defined group models, FFM showed a statistically significant constant decreasing trend of 0.670 kg;
- with the reduction in physical activity/exercise relative to the defined group models, FFMI showed a statistically significant constant decreasing trend of 0.097 kg•m^{-2}.

In the women sample, the results for the dependence between the change in the analyzed body constitution variables and different levels of physical activity/exercise showed the following model characteristics:

An increasing trend was established –

- with the reduction in physical activity/exercise relative to the defined group models, BM showed a statistically significant constant increasing trend of 2.15 kg;
- with the reduction in physical activity/exercise relative to the defined group models, BMI showed a statistically significant constant increasing trend of 0.957 kg•m^{-2};
- with the reduction in physical activity/exercise relative to the defined group models, BFMI showed a statistically significant constant increasing trend of 1.049 kg•m^{-2};
- with the reduction in physical activity/exercise relative to the defined group models, BFM showed a statistically significant constant increasing trend of 2.806 kg;
- with the reduction in physical activity/exercise relative to the defined group models, PBF showed a statistically significant constant increasing trend of 3.058%;

A decreasing trend was established –

- with the reduction in physical activity/exercise relative to the defined group models, FFM showed a statistically significant constant decreasing trend of 0.636 kg;
- with the reduction in physical activity/exercise relative to the defined group models, FFMI showed a statistically significant constant decreasing trend of 0.087 kg•m^{-2}.

CONCLUSION

The results obtained in this study can indicate that there were positive effects of an increase in physical activity and exercise on the body constitution. It was established that the positive effects were mainly manifested in a reduction of body mass and body mass index as indicators of the level of nutrition, followed by the reduction in body fat mass as an indicator of the balance between calorie intake and expenditure. Considering fat free mass, it was shown that it decreased with a reduction in physical activity/exercise in men, while it remained the same in women. Also, the results suggest that the minimal frequency of physical activity/exercise should be 4 sessions per week with the duration of between 274 and 307 min per week, i.e., 60 and 67 min per session in both men and women.

In addition, it was shown that there was a greater effect of physical activity/exercise on men than on women, relative to the change in body constitution. The results indicated that the average change trend for all variables was higher by 27.04% in men than in women, and that it ranged between 5.35% for FFM to 59.07% for BM. Obviously, several factors, such as women hormonal status, possibly different predominant forms of exercise and dieting, and various social and personal motives linked to the desirable body appearance, all contribute to a lower effect of exercising on the change in body composition in women than in men.

ACKNOWLEDGMENTS

This study was supported in part by the grants from Serbian Ministry of Education, Science and Technological Development (III47015).

REFERENCES

ACSM (American College of Sports Medicine) 2006. *Guidelines for Exercise Testing and Prescription.* 7th Edition. Baltimore: Lippincott Williams and Wilkins.

Adams, K., Schatzkin, A., Harris, T., Kipnis, V., Mouw, T., Ballard-Barbash, R., Hollenbeck, A. and Leitzmann, M. (2006). Overweight, obesity and mortality in a large prospective cohort of persons 50 to 71 years old. *New England Journal of Medicine, 355*(8), 763-778.

Ahmed, F., Waslien, C., Al-Sumaie, M.A. and Prakash, P. (2012). Secular trends and risk factors of overweight and obesity among Kuwaiti adults: National nutrition surveillance system data from 1998 to 2009. *Public Health Nutrition, 15*(11), 2124-30.

Blair, N.S. (2009). Physical inactivity: the biggest public health problem of the 21st century. *British Journal of sports Medicine, 43,* 1-2.

Boričić, K., Vasić, M., Grozdanov, J., Gudelj-Rakić, J., Živković-Šulović, M., Jaćović-Knežević, N., Jovanović, V., Kilibarda, V., Knežević, T., Krstić, M., Miljuš, D., Mickovski-Katalina, N. and Simić, D. (2014). *Rezultati istraživanja zdravlja stanovništva Srbija – 2013. godina.* Beograd: Institut za javno zdravlje Srbije "Dr Milan Jovanović Batut."(Results of research of population health Serbia - 2013. Belgrade: Institute for Public Health of Serbia "Dr Milan Jovanovic Batut.").

Caban, A., Lee, D., Fleming, L., Gómez-Marin, O., LeBlanc, W. and Pitman T. (2005). Obesity in US workers: The national health interview survey, 1986 to 2002. *American Journal of Public Health, 95,* 1614-1622.

De Lorenco, A., Bianchi, A., Maroni, P., Iannarelli, A., Di Daniele, N., Iacopino, L. and De Renzo, L. (2011). Adiposity rather than BMI determines metabolic risk. *International Journal of Cardiology, 166*(5), 111-117.

Dopsaj, M., Ilic, V., Djordjevic-Nikic, M., Vukovic, M., Eminovic, F., Macura, M. and Ilic, D. (2015). Descriptive model and gender dimorphism of body structure of physically active students of Belgrade University: Pilot study. *Anthropologist, 19*(1), 239-248.

Đorđevic-Nikic, M. and Dopsaj, M. (2013). Characteristics of eating habits and physical activity in relation to body mass index among adolescents. *Journal of American College of Nutrition, 32*(4), 224-33.

Đorđević-Nikić, M., Dopsaj, M., Rakić, S., Subošić, D., Prebeg, G., Macura, M., Mlađan, M. and Kekić, D. (2013). Morphological model of the population of working-age women in Belgrade measured using electrical multichanel bioimpedance model: Pilot study. *Physical Culture (Belgrade), 67*(2), 103-112.

Eiben, G., Dey, D., Rothenberg, E., Steen, B., Björkelund, C., Bengtsson, C. and Lissner, L. (2005). Obesity in 70-year-old Swedes: Secular changes over 30 years. *International Journal of Obesity, 29,* 810-817.

Gába, A and Přidalová, M. (2014). Age-related changes in body composition in a sample of Czech women aged 18-89 years: a cross-sectional study. *European Journal of Nutrition, 53,* 167-176.

Garrick-Ranson, G., Hasting, J., Bhella, P., Fujimoto, N., Shibata, S., Palmer, D., Boyd, K., Livingston, S., Dijk, E. and Levine, B. (2014). The effects of lifelong exercise dose on cardiovascular function during exercise. *Journal of Applied Physiology, 116,* 736-745.

Hair, J.F., Anderson, R.E., Tatham, R.L. and Black, W.C. (1998). *Multivariate Data Analysis.* 5th Edition. Upper Saddle River, NJ: Prentice Hall.

Hopman, W., Berger, C., Joseph, L., Barr, S., Gao, Y., Prior, J., Poliquin, S., Towheed, T. and Anastassiades, T. (2007). The association betwen body mass index and health-related quality of life: data from CAM*os*, a stratified population study. *Quality Life Research, 16,* 1595-1603.

InBody720 (2005). *The precision body composition analyser Users Manual.* 1996-2004 Biospace Co., Ltd. Seoul: Korea.

Kjonniksen, I., Anderssen, N. and Wold, B. (2009). Organized youth sports as a predictor of physical activity in adulthood. *Scandinavian Journal of Medicine and Science in Sports, 19,* 646-654.

Kolata, G. (1985). Obesity declared a disease. *Science, 227,* 1019-1020.

Lewis, C., Jacobs, D., McCreath, H., Kiefe, C., Schreiner, P., Smith, D. and Dale Williams, O. (2000). Weight gain continues in the 1990s: 10-year trend in weight and overweight from the CARDIA study. American Journal of Epidemiology, *151*(12), 1172-1181.

Moreno, L., Mesana, M., Fleta, J., Ruiz, J., Gonzáles-Gross, M., Sarría, A. and Marcos, A. (2005). Overweight, obesity and body fat composition in Spanis adolescents: The AVENA study. *Annals of Nutrition and Metabolism, 49,* 71-78.

Ogden, C., Carroll, M., Kit, B. and Flegal, K. (2012). *Prevalence of obesity in the United States, 2009-2010.* NCHS Data Brief, No. 82 (U.S. Department of Health and Human Services, Centers for Disease Control and Prevention, National center for health statistics).

Ostojic, S., Stojanovic, M., Stojanovic, V., Maric, J. and Njaradi, N. (2011). Correlation between fitness and fatness in 6-14-year old Serbian school children. *Journal of Healt Population and Nutrition, 29*(1), 53-60.

Palou, A., Serra, F., Bonet, M. and Pico, C. (2000). Obesity: molecular bases of a multifactorial problem. European Journal of Nutrition, *39*(4), 127-144.

Schutz, Y., Kyle, U.U.G. and Pichard, C. (2002). Fat-free mass index and fat mass index percentiles in Caucasians aged 18 – 98 y. *International Journal of Obesity, 26,* 953-960.

Starc, G. and Strel, J. (2011). Tracking excess weight and obesity from childhood to young adulthood: a 12-year prospective cohort study in Slovenia. *Public Health Nutrition, 14*(1), 49-55.

Sun, G., French, C. R., Martin, G. R., Younghusband, B., Green, R. C., Xie, Y., Mathews, M., Barron, J. R., Fitzpatrick, D. G., Gulliver, W. and Zang, H. (2005). Comparison of multifrequency bioelectrical impedance analysis with dualenergy x-ray absorptiometry for assessment of percentage body fat in a large, healthy population. *The American Journal of Clinical Nutrition, 81,* 74–78.

Tremblay, M. and Willms, D. (2000). Secular trends in the body mass index of Canadian children. *Canadian Medical Association Journal (CMAJ), 163*(11), 1429-1433.

Wang, Y., Monteiro, C. and Popkin, B. (2002). Trends of obesity and underweight in older children and adolescents in the United States, Brazil, China, and Russia. *American Journal of Clinical Nutrition, 75,* 971-97.

WHO, Consultation on Obesity. (2000). Obesity: Preventing and managing the global epidemic. *WHO Technical Report Series 894.* Geneva: WHO.

In: Physical Activity Effects on the Anthropological Status ...   ISBN: 978-1-63484-782-7
Editors: Fadilj Eminović and Milivoj Dopsaj   © 2016 Nova Science Publishers, Inc.

Chapter 12

THE EFFECTS OF SEDENTARY BEHAVIOR ON PHYSIOLOGICAL FUNCTION

Bryan P. McCormick, *PhD, FALS, FDRT

School of Public Health-Bloomington, Indiana University, Indiana, US

ABSTRACT

The benefits of a physically active lifestyle to health and functioning have been recognized for centuries. A physically inactive, or sedentary lifestyle, was thought to be unhealthy simply because it was not physically active. Only in the last few decades have investigators begun to examine sedentary behavior as a form of human behavior with health impacts. Initial research focused on behaviors producing less than 1.5 metabolic equivalents (METs); however, recent refinement of this definition has come to include only those behaviors performed in a seated or reclining position should be considered as sedentary. Findings have indicated that time spent in sedentary behavior has deleterious health outcomes even when people engage in adequate amounts of physical activity for health benefits. Sedentary behavior has been conceptualized as a distinct class of behavior as the approaches to reducing sedentary behavior are different from those to increase physical activity. In addition, physiological responses to sedentary behavior distinguish it from physiological responses to moderate to vigorous physical activity (MVPA). Finally, the measurement of sedentary behavior requires different approaches from the measurement of physical activity. The strongest evidence for the impact of sedentary behavior on physiological function is through insulin sensitivity and lipoprotein expression. Systematic meta-analyses have found that sedentary behavior increases hazard ratios particularly for the development of type 2 diabetes, all cause mortality, cardiovascular mortality and cancer mortality. Future research is needed to more clearly identify the physiological mechanisms through which sedentary behavior impacts physiological function, which will require greater refinement of the measurement of sedentary behavior.

Keywords: adults, physical activity, lifestyle, sedentary

---

* Corresponding author: Bryan P. McCormick. E-mail: bmccormi@indiana.edu.

INTRODUCTION

While the health beneficial effects of moderate to vigorous physical activity (MVPA) are well documented, the effects of sedentary behavior have only begun to be examined as a health determinant. Current research has increasingly demonstrated that the effects of sedentary behavior may be independent of MVPA. This chapter will review the current body of knowledge on sedentary behavior and the physiological health outcomes identified.

Defining Sedentary Behavior

A single consensus definition of sedentary behavior (SB) has yet to be identified (Boyington et al., 2015); however there are some consistencies in the way most investigators have characterized SB. First, most definitions of SB include some element of intensity of physical activity (PA) that is either measured directly, or collected via self-report. Considering intensity alone, there is general consensus that waking behavior or activities generating less than 1.5 metabolic equivalents (METs) can be considered as sedentary in nature (Pate et al., 2008). Included in this range of energy expenditure are such activities as lying down, sitting, quietly standing, and watching television or other screen-based entertainment. The advantage of such a definition is that it can be readily measured by accelerometer or by self-report of activities that fall within this energy expenditure range. However, there has recently been a suggestion that energy expenditure alone may not adequately distinguish among different types of low energy expenditure behaviors (Gibbs et al., 2015). Specifically, although a variety of behaviors may result in low energy expenditure, those performed in a seated or reclining position are most characteristic of SB. Thus, a recent characterization offered by the Sedentary Behavior Research Network is that "sedentary behaviour refers to any waking activity characterized by an energy expenditure ≤1.5 metabolic equivalents *and* a sitting or reclining posture" (2012).

The Study of Sedentary Behavior

Discussions of the value of a physically active lifestyle to one's health have been present throughout much of Western philosophy and science. In this vein, sedentary behavior was implicitly presumed to have a negative effect on one's health due to the absence of physical activity. Only recently has the effect of sedentary behavior been considered as an independent determinant of health, distinguishable from physical activity. For example, Owen and colleagues (2000) were among the first to assert that sedentary behavior was a distinct concept in health research stating "although sedentary behavior may arguably be conceptualized as no more than the other side of the physical activity coin, we see it as a class of behaviors that can coexist with and also compete with physical activity" (p. 156). Work in this area has developed relatively rapidly over the past two decades. A search of the US National Library of Medicine (PubMed) using the term "sedentary behavior" found more than 1,000 articles published from 1988 to 2014. Yet, 75% of these publications have appeared since 2010 (Figure 1).

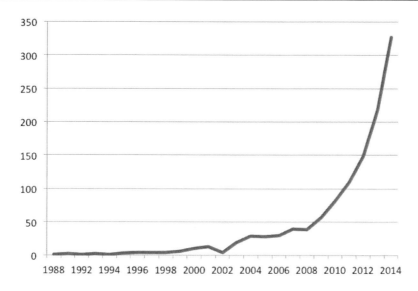

Figure 1. Sedentary Behavior Publications in PubMed 1998-2014.

In addition, most early research on sedentary behavior focused on its contribution to obesity (e.g., Epstein and Roemmich, 2001) although there are some early studies that considered its contribution to metabolic diseases (e.g., Hu et al., 2001).

Tremblay and coworkers (2010) offered that there are three important reasons for considering sedentary behavior as distinct from a lack of physical activity. First, sedentary behavior is unique from physical activity. This can be seen in the fact that approaches to increasing physical activity may differ from those to reduce sedentary behavior. For example (Tremblay et al., 2007), found that while sedentary behavior could be reduced by multiple approaches, increasing physical activity and exercise faced considerably more constraints. In addition, both physical activity and sedentary behavior can exist at the same time. While current recommendations are to accumulate at least 300 minutes of moderate or higher levels of physical activity over the week (World Health Organization, 2010), this leaves a considerable amount of the approximately 15.2 hours of waking time than can be spent in sedentary behaviors (Hamilton et al., 2008).

Second, physiological responses to sedentary behavior distinguish it from responses to physical activity. Empirically, Hamilton and colleagues (2004) were among the first to seek to distinguish the effects of inactivity from exercise in terms of physiological function due to the high disease risk associated with inactivity. In reviewing evidence to that point, Hamilton and colleagues pointed to a potential mechanism for the negative health effects of inactivity through a disruption of the enzyme lipoprotein lipase (LPL) widely regarded as having a relationship to coronary heart disease (CHD) through vascular function. They concluded that the reduced LPL activity could be attributed to the inactivity of weight-bearing skeletal muscles, and that even non-fatiguing muscle use (such as walking) resulted in significant increases in LPL activity.

The final reason for considering sedentary behavior as distinct from physical activity is that assessing and measuring sedentary behavior may require different metrics and indicators (Tremblay et al., 2010). For example, as noted above, initial definitions of sedentary behavior were based on energy expenditure alone; however, more recently this has been modified to only apply to a seated position. This measurement challenge may undermine findings linking health outcomes to sedentary behavior as some studies may not actually be measuring sedentary behavior (Pate et al., 2008).

Sedentary Behavior Physiology

Sedentary behavior appears to be consistently related to all-cause and cardiovascular disease (CVD) mortality (Biswas et al., 2015), as well as risk of Type 2 diabetes. In addition, while some reviews have found linkages to cancer incidence and mortality (Biswas et al., 2015), others have failed to find such a relationship (Proper et al., 2011). Thus, the currently best understood mechanisms through which sedentary behavior negatively affects health are through metabolic and cardiovascular functions. This risk has been found to be relatively large, such that higher levels of sedentary behavior are associated with a 112% increase in risk for diabetes, 149% increase in risk for cardiovascular disease, as well as a 90% increase in the risk of cardiovascular mortality (Wilmot et al., 2012).

One linkage of sedentary behavior to metabolic dysfunction appears to be through the connection to insulin sensitivity. In one of the earliest studies to identify this connection, Heath et al. (1983) identified that among highly trained athletes, a significant reduction in physical activity level resulted in significant decreases in insulin sensitivity even when overall fitness remained unchanged. Although this early work did not specifically examine sedentary behavior, a recent study found that daily displacement of 30 minutes of sedentary behavior with light physical activity conferred a 5% increase in insulin sensitivity, while daily displacement of 30 minutes of sedentary behavior with MVPA conferred 15%-18% increase in insulin sensitivity among adults with increased risk of type 2 diabetes (Yates et al., 2015). Additionally, in an experimental study of recreationally active young adults, Lyden and coworkers (2015) found that a seven day sedentary condition resulted in significant increases in 2-h plasma insulin. Interruptions in sedentary behavior may have benefits in improving insulin sensitivity in adults, although the findings are somewhat inconsistent. For example, Peddie et al. (2013) found that interrupting prolonged periods of sitting with light physical activity lowered plasma glucose and improved insulin sensitivity; however, Thorp et al. (2014) found that among obese adults only plasma glucose levels improved. In addition, such a benefit from interruptions in sedentary time has been found among children in observational studies (Saunders et al., 2013), but not in an experimental design (Travis J. Saunders et al., 2013). The effects of sedentary behavior on insulin sensitivity also may also be sex-linked. For example, Henderson et al. (2012) found that self-reported screen time was negatively associated with insulin sensitivity among girls, but not boys and the same female-only associations have been found in a population study of adults (Dunstan et al., 2007).

Another mechanism linking sedentary behavior to physiological outcomes has been proposed through the activity and expression of lipoproteins including lipoprotein lipase (LPL) as well as low-density lipoprotein cholesterol (LDL-C) and high-density lipoprotein cholesterol (HDL-C). As LPL plays a key role in lipid metabolism, it is implicated in such processes as changes in muscle glucose, local uptake of plasma triglycerides, fatty acid metabolism and high-density lipoprotein cholesterol (HDL-C) (Ekblom-Bak et al., 2010). Using a rodent model, Bey and Hamilton (2003) found that restrained muscular activity, consistent with sedentary behavior, resulted in significantly lower LPL activity, resulting in less triglyceride uptake into skeletal muscle as well as reduced plasma HDL-C concentrations. Importantly, LPL activity during non-exercise activity did not differ significantly between rats in the high-exercise versus muscular inactivity conditions. They interpreted this as highlighting the importance of local muscle contraction as opposed to the intensity of the contraction in LPL activity. This is also consistent with the recent clarification of sedentary behavior as only taking place in a seated or reclined position. Although quietly standing results in METs <1.5, muscle contraction is necessary to remain standing. The work in this area remains far from complete as there are multiple regulatory influences on LPL activity (Kersten, 2014). The relationship of sedentary time (measured as screen-time) to low-density lipoprotein cholesterol (LDL-C) was found to be significantly associated among women after controlling for MVPA and BMI; however, there was no significant association among men (Frazier-Wood et al., 2014). When plasma lipids have been examined among children, sedentary behavior has been found to be negatively associated with HDL-C levels regardless of sex or MVPA (Cliff et al., 2014; Cliff et al., 2013).

A final mechanism through which sedentary behavior may be linked with negative health outcomes is through increases in visceral adiposity (Thyfault and Krogh-Madsen, 2011). Both insulin resistance and visceral adiposity have been hypothesized to be interrelated precursors to type 2 diabetes. To date, most studies examining the relationship of activity level to adiposity are most accurately characterized as physical inactivity studies as opposed to sedentary behavior studies. These studies have consistently found that physical inactivity is associated with higher levels of adiposity (e.g., Philipsen et al., 2015). Research examining objectively measured sedentary behavior and visceral adiposity remains in its infancy; however, Henson et al. (2015) have documented the association of time spent in sedentary behavior with higher levels of heart, liver and visceral fat among individuals at high risk for type 2 diabetes.

Sedentary Behavior in Children and Youth

Research examining sedentary behavior in young children is still developing. One of the challenges of measurement, particularly among young children, has been the use of parental reports of *screen time* (e.g., on computer or watching television) as an indicator of sedentary behavior (Downing et al., 2015). The difficulty is that screen time alone may not adequately capture sedentary behavior. Engelen et al. (2015) found that while 51% of primary school children's after-school time was classified as sedentary behavior, only 22% of after-school time was engaged in screen time. They concluded that screen time was not a suitable proxy for sedentary behavior in primary school children. In addition, others have questioned if the criterion for METs (≤1.5 METs) signaling sedentary behavior among adults is appropriate among children (Saint-Maurice et al., 2015).

Measurement challenges not withstanding, the role of sedentary behavior in children's health may not mirror that of adults. For example, Carson, Stone, and Faulkner (2014) found that sedentary behavior was associated with body mass index (BMI), but only among children with the least amount of moderate to vigourous physical activity. Similarly, Byun and associates (2013) found no relationship of sedentary behavior to BMI among children, when controlling for MVPA. Thus, among children, sedentary behavior and MVPA may not be independent contributors to health outcomes.

Findings among adolescents also present a pattern that is somewhat inconsistent. For example in one longitudinal study sedentary behavior was significantly associated with the development of type 2 diabetes (Lee, 2014); whereas a prospective study of adolescents found that sedentary behavior in late childhood was unrelated to cardiometabolic risk in adolescence (Stamatakis et al., 2015). In addition, the effects of sedentary behavior among boys and girls appears to differ. Among boys, increasing use of screen based media and other sedentary behavior has been found to be associated with increased adiposity (Carson et al., 2014; Costigan et al., 2013); however, this relationship has not been consistently found among girls (Barnett et al., 2010). In summarizing research evidence to 2013, de Rezende and coworkers (2014) concluded that there was strong evidence linking sedentary to obesity among adolescents, with moderate evidence linking sedentary behavior to blood pressure and overall cholesterol.

Sedentary Behavior in Adults

The often-cited origin of sedentary behavior research is the study by Morris and Crawford (1958) of London bus drivers and conductors. Their findings of differences in cardiac risk between the predominantly sedentary drivers and predominantly active conductors provided a basis for considering sedentary behavior as a form of behavior, but at the time of its publication it was simply seen as the low energy pole of a physical activity continuum. Although estimates of the amount of time adults spend in sedentary behavior varies, there is evidence to suggest that sedentary time is increasing in many of the world's largest countries. Through an examination of country-level time use data Ng and Popkin (2012) found that weekly time in sedentary behavior increased annually by 1.3 hrs/week in the US, 1.4 hrs/week in the UK, and 1.8 hrs/week in China through the first decade of the 21st century.

Based on a recent systematic review, after adjustment for physical activity, sedentary behavior among adults confers greatest risk of the development of type 2 diabetes (HR 1.91; 95% CI 1.64-2.22), followed by all cause mortality (HR 1.24; CI 1.09-1.41), cardiovascular disease mortality (HR 1.179; CI 1.106-1.257), cancer mortality (HR 1.173; CI 1.108-1.242), cardiovascular disease incidence (HR 1.143; CI 1.002-1.729), and cancer incidence (HR 1.130; CI 1.053-1.213) (Biswas et al., 2015). This systematic review appears to present stronger evidence than previous reviews (e.g., Thorp et al., 2014; Wilmot et al., 2012) due to prior reviews inclusion of studies using largely self-report data and without control for physical activity.

As with children and adolescents, there remain concerns about the measurement of sedentary behavior (Gibbs et al., 2015), as much of the research is based on self-reported behavior as opposed to empirically measured. Additionally, not all studies have controlled for the joint effects of MVPA and sedentary behavior, which may have resulted in overestimation of sedentary behavior effects. Finally, the majority of published studies have been conducted among English speaking subjects, thus raising some questions about cultural effects.

CONCLUSION

Knowledge of the role of sedentary behavior in health continues to develop. Among adults, there is strong evidence that sedentary behavior affects cardiometabolic health independently of health enhancing physical activity. Although the picture is still developing, the role of sedentary behavior in the health and functioning of children and adolescents has clear health implications. That is, for most children and adolescents, baseline levels of sedentary behavior generally increase with age. Thus those children and adolescents who begin with high levels of sedentary behavior are more likely to become highly sedentary adults, with attendant health risks.

There remain a number of important questions to fully understand the impact of sedentary behavior on physiological function. Principal among these is identifying the biological mechanism through which certain forms of inactivity result in cardiometablic changes conferring health risks. Related to this question, there remain questions about the best definition and methods for capturing sedentary behavior. While postural conditions (e.g., sitting or reclining postures) have been proposed as a key criterion of sedentary behavior, it remains to be seen if this is in fact a measurable determinant that distinguishes a class of behaviors with specific health risks.

REFERENCES

Barnett, T.A., O'Loughlin, J., Sabiston, C.M., Karp, I., Belanger, M., Van Hulst, A., and Lambert, M. (2010). Teens and Screens: The Influence of Screen Time on Adiposity in Adolescents. *American Journal of Epidemiology*, 172(3), 255-262.

Bey, L., and Hamilton, M.T. (2003). Suppression of skeletal muscle lipoprotein lipase activity during physical inactivity: a molecular reason to maintain daily low-intensity activity. *Journal of Physiology-London*, 551(2), 673-682.

Biswas, A., Oh, P.I., Faulkner, G.E., Bajaj, R.R., Silver, M.A., Mitchell, M.S., and Alter, D.A. (2015). Sedentary time and its association with risk for disease incidence, mortality, and hospitalization in adults: a systematic review and meta-analysis. *Annals of Internal Medicine*, 162(2), 123-132.

Boyington, J., Joseph, L., Fielding, R., and Pate, R. (2015). Sedentary Behavior Research Priorities-NHLBI/NIA Sedentary Behavior Workshop Summary. *Medicine and Science in Sports and Exercise*, 47(6), 1291-1294.

Byun, W., Liu, J., and Pate, R.R. (2013). Association between objectively measured sedentary behavior and body mass index in preschool children. *International Journal of Obesity*, 37 (7), 961-965.

Carson, V., Stone, M., and Faulkner, G. (2014). Patterns of sedentary behavior and weight status among children. *Pediatric Exercise Science*, 26(1), 95-102.

Cliff, D.P., Jones, R.A., Burrows, T.L., Morgan, P.J., Collins, C.E., Baur, L.A., and Okely, A.D. (2014). Volumes and bouts of sedentary behavior and physical activity: Associations with cardiometabolic health in obese children. *Obesity*, 22(5), E112-E118.

Cliff, D.P., Okely, A.D., Burrows, T.L., Jones, R.A., Morgan, P.J., Collins, C.E., and Baur, L.A. (2013). Objectively measured sedentary behavior, physical activity, and plasma lipids in overweight and obese children. *Obesity,* 21(2), 382-385.

Costigan, S.A., Barnett, L., Plotnikoff, R.C., and Lubans, D.R. (2013). The health indicators associated with Screen-Based sedentary behavior among adolescent girls: A Systematic review. *Journal of Adolescent Health,* 52, 382-392.

de Rezende, L.F.M., Lopes, M.R., Rey-Lopez, J.P., Rodrigues Matsudo, V.K., and Luiz, O.D.C. (2014). Sedentary behavior and health outcomes: An overview of systematic reviews. *Plos One,* 9(8).e105620.

Downing, K.L., Hnatiuk, J., and Hesketh, K.D. (2015). Prevalence of sedentary behavior in children under 2 years: A systematic review. *Preventive Medicine,* 78, 105-114.

Dunstan, D.W., Salmon, J., Healy, G.N., Shaw, J.E., Jolley, D., Zimmet, P.Z., Steering, C. (2007). Association of television viewing with fasting and 2-h postchallenge plasma glucose levels in adults without diagnosed diabetes. *Diabetes Care,* 30(3), 516-522.

Ekblom-Bak, E., Hellenius, M.L., and Ekblom, B. (2010). Are we facing a new paradigm of inactivity physiology? *British Journal of Sports Medicine,* 44(12), 834-835.

Engelen, L., Bundy, A.C., Bauman, A., Naughton, G., Wyver, S., and Baur, L. (2015). Young children's after-school activities – There's more to it than screen time: A cross-sectional study of young primary school children. *Journal of Physical Activity and Health,* 12(1), 8-12.

Epstein, L.H., and Roemmich, J. N. (2001). Reducing sedentary behavior: Role in modifying physical activity. *Exercise and Sport Sciences Reviews,* 29(3), 103-108.

Franks, P.W., Ekelund, U., Brage, S., Wong, M.Y., and Wareham, N.J. (2004). Does the association of habitual physical activity with the metabolic syndrome differ by level of cardiorespiratory fitness? *Diabetes Care*, 27(5), 1187-1193.

Frazier-Wood, A.C., Borecki, I.B., Feitosa, M.F., Hopkins, P.N., Smith, C.E., and Arnett, D.K. (2014). Sex-specific associations between screen time and lipoprotein subfractions. *International Journal of Sport Nutrition and Exercise Metabolism*, 24(1), 59-69.

Gibbs, B.B., Hergenroeder, A.L., Katzmarzyk, P.T., Lee, I.M., and Jakicic, J.M. (2015). Definition, measurement, and health risks associated with sedentary behavior. *Medicine and Science in Sports and Exercise,* 47(6), 1295-1300.

Hamilton, M.T., Hamilton, D.G., and Zderic, T.W. (2004). Exercise physiology versus inactivity physiology: An essential concept for understanding lipoprotein lipase regulation. *Exercise and Sport Sciences Reviews,* 32(4), 161-166.

Hamilton, M.T., Healy, G.N., Dunstan, D.W., Zderic, T.W., and Owen, N. (2008). Too little exercise and too much sitting: Inactivity physiology and the need for new recommendations on sedentary behavior. *Current Cardiovascular Risk Reports* (4), 292.

Heath, G.W., Gavin, J.R., Hinderliter, J.M., Hagberg, J.M., Bloomfield, S.A., and Holloszy, J.O. (1983). Effects of exercise and lack of exercise on glucose-tolerance and insulin sensitivity. *Journal of Applied Physiology,* 55(2), 512-517.

Henderson, M., Gray-Donald, K., Mathieu, M.-E., Barnett, T.A., Hanley, J.A., O'Loughlin, J., Lambert, M. (2012). How are physical activity, fitness, and sedentary behavior associated with insulin sensitivity in children? *Diabetes Care,* 35(6), 1272-1278.

Henson, J., Edwardson, C.L., Morgan, B., Horsfield, M.A., Bodicoat, D.H., Biddle, S.J.H., Yates, T. (2015). Associations of sedentary time with fat distribution in a high-risk population. *Medicine and Science in Sports and Exercise,* 47(8), 1727-1734.

Hu, F.B., Leitzmann, M.F., Stampfer, M.J., Willett, W.C., Rimm, E. B., and Colditz, G. A. (2001). Physical activity and television watching in relation to risk for type 2 diabetes mellitus in men. *Archives of Internal Medicine,* 161(12), 1542-1548.

Kersten, S. (2014). Physiological regulation of lipoprotein lipase. *Biochimica et Biophysica Acta-Molecular and Cell Biology of Lipids,* 1841(7), 919-933.

Lee, P.H. (2014). Association between adolescents' physical activity and sedentary behaviors with change in BMI and risk of type 2 diabetes. *Plos One,* 9(10), e110732.

Lyden, K., Keadle, S.K., Staudenmayer, J., Braun, B., and Freedson, P.S. (2015). Discrete features of sedentary behavior impact cardiometabolic risk factors. *Medicine and Science in Sports and Exercise,* 47(5), 1079-1086.

Morris, J.N., and Crawford, M.D. (1958). Coronary heart disease and physical activity of work - evidence of a national necropsy survey. *British Medical Journal*, 2(DEC20), 1485-1496.

Owen, N., Leslie, E., Salmon, J., and Fotheringham, M. J. (2000). Environmental determinants of physical activity and sedentary behavior. *Exercise and Sport Sciences Reviews,* 28(4), 153-158.

Pate, R.R., O'Neill, J.R., and Lobelo, F. (2008). The evolving definition of "sedentary." *Exercise and Sport Sciences Reviews*, 36(4), 173-178.

Peddie, M.C., Bone, J.L., Rehrer, N.J., Skeaff, C.M., Gray, A.R., and Perry, T.L. (2013). Breaking prolonged sitting reduces postprandial glycemia in healthy, normal-weight adults: a randomized crossover trial. *American Journals of Clinical Nutrition,* 98(2), 358-366.

Philipsen, A., Hansen, A.-L.S., Jkrgensen, M. E., Brage, S., Carstensen, B., Sandbaek, A., Witte, D.R. (2015). Associations of objectively measured physical activity and abdominal fat distribution. *Medicine and Science in Sports and Exercise,* 47(5), 983-989.

Proper, K.I., Singh, A.S., van Mechelen, W., and Chinapaw, M.J.M. (2011). Sedentary Behaviors and Health Outcomes Among Adults A Systematic Review of Prospective Studies. *American Journal of Preventive Medicine,* 40(2), 174-182.

Saint-Maurice, P.F., Kim, Y., Welk, G.J., and Gaesser, G.A. (2015). Kids are not little adults: what MET threshold captures sedentary behavior in children? *European Journal of Applied Physiology*, 10p. doi: 10.1007/s00421-015-3238-1.

Saunders, T.J., Chaput, J.-P., Goldfield, G.S., Colley, R.C., Kenny, G.P., Doucet, E., and Tremblay, M.S. (2013). Prolonged sitting and markers of cardiometabolic disease risk in children and youth: A randomized crossover study. *Metabolism-Clinical and Experimental*, 62(10), 1423-1428.

Saunders, T.J., Tremblay, M.S., Mathieu, M.È., Henderson, M., O'Loughlin, J., Tremblay, A., and Chaput, J.P. (2013). Associations of sedentary behavior, sedentary bouts and breaks in sedentary time with cardiometabolic risk in children with a family history of obesity. *PLoS ONE,* 8(11), e79143-e79143.

Sedentary Behavior Research Network. (2012). Letter to the Editor: Standardized use of the terms "sedentary" and "sedentary behaviours." *Applied Physiology Nutrition and Metabolism,* 37(3), 540-542.

Stamatakis, E., Coombs, N., Tiling, K., Mattocks, C., Cooper, A., Hardy, L.L., and Lawlor, D. A. (2015). Sedentary Time in Late Childhood and Cardiometabolic Risk in Adolescence. *Pediatrics,* 135(6), E1432-E1441.

Thorp, A.A., Kingwell, B.A., Sethi, P., Hammond, L., Owen, N., and Dunstan, D.W. (2014). Alternating Bouts of Sitting and Standing Attenuate Postprandial Glucose Responses. *Medicine and Science in Sports and Exercise*, 46(11), 2053-2061.

Thyfault, J.P., and Krogh-Madsen, R. (2011). Metabolic disruptions induced by reduced ambulatory activity in free-living humans. *Journal of Applied Physiology*, 111(4), 1218-1224.

Tremblay, M.S., Colley, R.C., Saunders, T.J., Healy, G.N., and Owen, N. (2010). Physiological and health implications of a sedentary lifestyle. *Applied Physiology Nutrition and Metabolism-Physiologie Appliquee Nutrition Et Metabolisme*, 35(6), 725-740.

Tremblay, M.S., Esliger, D.W., Tremblay, A., and Colley, R. (2007). Incidental movement, lifestyle-embedded activity and sleep: new frontiers in physical activity assessment. *Canadian Journal of Public Health.*, 98, S208-S217.

Wilmot, E.G., Edwardson, C.L., Achana, F.A., Davies, M.J., Gorely, T., Gray, L.J., Biddle, S.J.H. (2012). Sedentary time in adults and the association with diabetes, cardiovascular disease and death: systematic review and meta-analysis. *Diabetologia*, 55(11), 2895-2905.

World Health Organization. (2010). *Global recommendations on physical activity for health*. Geneva, Switzerland: World Health Organization.

Yates, T., Henson, J., Edwardson, C., Dunstan, D., Bodicoat, D. H., Khunti, K., and Davies, M. J. (2015). Objectively measured sedentary time and associations with insulin sensitivity: Importance of reallocating sedentary time to physical activity. *Preventive Medicine*, 79. doi: 10.1016/j.ypmed.2015.04.005.

In: Physical Activity Effects on the Anthropological Status …   ISBN: 978-1-63484-782-7
Editors: Fadilj Eminović and Milivoj Dopsaj   © 2016 Nova Science Publishers, Inc.

Chapter 13

THE ROLE OF EXERCISE IN PREVENTING AND TREATING HIV INFECTION AND CANCER

Nevena Veljković, Sanja Glisić, Branislava Gemović
and Veljko Veljković[*]

Center for Multidisciplinary Research, University of Belgrade,
Institute of Nuclear Sciences VINCA, Belgrade, Serbia

ABSTRACT

There is convincing evidence from numerous clinical and epidemiological studies that physical activity can reduce the risk for breast and prostate cancer. The biological mechanisms underlying this phenomenon remain elusive. Herein we suggest a role for naturally produced antibodies reactive with the vasoactive intestinal peptide (VIP) in the suppression of breast and prostate cancer and in control of the HIV disease progression. The proposed molecular mechanism suggests that targeting of VIP pathway with natural antibodies elicited by the physical exercise represents a promising approach in supportive treatment of the breast and prostate cancer and AIDS.

Keywords: physical exercise, vasoactive intestinal peptide, natural autoantibodies, breast cancer, prostate cancer, AIDS

INTRODUCTION

Thirty-five years after its discovery, the human immunodeficiency virus (HIV) and its constantly increasing prevalence continue to represent a growing worldwide public health problem. According to recent estimates, over 35 million people are living with HIV all over the world (UNAIDS World AIDS Day Report, 2014). Vaccination as the best strategy to protect against infection seems not to be an attainable goal. To the present, the only one candidate HIV vaccine progressed to large phase III clinical trial (Francis et al., 1998), but it

---

[*] Corresponding author: Email: vv@vinca.rs.

failed to substantially protect the vaccinated (Cohen, 2008; Veljkovic et al., 2008). Despite of that, the success of drug cocktail, highly active antiretroviral therapy (HAART) has brought to life the new concept in infectious diseases management. However, the HAART is not curative, meaning that those who acquire HIV will need to take antiretrovirals lifelong. The major drawback is that HIV easily acquires resistance to individual HAART components, which produces constant demands for new drugs.

Clearly other less toxic, inexpensive, non-drug modalities must be pursued in order to slow the spread of HIV and decrease the disease burden related to HIV disease and treatment. Previously we proposed exercise as an important solution to these vexing problems. Exercise has been shown to promote the development of antibodies (anti-VIP/NTM) in both normal and HIV individuals with a specific affinity (or cross reactivity) to the HIV-1 envelope protein (gp120 surface antigen) of HIV. Evidence in the literature also supports the idea that increasing the titer of this unique antibody (either by passive immunization or exercise) may slow HIV disease progression and reconstitute the damaged immune system (Veljkovic et al., 2001; Veljkovic et al., 2010). The molecular mechanism connecting physical activity with augmenting immune system function in HIV is detailed. Further we will describe a mechanism of interaction between anti-VIP autoantibodies and tumor marker highly homologous with HIV-1 envelope protein expressed on > 90% breast, gynecological and prostate tumor cells, pointing out exercise as useful supportive cancer therapy.

EXERCISE AS SOURCE OF VIP/NTM-REACTIVE AUTOANTIBODIES

The virus entry begins with the specific binding of HIV-1 Env subunit gp120 (HIV-1 gp120) to the primary host receptor CD4, which is expressed mainly on T-lymphocytes and macrophages. C-terminus of the second conserved domain (C2) of HIV-1 Env protein encompasses residues directly involved in binding to the CD4 receptor and in post-receptor binding events. However, this important target for HIV-1 neutralization is not immunogenic in humans. Structural similarity and strong immunological crossreactivity with gp120 point out vasoactive intestinal peptide (VIP) as a natural mimetic which can elicit antibodies reactive with this critical region of HIV-1 Env protein (Veljkovic et al., 1992). VIP is a 28-amino-acid pleiotropic peptide with broad biological actions including potent vasodilatator and brochodilatator activity. It is also neurotransmitter and immunomodulator which plays an important role immune homeostasis.

Several studies demonstrated increase in plasma VIP concentration as reaction on exercise. Marked increases in peripheral plasma concentration of VIP [1.8 (rest) vs. 22.3 pmol/l (3 h)] during 3-h period of mild bicycle exercise were reported (Galbo et al., 1979; Hilsted et al., 1980). Another study of twenty-four military cadets went through a 5-day period of heavy physical exercise (35% of VO2 max) demonstrated that plasma concentration of VIP increased two- to five-fold during the course, with the highest increase on day 2 (Oktedalen et al., 1983). Similar study performed during a ranger training course lasting for five days with almost continuous physical activity demonstrated increase of the plasma VIP concentration from 8.8 pmol/l to a maximum of 23.4 pmol/l on the second day of the course (Wiik et al., 1988). The same researchers have investigated effect of exercise in twelve subjects participating in a 90-km cross-country ski race lasting 4.45 – 6.50 h. Plasma concentration of VIP was greatly increased immediately after the race, and the level was not normalized within 140 minutes, though there was a significant decrease after 80 minutes with rest (Oktedalen et al., 1983a). Oektedalen and co-workers have reported that VIP increased 2-fold in twenty young men participated in a five day training course with prolonged and heavy physical exercise (Oktedalen et al., 1983b). In seven subjects with exercise-induced asthma, plasma VIP rose significantly 5 min after the test compared with the controls (Hvidsten et al., 1986). Study of healthy subjects performing ergometer exercise with progressive increases in workload until exhaustion, lasting from 16 to 32 minutes and with a corresponding maximum energy output of 1500 to 5100 W, showed an increase in plasma VIP concentration from a pre-stimulatory level of 3.3 pmol/l to 5.6 pmol/l (Woie etal., 1986). Opstad reported that plasma VIP increased during physical exercise lasting from more than 20 minutes with a workload of more than 50% of VO2 max (Opstad, 1987). According to this study a further increase took place in the early recovery period to a maximum level 5 − 10 minutes after the exercise. Significant increase in plasma concentration of VIP during exercise was also demonstrated by Paul and co-workers (Paul et al., 1987). Plasma concentrations of VIP was analyzed in six male endurance runners and six male hockey players before during and 15 min after 90 min treadmill running at 65% maximum oxygen uptake (MacLaren et al., 1995). Plasma VIP level increased significantly beyond resting levels for both groups (endurance runners, 76.1 ng/l; hockey players 155.6 ng/l).

The above overview of experimental data demonstrates significant increase of the plasma VIP concentration during and after exercise. Strong and consistent evidences from number of studies conducted worldwide support the hypothesis that regular physical activity reduces breast cancer risk by 20% to 30% in a dose–dependent manner (Friedenreich, 2011). Long-term athletic training during the college and pre-college years lowers the risk of breast cancer throughout the life span (Frisch et al., 1987; Wyshak and Frisch, 2000). For tertiary cancer prevention, observational studies suggest that breast cancer survivors performing exercise (e.g., 2–3 h of brisk walking/week) have a 40–67% reduction in breast cancer recurrence and all-cause mortality compared with inactive survivors (Irwin et al., 2008; Cheema et al., 2008; McTiernana et al., 2010). Similar data about the average risk reduction were reported for prostate cancer (Kenfield et al., 2011; Richman et al., 2011; Forbes et al., 2015). However, the potential biologic mechanisms through which physical activity may decrease the risk of breast and prostate cancer are still not known. Several putative etiologic pathways, such as those involving steroid hormones, chronic inflammation, growth factors, lymphokines and insulin resistance were suggested (reviewed in Friedenreich, 2011). On the other hand, there are mounting evidences that VIP pathway plays an important role in pathogenesis of breast and prostate cancer, indicating that elevated concentration of VIP, a facilitator of breast and prostate cancer, in the circulation may contribute to these diseases and that suppression of this peptide could have positive effect (Veljkovic et al., 2011a and references herein). We hypothesized that suppressive anti-VIP antibodies could contribute to a better control of breast and prostate cancer and that lack of these antibodies could contribute to the progression of these diseases. This is due to interaction between anti-VIP antibodies and tumor marker highly homologous with NTM peptide derived from HIV-1 gp120 which is expressed on > 90% breast, gynecological and prostate tumor cells. In order to test this assumption we compared NTM reactivity of sera collected from cancer patients and healthy controls and showed that this reactivity is significantly lower in cancer patients. This pointed out anti-VIP antibodies and exercise as a non-drug modality for cancer management (Veljkovic et al., 2011b).

Paul and co-workers proposed that autoantibodies directed against VIP are potent modifiers of its biological actions (Paul et al., 1985). They demonstrated the existence in normal human plasma of autoantibodies that bind VIP (Paul et al., 1985). Based on evaluation of the histories of VIP-antibody positive subjects, Paul and Said have suggested that muscular exercise may be a factor influencing the incidence of these antibodies (Paul and Said, 1988). According to their results specific autoantibodies to VIP were present in plasma from 29.6% healthy human subjects who habitually performed muscular exercise, compared to 2.3% healthy subjects who did not (Paul and Said, 1988). We have demonstrated in prior publications that natural anti-VIP antibodies which recognize the C2 domain of HIV-1 gp120, encompassing peptides NTM and NTM1, could represent an important host factor in control of the HIV disease progression (Veljkovic et al., 2003; Veljkovic et al., 2004; Djordjevic et al., 2007). Besides, we demonstrated that sera from well-trained athletic (HIV-negative) subjects showed high reactivity with HIV-1 gp120-derived peptide NTM1 (FTDNAKTI) and confirmed that aerobic exercise training stimulates production of these natural autoantibodies (Veljkovic et al., 2010).

These results open the question concerning possible effect of VIP on immune system during the exercise. In order to answer this important question, we will briefly summarize some immunomodulatory properties of this peptide.

The evidence supports the theory that VIP acts not as an inhibitor, but as modulator of immune function, modulating the mobility and adherence of lymphocytes and macrophages, phagocytic cell functions (phagocytosis and free radical production), the lymphocyte proliferative response, lymphokine and immunoglobulin production and the NK cell activity (Delafuente et al., 1996). VIP participates in the intricate cytokine network controlling local immune responses by down-regulation of the expression of IL-2 and IL-10 mRNA in T cells stimulated through the TCR associated CD3 complex, and by significant reduction of the stability of the newly synthesized IL-4 protein (Wang et al., 1996). It also modulates the inflammatory functions through down-regulation of the expression of proinflammatory cytokines as TNF-□, IL-12, IL-1, IL-6 and NO (nitric oxide). Acting as a physiological cytoprotective molecule VIP modulats the inflammatory cell functions through the down-regulatory effects on the expression of various key cytokines (Pozo et al., 2000). Existence on lymphocytes of different receptors for prepro-VIP-derived peptides, suggests that VIP may be considered as important immunoregulatory molecule (Yiangoa et al., 1990). VIP stimulates IL-2 release at low concentrations with a marked effect at 10(-14) M that gradually returned to control levels by 10 (-7) M (Nio et al., 1993). On the other hand, it also can inhibit IL-2 production by either unfractionated spleen cells, or by purified CD4+ T cells in a dose-dependent manner. The effect is specific, since structurally related peptides such as secretin and glucagon have little or no inhibitory effect. VIP induces a rapid increase in intracellular cAMP in CD4+ T cells. This results suggests that the inhibitory effect of VIP could be mediated through the induction of cAMP. Investigations of this phenomenon by northern blots showed that VIP downregulated IL-2 mRNA, indicating the occurrence of a transcriptional regulatory event (Ganea and Sun, 1993). This conclusion is supported by another study which showed that VIP inhibits IL-2 and IL-4 production through different molecular mechanisms. IL-2 production was regulated at a transcriptional level through the downregulation of IL-2 mRNA, whereas the production of IL-4 was modulated at a posttranscriptional level (Sun and Ganea, 1993). Through its downregulatory effect on IL-2 and IL-4 production, locally released VIP could potentially affect T cell development within the thymus (Xin et al., 1994).

The CD4 and CD8 spleen cells represent at least two of the cellular targets for VIP inhibition of proliferation [44]. VIP also up-regulates the costimulatory activity of macrophages for Ag-primed CD4+ T cells. VIP-treated macrophages gain the ability to induce Th2-type cytokines such as IL-4 and IL-5 and reduce Th1-type cytokines such as IFN-gamma and IL-2. One of the consequences of the VIP-induced shift in cytokine profile is a change in the Ag-specific Ig isotype, increasing IgG1 and decreasing IgG2a levels (Delgado et al., 1996). It was demonstrated that in the presence of costimulators (e.g., the anti-CD40 MoAb plus other neuropeptides) VIP may induce IgA1 and IgA2 production by isotype switching (Kimata and Fujimoto, 1995).

Depending on interactions with the local cytokine network, VIP may contribute significantly to controlling the amplitude and timing of the inflammatory response to foreign antigens. Presence of VIP and VIP-receptors in the thymus, and their effect on thymic cytokine production, suggests that VIP released locally within the thymic environment could also affect T cell development, and therefore participate in the generation and maturation of immune cells (Ganea, 1996).

In B cell lines, GM-1056, IM-9, and CBL, VIP enhanced IgA1, IgG1 and IgM production, respectively, in a dose-dependent fashion, while the other neuropeptides somatostatin or substance P failed to do so. Among the various cytokines examined including IL-1 beta, IL-2, IL-4, IL-5, IL-6, IL-8, IL-10, IL-13, and G-CSF. IL-6 and IL-10 also enhanced Ig production. However, VIP-induced enhancement of Ig production was specific, and was not mediated via these cytokines, since enhancement was blocked by the VIP antagonist (Kimata, 1996).

VIP induces increased levels of IL-10 in both serum and peritoneal fluid, and increases expression of the IL-10 mRNA in peritoneal exudate cells. The stimulation of IL-10 production in activated macrophages represents a novel anti-inflammatory activity of VIP, which presumably acts in vivo in conjunction with the inhibition of proinflammatory cytokines such as IL-6 and TNF-alpha to reduce the magnitude of the immune response (Delgado et al., 1999a).

VIP inhibits the production of IL-12, IL-6, tumor necrosis factor alpha (TNFalpha), and interferon gamma (IFNgamma) in vivo in endotoxemic mice. The presence of VIP in the lymphoid organs and the specific effects on cytokine production offer a physiological basis for their immunomodulatory role in vivo (Delgado et al., 1999b). It also inhibits cytokine production in stimulated CD4+ T cells through two separate mechanisms, which involve both cAMP-dependent and cAMP-independent transduction pathways (Wang et al., 1999).

Especially is important bimodal (stimulatory and inhibitory) effect of VIP on the NK cell activity. VIP, either preincubated or coincubated with human lymphocytes and hepatitis B surface antigen (HBsAg) strongly restores NK cell activity depressed by viral antigen. This study revealed that VIP represents a strong activator of NK cell activity (Azzari et al., 1992). VIP is also able to decrease NK cell activity of human large granular lymphocytes (LGL), showing maximal inhibition as dose ranging from 10^{-8} to 10^{-6} M. VIP -antagonist (4C1-D-Phe6-Leu17) was able to complete reverse the inhibitory effect of VIP on NK activity. This study confirmed the presence of a receptor for VIP on human LGL with NK activity (Siriani et al., 1992).

Inhibitory effect of VIP on NK effector function has been also reported (Rola-Pleszczynski et al., 1985). However, when lymphocytes were preincubated with VIP, than washed and added to target cells, a significant augmentation of NK activity ensued. Binding studies revealed that preincubation with VIP resulted in increased numbers of efector-target conjugates, whereas cytotoxic activity was not affected at the single cell level (Rola-Pleszczynski et al., 1985). In concentration of 10^{-6} M, VIP significantly inhibits the NK cell activity of normal human peripheral blood mononuclear cells (PBMC) on K562 target cells (Drew and Shearman, 1985).

CONCLUSION

In summary, results presented above strongly suggest that VIP produced during exercise could play an important role in modulation of activities of the immune system. Strong evidences about beneficial roles of VIP/NTM-reactive antibodies imply physical exercise as inexpensive and non-toxic approach in control of cancer and HIV disease, but an additional research is warranted before clear conclusions can be reached.

ACKNOWLEDGMENTS

This work was supported by the Ministry of Education, Science and Technological Development of the Republic of Serbia (Grant no. 173001).

REFERENCES

Azzari, C., Rossi, M. E., Resti, M., Caldini, A. L., Ciappi, S. and Vierucci, A. (1992). VIP restores natural killer cell activity depressed by hepatitis B surface antigen. *Viral Immunology*, *5*(3), 195-200.

Cohen, J. (2008). AIDS vaccine research. Thumbs down on expensive, hotly debated trial of NIH AIDS vaccine. *Science*, *321*(5888), 472.

Cheema, B., Gaul, C. A., Lane, K., Fiatarone, A. and Singh, M. A. (2008). Progressive resistance training in breast cancer: a systematic review of clinical trials. *Breast Cancer Research and Treatment*, *109*(1), 9-26.

Delgado, M., Munoz-Elias, E. J., Gomariz, R. P. and Ganea, D. (1999). Vasoactive intestinal peptide and pituitary adenylate cyclase-activating polypeptide enhance IL-10 production by murine macrophages: *in vitro* and *in vivo* studies. *Journal of Immunology*, *162*(3), 1707-1716.

Delgado, M., Munoz-Elias, E. J., Gomariz, R. P. and Ganea, D. (1999). VIP and PACAP inhibit IL-12 production in LPS-stimulated macrophages. Subsequent effect on IFNgamma synthesis by T cells. *Journal of Neuroimmunology*, *96*(2), 167-181.

Delgado, M., Leceta. J., Gomariz, R. P. and Ganea, D. (1999). Vasoactive intestinal peptide and pituitary adenylate cyclase-activating polypeptide stimulate the induction of Th2 responses by up-regulating B7.2 expression. *Journal of Immunology*, *163*(7), 3629-3635.

Drew, P. A. and Shearman, D. J. (1985). Vaso-active intestinal peptide: a neurotransmitter which reduces human NK cell activity and increases Ig synthesis. *Australian Journal of Experimental Biology and Medical Science*, *63*(Pt 3), 313-318.

Djordjevic, A., Veljkovic, M., Antoni, S., Sakarellos-Daitsiotis, M., Krikorian, D., Zevgiti, S., Dietrich, U., Veljkovic, N. and Branch, D. R. (2007). The presence of antibodies recognizing a peptide derived from the second conserved region of HIV-1 gp120 correlates with non-progressive HIV infection. *Current HIV Research*, *5*(5), 443-448.

Delafuente, M., Delgado, M. and Gomeriz, R. P. (1996). VIP modulation of immune cell functions. *Advances in Neuroimmunology*, *6*, 75-91.

Forbes, C. C., Blanchard, C. M., Mummery, W. K. and Courneya, K. (2015). Prevalence and correlates of strength exercise among breast, prostate, and colorectal cancer survivors. *Oncology Nursing Forum*, *42*(2), 118-27.

Francis, D. P., Gregory, T., McElrath, M. J., Belshe, R. B., Gorse, G. J., Migasena, S., Kitayaporn, D., Pitisuttitham, P., Matthews, T., Schwartz, D. H. and Berman, P. W. (1998). Advancing AIDSVAX to phase 3. Safety, immunogenicity, and plans for phase 3. *AIDS Research and Human Retroviruses*, *14*(Suppl 3), S325-331.

Friedenreich, C. M. (2011). Physical activity and breast cancer: Review of the Eepidemiologic evidence and biologic mechanisms. *Recent Results of Cancer Research*, *188*, 125-139.

Frisch, R. E., Wyshak, G., Witschi, J., Albright, N. L., Albright, T. E. and Schiff, I. (1987). Lower lifetime occurrence of breast cancer and cancers of the reproductive system among former college athletes. *International Journal of Fertility*, *32*(3), 217-225.

Galbo, H., Hilsted, J., Fahrenkrug, J. and Schaffalitzky De Muckadell, O. B. (1979). Fasting and prolonged exercise increase vasoactive intestinal polypeptide (VIP) in plasma. *Acta Physiologica Scandinavica*, *105*(3), 374-377.

Ganea, D. (1996). Regulatory effects of vasoactive intestinal peptide on cytokine production in central and peripheral lymphoid organs. *Advances in Neuroimmunology*, *6*(1), 61-74.

Ganea, D. and Sun, L. (1993). Vasoactive intestinal peptide downregulates the expression of IL-2 but not of IFN gamma from stimulated murine T lymphocytes. *Journal of Neuroimmunology*, *47*(2), 147-158.

Hvidsten, D., Jenssen, T. G., Bolle, R. and Burhol, P. G. (1986). Plasma gastrointestinal regulatory peptides in exercise-induced asthma. *European Journal of Respiratory Diseases*, *68*(5), 326-331.

Hilsted, J., Galbo, H., Sonne, B., Schwartz, T., Fahtenkrug, J., de Muckadell, O. B., Lauritsen, K. B. and Tronier, B. (1980). Gastroenteropancreatic hormonal changes during exercise. *American Journal of Physiology*, *239*(3), G136-140.

Irwin, M. L., Smith, A. W., McTiernan, A., Ballard-Barbash, R., Cronin, K., et al. (2008). Influence of pre- and postdiagnosis physical activity on mortality in breast cancer survivors: the health, eating, activity, and lifestyle study. *Journal of Clinical Oncology*, *26*(24), 3958-3964.

Kenfield, S. A., Stampfer, M. J., Giovannucci, E. and Chan, J. M. (2011). Physical activity and survival after prostate cancer diagnosis in the health professionals follow-up study. *Journal of Clinical Oncology*, *29*(6), 726-732.

Kimata, H. (1996). Vasoactive intestinal peptide differentially modulates human immunoglobulin production. *Advances in Neuroimmunology*, *6*(1), 107-115.

Kimata, H. and Fujimoto, M. (1995). Induction of IgA1 and IgA2 production in immature human fetal B cells and pre-B cells by vasoactive intestinal peptide. *Blood*, *85*(8), 2098-2104.

MacLaren, D. P., Raine, N. M., O'Connor, A. M. and Buchanan, K. D. (1995). Human gastrin and vasoactive intestinal polypeptide responses to endurance running in relation to training status and fluid ingested. *Clinical Science (Colch)*, *89*, 137-143.

McTiernan, A., Irwin, M. and Vongruenigen, V. (2010). Weight, physical activity, diet, and prognosis in breast and gynecologic cancers. *Journal of Clinical Oncology*, *28*(26), 4074-4080.

Nio, D. A., Moylan, R. N. and Roche, J. K. (1993). Modulation of T lymphocyte function by neuropeptides. Evidence for their role as local immunoregulatory elements. *Journal of Immunology*, *150*(12), 5281-5288.

Opstad, P. K. (1987). The plasma vasoactive intestinal peptide (VIP) response to exercise is increased after prolonged strain, sleep and energy deficiency and extinguished by glucose infusion. *Peptides*, *8*(1), 175-178.

Oektedalen, O., Opstad, P. K., Schaffalitzky de Muckadell, O. B., Fausa, O. and Flaten, O. (1983). Basal hyperchlorhydria and its relation to the plasma concentrations of secretin, vasoactive intestinal polypeptide (VIP) and gastrin during prolonged strain. *Regulatory Peptides*, *5*(3), 235-244.

Oktedalen, O., Opstad, P. K. and de Muckadell, O. B. (1983). The plasma concentration of secretin and vasoactive intestinal polypeptide (VIP) after long-term,strenuous exercise. *European Journal of Physiology and Occupational Physiology*, *52*, 5-8.

Oktedalen, O., Opstad, P. K., Fahrenkrug, J. and Fonnum, F. (1983). Plasma concentration of vasoactive intestinal polypeptide during prolonged physical exercise, calorie supply deficiency, and sleep deprivation. *Scandinavian Journal of Gastroenterology*, *18*(8), 1057-1062.

Paul, S. and Said, S. I. (1988). Human autoantibody to vasoactive intestinal peptide: increased incidence in muscular exercise. *Life Science*, *43*(13), 1079-1984.

Paul, S. (1987). Elevated levels of atrial natriuretic peptide and vasoactive intestinal peptide in exercising man. *Clinical Research*, *35*, 112A.

Paul, S., Heinz-Erian, P. and Said, S. I. (1985). Autoantibody to vasoactive intestinal peptide in human circulation. *Biochemical and Biophysical Research Communications*, *130*(1), 479-485.

Pozo, D., Delgado, M., Martinez, C., Guerrero, J. M., Receta, J., Gomariz, R. P. and Calvo, J. R. (2000). Immunobiology of vasoactive intestinal peptide (VIP). *Immunology Today*, *21*(1), 7-11.

Richman, E. L., Kenfield, S. A., Stampfer, M. J., Paciorek, A., Carroll, P. R. and Chan, J. M. (2011). Physical activity after diagnosis and risk of prostate cancer progression: data from the cancer of the prostate strategic urologic research endeavor. *Cancer Research*, *71*(11), 3889-3895.

Rola-Pleszczynski, M., Boldue, D. and St-Pierre, S. (1985). The effects of vasoactive intestinal peptide on human natural killer cell function. *Journal of Immunology*, *135*(4), 2569-2573.

Sun, L. and Ganea, D. (1993). Vasoactive intestinal peptide inhibits interleukin (IL)-2 and IL-4 production through different molecular mechanisms in T cells activated via the T cell receptor/CD3 complex. *Journal of Neuroimmunology*, *48*, 59-69.

Sirianni, M. C., Annibale, B., Tagliaferri, F., Fais, S., De Luca, S., Pallone, F., Delle Fave, G. and Aiuti, F. (1992). Modulation of human natural killer activity by vasoactive intestinal peptide (VIP) family, VIP, glucagon and GHRF specifically inhibit NK activity. *Regulatory Peptides*, *38*(1), 79-87.

Teresi, S., Boudard, F. and Bastide, M. (1996). Effect of calcitonin gene-related peptide and vasoactive intestinal peptide on murine CD4 and CD8 T cell proliferation. *Immunology Letters*, *50*(1-2), 105-113.

UNAIDS World AIDS Day Report. (2014). Available from: http://www. unaids.org/en/resources/campaigns/World-AIDSDay-Report-2014/factsheet.

Veljkovic, M., Branch, D. R., Dopsaj, V., Veljkovic, V., Veljkovic, N., Glisic, S. and Colombatti, A. (2011). Can natural antibodies to VIP or VIP-like HIV-1 glycoprotein facilitate prevention and supportive treatment of breast cancer? *Medical Hypotheses*, *77*(3), 404-408.

Veljkovic. M., Dopsaj. V., Dopsaj, M., Branch, D. R., Veljkovic, N., Sakarellos-Daitsiotis, M. M., Veljkovic, V., Glisic, S. and Colombatti, A. (2011). Physical activity and natural anti-VIP antibodies: potential role in breast and prostate cancer therapy. *PLoS One*, *6*(11), e28304.

Veljkovic, M., Dopsaj, V., Stringer, W. W., Sakarellos-Daitsiotis, M., Zevgiti, S., Veljkovic, V., Glisic, S. and Dopsaj, M. (2010). Aerobic exercise training as a potential source of natural antibodies protective against human immunodeficiency virus-1. *Scandinavian Journal of Medicine and Science in Sports*, *20*(3), 469-474.

Veljkovic, V., Veljkovic, N., Glisic, S. and Ho, M. W. (2008). AIDS vaccine: efficacy, safety and ethics. *Vaccine*, *26*(24), 3072-3077.

Veljkovic, N., Branch, D. R., Metlas, R., Prljic, J., Manfred, i. R., Stringer, W. W. and Veljkovic, V. (2004). Antibodies reactive with C-terminus of the second conserved region of HIV-1gp120 as possible prognostic marker and therapeutic agent for HIV disease. *Journal of Clinical Virology*, *31*(Suppl. 1), S39-44.

Veljkovic, N., Branch, D. R., Metlas, R., Prljic, J., Vlahovicek, K., Pongor, S. and Veljkovic, V. (2003). Design of peptide mimetics of HIV-1 gp120 for prevention and therapy of HIV disease. *Journal of Peptide Research*, *62*(4), 158-166.

Veljkovic, V., Metlas, R., Jevtovic, D. and Stringer, W. W. (2001). The role of passive immunization in hiv-positive patients: a case report. *Chest*, *120*(2), 662- 6.

Veljkovic, V., Metlas, R., Raspopovic, J. and Pongor, S. (1992). Spectral and sequence similarity between vasoactive intestinal peptide and the second conserved region of human immunodeficiency virus type 1 envelope glycoprotein (gp120): possible consequences on prevention and therapy of AIDS. *Biochemical and Biophysical Research Communication*, *189*(2), 705-710.

Wang, H. Y., Jiang, X., Gozes, I., Fridkin, M., Brenneman, D. E. and Ganea, D. (1999). *Vasoactive intestinal peptide inhibits cytokine production in T lymphocytes through cAMP-dependent and cAMP-independent mechanisms. Regulatory Peptides*, *84*(1-3), 55-67.

Wang, H. F., Xin, Z., Tang, H. and Ganea, D. (1996). Vasoactive intestinal peptide inhibits IL-4 production in murine T cells by a post-transcriptional mechanism. *Journal of Immunology*, *156*, 3243-3253.

Wiik, P., Opstad, P. K., Knardahl, S. and Boyum, A. (1988). Receptor for vasoactive intestinal peptide (VIP) on human mononuclear leucocytes are upregulated during prolonged strain and energy deficiency. *Peptides*, *9*(1), 181-186.

Woie, L., Cada, B. and Opstad, P. K. (1986). Increase in plasma vasoactive intestinal polypeptide (VIP) in muscular exercise in humans. Relation to haemodynamic and hormonal changes. *General Pharmacology*, *18*(6), 577-587.

Wyshak, G. and Frisch, R. E. (2000). Breast cancer among former college athletes compared to non-athletes: a 15-year follow-up. *British Journal of Cancer*, *82*(3), 726-730.

Xin, Z., Tang, H. and Ganea, D. (1994). Vasoactive intestinal peptide inhibits interleukin (IL)-2 and IL-4 production in murine thymocytes activated via the TCR/CD3 complex. *Journal of Neuroimmunology*, *54*, 59-68.

Yiangou, Y., Serrano, R., Bloom, S. R., Pena, J. and Festenstein, H. (1990). Effects of prepro-vasoactive intestinal peptide-derived peptides on the murine immune response. *Journal of Neuroimmunology*, *29*(1-3), 65-72.

In: Physical Activity Effects on the Anthropological Status ...   ISBN: 978-1-63484-782-7
Editors: Fadilj Eminović and Milivoj Dopsaj   © 2016 Nova Science Publishers, Inc.

Chapter 14

PHYSICAL ACTIVITY AND COGNITION ACROSS THE LIFE SPAN

Dragan Pavlović

Faculty for Special Education and Rehabilitation,
Faculty of Philosophy, Department of Psychology,
University of Belgrade, Belgrade, Serbia

ABSTRACT

Animal studies showed positive impact of physical activity on cognitive abilities. In animal models, exercizing increases the plasticity of the nervous system, enhancing synaptic function, especially for learning. One of the main mechanisms is the increase of attentional capacities enabling faster information processing. Human trials confirmed these results in all ages. Aerobic training of pregnant women has favorable effects on brain development and cognition of their offspring. During the school period children who exercise more vigorously learn better and have better attention. In the adult period physical activity improves cognition and enhances neurogenesis in critical structures such as hippocampus and dorsal striatum. Midlife physical activity prevents cognitive loss in old age. Even if started late in life, aerobic training reduces brain tissue loss and has preventive effects on dementia of all types. There are indications that exercise also exerts influence on the human genome promoting epigenetic modifications. The pivotal factor in aforementioned processes is brain derived neurotrophic factor (BDNF) the molecule that influences energy homeostasis through control of feeding and physical activity. BDNF stimulates glucose transport, mitochondrial biogenesis, increases insulin sensitivity and parasympathetic tone, with positive effects on cognition, emotion, cardiovascular function, and peripheral metabolism. Lack of physical activity impairs BDNF. Exercise upregulates the expression of genes mediating synaptic modulation and signal transduction, increases the volume of gray matter in critical structures of frontal and temporal lobe as shown in neuroimaging studies. Exercise also has the effect of preventing cognitive decline and dementia in old age. Exercise has beneficial effects on cognition in many neuropsychiatric conditions such as stroke, multiple sclerosis, Parkinson's disease, various dementias, schizophrenia, affective diseases, and also in vascular diseases and diabetes mellitus. Across the lifespan physical activity improves attentional and executive processes, cognitive control, memory and learning, visuospatial abilities, thus improving activities of daily living and quality of life. The recommended types of physical activity are walking, hiking, jogging/running, bicycling, and dance, use of exercise machines, yoga, stretching, tennis, squash and lap-swimming.

Keywords: physical activity, cognition, brain derived neurotrophic factor (BDNF), aerobic exercise, synaptogenesis, sarcopenia

INTRODUCTION

Mobility is one of the main factors of quality of life (QoL). Unrestricted motion is almost a synonym for human health. It has been estimated that physical inactivity is responsible for 5-10% of deaths worldwide (World Health Organization, 2002). Regular exercise reduces morbidity and mortality even in patients with chronic diseases including the cardiovascular and cerebrovascular diseases, arterial hypertension, diabetes, obesity, osteoporosis, mental diseases and some types of cancer such as those of colon and breast (Haskell et al. 2007). In elderly, physical activity reduces risk of falls and cognitive decline (Nelson et al., 2007).

It has been found that aerobic fitness reduces brain tissue loss and improves cognition during aging (Gomez-Pinilla, Hillman, 2013). Extensive animal studies, investigations of humoral factors, neuropsychological testing, electrophysiological and neuroimaging studies yielded numerous evidence of favorable impact of exercise on cardiorespiratory fitness and cognitive functions (McKee et al., 2014). One of the main mechanisms of exercise influence is the enlargement of attentional resources enabling faster information processing. According to animal models, physical activity increases the plasticity of the nervous system, enhancing synaptic function, especially for learning. Adequate nutrition complements the effects of exercise, and both influence the energy metabolism mainly through mitochondrial functions. Exercise protects central nervous system (CNS) from neurological disorders, and also exerts influence on the human genome promoting epigenetic modifications. Brain derived neurotrophic factor (BDNF) influences energy homeostasis through control of feeding and physical activity (Marosi, Mattson, 2014). BDNF has favorable influence of energetic challenges on cognition, emotion, cardiovascular function, and peripheral metabolism through stimulation of glucose transport and mitochondrial biogenesis. Important effects of BDNF are increase of insulin sensitivity and parasympathetic tone. Three main factors impairing BDNF system are sedentary lifestyle, chronic stress and genetic factors.

Exercise has positive influence on cognitive processes from early childhood to senescence, reducing the rate of brain tissue loss (i.e., atrophy) and improving functions of many brain areas (Colcombe et al., 2006). The main regions that benefit from physical activity are those mediating cognition, memory, inhibition and attention. Less active individuals are incapable of assigning more attentional resources during stimulus engagement and less capable to accomplish tasks.

In the domain of pathology, physical activity has the potential to reduce the risk for Alzheimer, Huntington's and Parkinson's diseases and also to diminish functional decline if the neurodegeneration occurs, and reduces the risk of traumatic brain injury (McKee et al., 2014). Regular exercising is also therapeutic and protective in depression. One proposed mechanism is favorable impact of exercise on the hypothalamic-pituitary-adrenal axis known to control the stress response. Another benefit is the promotion of homeostasis after an immune challenge (Barrientos et al., 2011). Physical activity even reduces the genetic risk for dementia (Deeny et al., 2008). There are also indirect favourable effects of exercise on brain health through risk reduction of cardiovascular disease, type 2 diabetes, hypertension, obesity, stroke, elevated cholesterol levels, inflammation and oxydation (McKee et al., 2014).

ANATOMOFUNCTIONAL INTERFACE OF EXERCISE AND COGNITION

Many animal and human studies found that physical training enhances cognition through the processes of neurogenesis, synaptogenesis, angiogenesis and the release of neurotrophins (Hötting, Röder, 2013). These changes enhance the capacity of an individual to respond to new demands with behavioral adaptations and enhance survival. Recent animal studies revealed the importance of physical activity for synaptic plasticity and energy metabolism (Gomez-Pinilla, F., Hillman, C., 2013). All aforementioned processes have favorable effects on neuroplasticity, the process of changing functional and structural properties of the brain under the changing demands. Neuroplasticity is crucial for learning and attaining skills (Hötting, Röder, 2013).

Regular exercise leads to augmentation of synaptic information flow via the production of BDNF, especially in cognitive-crucial areas such as hippocampus (Vaynman et al., 2003). BDNF is coordinating other neurotrophic factors, neurotransmitters and hormones and with insulin-like growth factor 1 (IGF-1) mediates synaptic plasticity, neurogenesis and metabolism (Vaynman et al., 2004).

Adult neurogenesis is one of the most important factors of brain health. Several areas of adult mammalian brain, such as the olfactory bulb, hippocampal formation, certain parts of hypothalamus and periventricular area, retain the ability to produce new neurons, the process known as neurogenesis. In the adult rodent brain, exercise promotes neurogenesis which can be the core of positive influence of physical activity on cognition (Itoh et al., 2011). Furthermore, vascular endothelial growth factor (VEGF) mediates brain angiogenic effects of exercise (During, Cao, 2006). Neurovascular changes in the hippocampus imposed by exercise probably mediate effects on cognition (Clark et al., 2009). Antibodies against IGF-1 and VEGF block the effects of exercise (Ding et al., 2006; Fabel et al., 2003). Aerobic exercise and physical activity in general significantly increase the number of new neurons formed in the hippocampus, while mental training with challenging goals increases the numbers of neurons that survive (Curlik, Shors, 2013).

Exercise modulates BDNF at two levels: 1. at the transcriptional level by using mechanisms of epigenetic regulation, 2. at the translational level by using the tissue-type plasminogen activator (tPA) (Gomez-Pinilla, Hillman, 2013). BDNF system in the brain uses two molecules: the precursor (proBDNF) and its mature product (mBDNF), binding to different receptors and having different effects. tPA facilitate proBDNF cleavage into mBDNF and can have an important role in mediating favorable exercise effects on the brain.

Motor activity has the pivotal role in the evolution of the human brain. It is essential for the cognitive functions necessary for survival. These influences are particularly evident in hippocampus and hypothalamus, leading to more efficacious energy metabolism and enlargement of the brain. The physical activity also induces changes in networks involving the prefrontal cortex (Gomez-Pinilla, Hillman, 2013). Higher fitness correlates with larger bilateral hippocampal volume in older adults on functional magnetic resonance imaging (fMRI) (Erickson et al., 2010). Functional effects are, among others, better spatial memory performance and higher serum BDNF level. Animal model reveale that mice that exercise selectively, have upregulated dentate gyrus cerebral blood volume, correlating with increased neurogenesis. Human studies showed the same results with increased capacity for verbal learning (Pereira et al., 2007). It is of particular interest that the brain areas most affected by aging also show the greatest fitness-related sparing.

Aerobic training demonstrates increase in gray matter in the frontal lobes, including the dorsal anterior cingulate cortex (ACC), supplementary motor area, middle frontal gyrus, dorsolateral region of the right inferior frontal gyrus, the left superior temporal lobe, and white matter volume in the anterior third of the corpus callosum (Colcombe et al., 2006). These regions exert top-down control on cognition and behavior. Aerobic fitness training also changes blood flow and metabolic activity in the brain, including reduced activation in rostral ACC activity, leading to less behavioral conflict. Other systems that benefits from aerobic training are the default mode network (posterior cingulate cortex, frontal medial cortex, hippocampal and parahippocampal cortices), frontal executive and fronto-parietal networks (Voss et al., 2010). Exercise also increase functional connectivity leading to better cognition.

Genetic studies show that exercise upregulates the expression of genes mediating synaptic modulation and signal transduction such as synapsin I and II, synaptotagmin, syntaxin, CaM-KII, MAP-K/ERK, I and II, protein kinase C, PKC-δ and transcription factor cAMP response element binding protein (CREB) (Molteni et al., 2004; Gomez-Pinilla, F., Hillman, C., 2013). Another set of genes affected by aerobic training are those related to neurotransmitter systems with upregulation of N-methyl-D-aspartate (NMDA) glutamatergic receptor system and downregulation of GABAergic system, the two being mostly antagonistic. Majority of the abovementioned genes are associated with BDNF and IGF brain systems (Ding et al., 2006).

Adenosine monophosphate-activated protein kinase (AMPK) is a serine-threonine kinase that can sense low energy levels and is capable of reestablishing the energy balance by means of normalizing cellular metabolism (Hardie, 2004). Another molecule influencing energy balance is ghrelin. Ghrelin is secreted from an empty stomach increasing appetite and energy intake, and can bind to hippocampal receptors mediating hippocampal synaptic plasticity (McNay, 2007). There is also a central ghrelin production. Other important molecules are UmtCK, UCP2 and docosahexaenoic acid (DHA). UmtCK may influence cognition interacting with BDNF system while UCP2 is a mitochondrial uncoupling protein that supposedly play a role in the regulation of energy metabolism. DHA is an omega-3 fatty acid that is a primary structural component of the human brain, providing neuronal membranes with the fluidity enabling normal neuronal signaling (Teague et al., 2002). Humans are dependent on dietary consumption of DHA as they can not synthesize omega-3 fatty acids (Pavlović, 2012a). Exercise can preserve membrane DHA by acting on molecular systems in the hippocampus. Physical activity modifies syntaxin 3, a plasma membrane-bound protein linked to the function of DHA (Darios, Davletov, 2006). Aerobic training is necessary for maintenance of neurons so that lack of exercise may worsen the effects of numerous neurological illnesses (Gomez-Pinilla, 2008). Another molecular mechanism of aerobic training is change in the NR2B subunit of the NMDA receptor, allowing synaptic growth and plasticity. Physical activity exerts its influence also through monoaminergic, endorphinergic and endocannabinoid systems (Rossi et al., 2014).

Epigenetics is the discipline of genetics that study cellular and physiological trait variations that are not caused by changes in the deoxyribonucleic acid (DNA) sequence. Epigenetics explores environmental factors that affect gene functions. There is still controversy whether these transcriptional gene changes are heritable or not in mammals. These changes can be important in control of cognitive functions and emotions. Epigenetic mechanisms such as postreplication modifications of DNA and nuclear proteins have impact on BDNF gene, known as an interface between physical activity and cognition. BDNF can mediate synapse plasticity downstream, learning and memory and reduction of depression (Feng et al., 2007).

CHILDHOOD

Pregnancy

Exercise improves cognition, academic performance and overall health in children (Drollette et al., 2014). Physical activity is of utmost importance for young of all ages, and even before birth. Aerobic fitness workout of the mother during pregnancy can increase placental and fetal growth (Sibley, Etnier, 2003). The placenta may produce and/or permeate neurotrophic factors for the developing brain.

In a series of studies of Clapp and coworkers, pregnant women who performed aerobic exercise three or more times per week for at least 20 minutes or more, were included. Control subjects voluntarily stopped exercising during pregnancy. The children of active mothers showed better capacity of environmental stimulus orientation and self-regulation after sound and light stimuli, five days after birth (Clapp et al., 1999). One-year old children of active women had significantly higher scores on psychomotor scale of the Bayley Scales of Infant Development (Clapp et al., 1998). The offspring of active mothers were tested again five years after birth. These children showed better scores on tests of general intelligence and oral language (Clapp, 1996).

School Age

Improvement in scholastic performances is the ultimate goal of classical teaching, but counterintuitively more time of physical education and less time in the classroom leads to improvement in learning (Sallis, 2010). Metaanalysis of studies in school age children revealed that exercise correlated to perceptual skills, intelligent quotient (IQ), achievement, verbal tests, mathematics tests, and developmental level/academic readiness (Sibley, Etnier, 2003). Moreover, there is evidence that aerobic physical activity in childhood has favorable effects on cognition, academic achievement, and psychosocial function (Singh et al., 2012; Lees, Hopkins, 2013). In the random controlled study of Hillman et al. (2014) 221 children age 7 to 9 years were engaged in 9-month afterschool physical training program with matching control. Results showed significantly increased fitness measured by maximal oxygen consumption, attentional inhibition and cognitive flexibility, measures of executive control. A British random controlled study of Davis et al. (2011) in 171 sedentary, overweight

7- to 11-year-old children revealed dose-response benefits of exercise on executive function and mathematical achievement. There were signs of increased bilateral prefrontal cortex activity and reduced bilateral posterior parietal cortex activity. In the Irish study, 30 adolescents between the ages of 13 and 14 years, after acute exercise and after a period of relaxation, performed a modified Eriksen flanker task (Hogan M et al., 2013). Fit adolescents had significantly faster reaction times in the exercise then in resting condition. In a study with 18 preadolescent participants, exercise was found to improve spelling on Wide Range Achievement Test (WRAT 4) and arithmetic, but did not change sentence comprehension, independently from the intensity of exercise (Duncan, Johnson, 2013).

Moderate-intensity bout of aerobic exercise of treadmill walking in 40 preadolescent children showed improvement in event related potentials and a modified Eriksen flanker task (Drollette et al., 2014). The children to benefit most were those with lower inhibitory control capacity, one of the processes known as cognitive control. Cognitive control is the top-down brain activity responsible for self-regulation in selecting, scheduling, maintaining, and coordinating the computational processes that underlie perception, memory, and goal directed behavior (Norman, Shallice, 1986). This function overlaps with the concept of metacognition. Closely related to cognitive control are processes of inhibition, working memory, and cognitive flexibility (Diamond, 2006).

In a randomized controlled pilot study 64 healthy children (mean age 6.2 yrs. SD 0.3) were engaged in two hours of aerobically intense physical education per week for 10 weeks or standard physical education (Fisher et al., 2011). The neuropsychological battery applied consisted of Cambridge Neuropsychological Test Battery (CANTAB), the Attention Network Test (ANT), the Cognitive Assessment System (CAS) and the short form of the Connor's Parent Rating Scale (CPRS:S). In the experimental group significant improvement from baseline was found on spatial span and working memory on CANTAB and ANT Reaction Time and Accuracy.

Particular problem across all ages, but very prominent in childhood, is the association of energy consumption and storage as well as spending of energy, with cognitive and scholastic performances (Burkhalter, Hillman, 2011). Pattern of overconsumption of energy with increased body mass coupled with sedentary lifestyle is related to lower cognitive performance and academic achievement during school period. Present recommendations state that children should have 60 minutes or more of physical exercise daily, mostly moderate to strong intensity aerobic training (Strong et al., 2005).

Physical exercise reduces the risk of cardiovascular diseases, obesity, depression, and anxiety (Meeusen, 2014). Adequate nutrition can also prevent and protect against various diseases. Unfortunately, in developed and developing countries, there is increase in sedentary lifestyle among children leading to earlier onset of diabetes type 2 and obesity. Overweight is associated with reduced, and aerobic fitness with increased academic achievement (Davis, Cooper, 2011). Nutrition is also of utmost importance for the cognitive development, and formation of the optimal neuronal connections. Especially omega-3 fatty acids consumption improves synaptic function in contrast to intake of higher quantities of sugar and saturated fats that increase oxidative stress and decrease synaptic plasticity and cognition (Gomez-Pinilla, 2011). Physical activity augments effects of healthy diet on brain functioning.

Neuroimaging and Electrophysiology Studies

The volume of the hippocampus on MRI bilaterally was greater in physically fit preadolescent children in contrast to unfit controls according to Chaddock et al. (2010). The volume positively correlated to scores on memory tasks. Another brain structure that seems to benefit from exercise is dorsal striatum known to partake in cognitive control and inhibition. The dorsal striatum was larger in more physically fit children (Chaddock et al., 2010).

Cognitive control, as mentioned previously, is goal-directed cognitive process underlying perception, memory, and action, particularly prone to benefit from aerobic exercise (Hillman et al., 2011). Inhibitory aspect of cognitive control is the capacity to disregard the distractions and focus on task-important aspects of the environment. Potential electrophysiological measure of fitness-cognition association is P3 (P300 or P3b) wave of the event-related brain potential (ERP). The P3 is believed to represent the updating of memory once sensory information has been analyzed (Donchin, 1981). The amplitude of P3 is proportional to the quantity of attentional resources for the period of stimulus processing (Polich, 2007) while the latency is proportional to stimulus evaluation time (Duncan-Johnson, 1981). Comparison of P3 between higher-fit and lower-fit children (M = 9.6 years) was done in a study of Hillman et al. (2005). ERPs were recorded during a cognitive task of responding to rare stimuli ("oddballs") immerged in frequent non-target stimuli. Children that were fit showed larger P3 amplitude, shorter P3 latency and better task performance than unfit controls. In a study with 9–10 year old children with a modified flanker task higher-fit children displayed more correct responses and larger P3 amplitudes than lower-fit children (Hillman et al., 2009).

ADULTHOOD

The majority of studies of association of physical activity and cognitive abilities explored these factors in older adults, especially demented, and to a lesser extent children and adults. In a study of 144 community members aged 19 to 93, working memory and momentary affect experience were examined after exercise or neutral activity (Hogan CL et al., 2013). Physical activity was associated with increased levels of high-arousal positive affect (HAP) and decreased levels of low-arousal positive affect (LAP), and also led to faster reaction times on a working memory task, across ages.

In a counterbalanced, crossover, randomized controlled study, 87 young adults (mean age, 21.4 years) were tested cognitively, preceded or not, with 30 minutes of three grades of exercise (Loprinzi, Kane, 2015). Questionnaires were applied assessing sedentary or active lifestyles. After a 30-minute acute bout of moderate-intensity exercise, concertation was significantly better than with no exercise. Visual attention and task switching were worse in individuals with sedentary behavior. Cardiorespiratory fitness was insignificantly associated with reasoning-related cognitive function.

A study conducted in 67 adolescents from Spain examined effects of increasing the time and intensity of physical education on cognitive performance and academic achievement

(Ardoy et al., 2014). The experimental group that was on intensive physical education four times a week, showed increase in non-verbal and verbal ability, abstract reasoning, spatial ability, and numerical ability but not on verbal reasoning, compared to control group (two regular classes a week). Measures of school achievement revealed that mean school grades increased more in experimental than in control group. The group of slightly increased physical education (four times a week of regular training) did not show any difference from control group having two regular classes a week.

A single bout of exercise was shown to improve motor memory and motor skill learning in a Danish study on 48 young subjects (Roig et al., 2012). The instrument used was visuomotor accuracy-tracking task. A bout of intense cycling or rest was applied before or after testing. A single session of intense training immediately after practicing (in the early phase of memory consolidation) showed the best long-term retention of the motor skill, but not an immediate effect. On the contrary, a bout of moderate to high intensity ergobycicle training was associated with harmful effects on the executive component of the computerized modified-Stroop task during exercise (Labelle et al., 2014).

An important question is weather midlife exercise has long-lasting cognitive effects in the older age. The Age Gene/Environment Susceptibility—Reykjavik Study addressed this problem in a population-based cohort of men and women (Chang et al., 2010). The time elapsed from physical activity in midlife to measurements in older age was 26 years. Subjects were tested with neuropsychological battery and the presence of dementia was assessed according to current criteria. Screening for dementia was done with Mini-Mental State Examination (Folstein et al., 1975) and the digit symbol substitution test (Wechsler, 1955) and further supplemented with other tests if needed. The number of nondemented individuals was 4,761, and of demented 184 (3.7%). No midlife exercise reported 68.8% of participants, equal or less than 5 hours 26.5%, and more than 5 hours 4.5%. Nondemented participants from both active groups had significantly faster speed of processing, better memory and executive function. The ≤5 hours exercise group was significantly less prone to dementia in late life after adjusting for confounders.

The impact of regular physical training as opposed to a single bout of training on cognition and emotions were assessed in a study in 75 young adults (ages 18–36) (Hopkins et al., 2012). The group consisted of healthy, sedentary young adults. They were genetically evaluated to determine BDNF allelic status (Val-Val or Val-Met polymorphism). Subjects were neuropsychologicaly assessed with novel object recognition (NOR) memory and a battery of surveys and questionnaires, between the acquisition and recall on memory test. Testing was done on the baseline and after a four-week exercise program, with or without exercise on the final day, or with exercise on the final test day only, or remaining sedentary for the same period. Pedometers were given to observe their daily activity. Subjects who were physicaly active showed better object recognition memory and diminution in perceived stress, only in participants who trained for four weeks including the final day of testing. Interestingly, improvements on the NOR test were observed exclusively in subjects homozygous for the BDNF Val allele. Exercise-induced changes in cognition were not correlated with changes in emotions.

AGING

Introduction

Several reports found that older adults, between 65 and 74 years of age, are the least physically active portion of the population (Tyndall et al., 2013). Numerous studies have demonstrated that physical activity increase cognitive functions in older adults improves physical capacity and quality of life, and prevent, or at least reduce cognitive deterioration (Chang et al., 2012; Bherer, 2015). It is important that physical activity is performed safely and in that case it can reduce morbidity and mortality even in old age (Lautenschlager et al., 2012). There is a body od evidence that exercise can contribute to healthy brain aging and have protective effects against cognitive deterioration and dementia.

Studies

Level of improvement of cognition is much higher after exercise than after cognitive training, even in frail individuals and those at risk of cognitive impairment. A systematic review of relevant studies examining the effects of exercise on cognitive functions in older adults found that 26 out of 27 studies reported a positive correlation between physical activity and maintenance or enhancement of cognitive function (Carvalho et al., 2014).

The randomized controlled trial conducted by Linde and Alfermann (2014) assessed effects of physical, cognitive, and combined physical plus cognitive activity on 70 healthy senior individuals (age 60-75). The three experimental groups showed enhanced concentration immediately after intervention opposed to the control group. Only the two exercise groups had improvement in concentration 3 months later. The cognitive training group displayed better cognitive speed 3 months after intervention while combined training group improved both immediately and three months after intervention. Short-term memory, spatial relations and reasoning were not affected. The best results were obtained with combined paradigm.

Frailty, Sarcopenia and Wellness

An almost unavoidable condition in older individuals is frailty, defined as an age-associated syndrome of reduced functional reserve and withstanding of stress because of decline in several physiological systems (Casas-Herrero et al., 2013). Frailty is the effect of cumulative declines across multiple physiologic systems (Landi et al., 2010). Frailty leads to functional decline, falls, institutionalization and increased mortality.

Among most important contributing factors is sarcopenia – the loss of muscle mass. Reduced exercise further augments muscle loss. Sarcopenia almost inevitably leads to frailty (Morie et al., 2010). Frailty is associated with muscle atrophy and cognitive decline as they share some pathophysiological mechanisms (Garcia-Garcia et al., 2011). People with dementia in general have impaired gait and a low level of physical activity, the characteristics shared with frailty (Garcia-Garcia et al., 2011). People with cognitive loss have difficulties in simultaneous talking or counting while walking ("stops walking while talking") and are more prone to falls (Uemura et al., 2012). These findings lead to development of assessment of interaction between cognition (mostly executive function) and gait based on walking while performing a secondary task (the dual-task paradigm) (Casas-Herrero et al., 2013). Regular physical activity has been shown to protect against diverse components of the frailty syndrome and importantly, frailty is not a contra-indication to physical activity (Landi et al., 2010).

The Toledo Study tested the neuromuscular and functional performance in 43 frail oldest old with and without mild cognitive impairment (MCI) and relations between functional capacities, muscle mass, strength, and power output of the leg muscles (Casas-Herrero et al., 2013). The study showed that the frail oldest old, with and without MCI, have similar functional and neuromuscular results compared to non frail subjects. Functional outcomes and incidences of falls were associated with muscle mass, strength, and power in the frail elderly population. The systematic review of trials examining the usefulness of physical activity on improving cognitive function in older people found 12 medium- to high-quality randomized controlled trials (Tseng et al., 2011). The analysis demonstrated that an exercise of 6 weeks and at least 3 times per week for 60 minutes had a favorable effect on cognition.

Another concept important in maintaining good cognition and quality of life in senescence is wellness. The wellness is divided in six dimensions: occupational, social, intellectual, physical, emotional, and spiritual (Strout, Howard, 2012). Studies so far revealed that midlife occupation complexity, marriage, social networks, formal education, intellectual activities, physical activity, healthy nutrition, motivational ability, purpose in life, and spirituality have protective effects on cognition. Not all dimensions are necessary to be highly represented as even one can at least partially compensate for low wellness in other dimensions. The more dimensions are developed, the higher is the benefit.

Biological and Neuroimaging Data

In 62 older healthy individuals, a six months regime of medium or low-intensity exercise, or control regime, resulted in increase in memory scores, local gray matter volume in prefrontal and cingulate cortex, and BDNF levels, without significant differences between intensity groups (Ruscheweyh et al., 2011). Catecholamine levels were not changed significantly among experimental and control groups. Another trial addressed effects of weight loss and exercise on cognition, mood, and quality of life in 107 frail obese older adults. Weight loss and exercise improve cognition and quality of life, but their combination may offer benefits similar to physical activity alone.

Physical training has beneficial influence on preservation of gray matter in late adulthood. In Pittsburgh component of the Cardiovascular Health Study Cognition Study (CHS-CS) trial in 299 adults (mean age 78 years), grey matter volume and cognition were measured 9 years after the initial assessment. Physical activity was assessed by quantity of walking, and MRI has been done on both occasions (Erickson et al., 2010). Study showed greater preservation of volumes of frontal, occipital, entorhinal, and hippocampal regions on

MRI and reduction on cognitive decline in individuals that walked 72 blocks a week. At the initial evaluation, females stated less than males.

A diffusion tensor imaging study of brain areas mediating memory and executive function was conducted in 276 subjects, mean age = 83.0 years (Tian et al., 2014). Participants were divided in three levels of physical activity: sedentary, lifestyle active, and exercise active. This study examined whether higher physical activity would be longitudinally associated with greater microstructural integrity in memory- and executive function-related networks and whether these associations would be independent of physical function and chronic diseases. The exercise active group had lower mean diffusivity in the medial temporal lobe and the cingulate, independent of age, sex, and race. These results reflex greater memory-related microstructural integrity in elderly.

There are biological factors that modify exercise-cognition interaction such as Apolipoprotein E (APOE) genotype. In a cross-sectional study of 1799 older individuals examined in the Third National Health and Nutrition Examination Survey (NHANES-III; 1988–1994), physical activity positively correlated with better cognition on a short mental status examination (SMSE) (Obisesan et al., 2012). Participants were a representative sample of US noninstitutionalized population. The effect was better in non-ε4 carriers regardless of ethnicity, education, income, and history of serious chronic illness. The presence of APOE allele ε4 is the most frequently present nondeterministic genetic risk factor for late-onset Alzheimer's dementia. With corrections for mobility limitations, all allele carriers benefit from physical activity. These findings open the opportunity for broad implementation of exercise as an important primary intervention strategy in dementia.

In a portion of subjects from the Pittsburgh Cardiovascular Health Study-Cognition Study, tensor-based morphometry to high-resolution brain MRI was used to discern the impact of education and physical activity on brain tissue volumes in the elderly (Ho et al. 2011). Brain tissue volumes of target areas were related to educational level and physical activity. Higher educational levels were associated with ~2–3% greater tissue volumes in the temporal gray matter, while more exercise was associated with ~2–2.5% greater average tissue volumes in the white matter of the corona radiata. Also body mass index (BMI) highly correlated with education and physical activity.

DEMENTIA

Dementia is a syndrome of acquired cognitive decline with reduced activities of daily living and behavior changes, caused by more than 200 etiologies, the most frequent being Alzheimer's disease (AD), vascular dementias (VaD), Lewy body dementia (LBD) and frontotemporal dementias (FTD), comprising around 95% of all cases (Pavlović, Pavlović, 2014). Alzheimer's disease is the most frequent dementia, of epidemic proportions (Winchester et al., 2013). Exercise is a lifestyle intervention shown to benefit patients with dementia (Stubbs et al., 2015).

Regular exercise, has been shown to improve cognition, emotions and activity. In 104 early-stage AD patients, lack of physical activity positively correlated with severity of dementia measured with the Mini-Mental State Examination (MMSE), and negative emotions assessed with Profile of Mood States (POMS). Active patients had an attenuation in global cognitive decline. Intervention of implementation of walking activities, more than 2 hours per week over 1 year, had a significant improvement of MMSE scores. Another option for AD patients is treadmill training. In a study of elderly with mild dementia, a neuropsychological battery was applied before the treadmill training and after 16 weeks (Recovered et al., 2014). Experimental group showed improvement in Cambridge Cognitive Examination (CAMCOG) while controls declined. Also the experimental group had significant improvement on the functional capacity. The recent rigorous systematic review of the efficacy of combined cognitive and exercise training in older adults with or without cognitive impairment revealed the efficacy of combined intervention in improving cognitive and functional status (Law et al., 2014). When it comes to the whole spectrum of dementia, a cross-sectional study with 134 individuals, mean age 82 years, showed that strength, aerobic fitness, and balance are significantly associated with working memory (Volkers, Scherder, 2014).

The latest Cochrane Database meta analysis of exercise programs for people with dementia found high heterogeneity of studies in regard to type and severity of dementia and intensity of physical activity (Forbes et al., 2013). In spite of methodological variability of eligible studies, authors of the review concluded that exercise programs might have a significant impact on improving activities of daily living (ADLs) and possibly in improving cognition in people with dementia, but not on depression. A systematic review of longitudinal studies, with a follow-up time of at least 2 years revealed that a protective effect of mental activity on cognitive function has been consistently reported (Wang et al., 2012). The same review found that the protective effect of physical activity on the risk of dementia has been reported in majority of observational studies, but less evident in interventional studies. The non-aerobic exercise program of 6 weeks in a group of 27 AD patients exhibited significant improvements in sustained attention, visual memory but only a trend in working memory (Yágüez et al., 2011). Patients were tested with six computerized tests from the CANTAB, pre and post training. During six weeks of follow up subjects from control group (N = 12) significantly deteriorated in attention.

Preventive measures are urgently needed to reduce the growing epidemic of dementia. There are substantial evidence that physical activity, mostly aerobic training may decrease dementia risk (Ahlskog et al., 2011). A meta-analyses of prospective studies revealed a significant reduce of risk of dementia related to midlife exercise. Physical activity, short and long-term, have beneficent effect on cognition in all ages opposed to sedentary lifestyle in healthy subjects but also in those with cognitive decline. Aerobic training also has favorable effects on brain circulation. In older adults exercise is related to larger hippocampal and cortical gray matter volumes, improved function of various brain networks, and better spatial memory compared with unfit seniors.

Community based physical training programs would be the best approach because of the widest availability. A four month intervention randomized controlled study from Tasmania included 40 community-dwelling AD patients mean age of 74.1 years (Vreugdenhil et al., 2012). They were diagnosed with mild to moderate dementia. In the experimental group subjects had a program of daily workouts and walking under the supervision of their informal carers. After four months of exercise, patients showed improved cognition significantly increased MMSE scores by 2.6 points, better mobility and increased Instrumental Activities of Daily Living scores. Another approach is implementation of widely popular systems of training such as yoga or Tai Chi. In a randomized controlled study with 389 older persons with mild dementia or amnestic mild cognitive impairment (MCI), participants engaged in a

24 forms simplified Tai Chi program or stretching and toning exercise for one year at least three times per week (Lam et al., 2011). Both experimental and control group exhibited improvement in global cognitive function, delayed recall and subjective cognitive complaints after 5 months. Progression to dementia occurred in 2.2% subjects from Tai Chi group and 10.8% from control group.

As subjective self report about physical activity is not reliable, objective actigraphic measures can be applied. A portable actigraph is usually a battery-operated activity monitor worn on the wrist, waist or leg. In a study of community-dwelling elderly subjects from the Rush Memory and Aging Project, 70 with and 624 without dementia, total daily activity was measured for 2-16 days (James et al., 2012). Muscle strength and motor performance were measured. Cognition was evaluated using a battery of 19 tests. When controlling for age, sex, and education, total activity per day related with global motor scores, regardless of dementia status.

OTHER NEUROPSYCHIATRIC DISEASES

Stroke

Stroke is one of the leading causes of morbidity, disability and mortality, encroaching also cognitive disturbances of various severity (Pavlović, 2012b). Cerebrovascular diseases are an important health hazard worldwide leading to various neurological sequels including impairments in cognition, mood and QoL. There is the reciprocal connection between motor activity and cognition in stroke. Cognitive impairment due to brain infarction can affect walking, motion control, and proper conduct during the walk. In a Serbian study 50 stroke patients with hemiparesis, and 50 controls during the rehabilitation were tested with Trail Making (TMT A B) and MMSE and Functional Ambulation Category (FAC) test and STEP test (Arsić et al., 2015). In stroke patients, performance on MMSE test was positively associated with the frequency and length of stride in walking.

Finding ways for improving cognition is of utmost importance in this population. A small pilot study in 12 patients with chronic stroke showed that a 12-week aerobic and strengthening exercise, 3 days per week, has favorable effects on cognition (Kluding et al., 2011). All subjects improved on measures of executive function (Digit Span Backwards and Flanker tests). Another trial included 41 poststroke patients with motor impairments (Marzolini et al., 2013). Patients were engaged in a 6-month aerobic and resistance training 10 weeks or more after the stroke. There were significant improvements of cognition on Montreal Cognitive Assessment (MoCA) overall scores and scores on subdomains of attention/concentration and visuospatial/executive function. Moreover, a significant number of treated patients ceased to fulfill the criteria for MCI.

Parkinson's Disease

Another important neuropsychiatric illness is Parkinson's disease (PD). A small study with 28 PD patients examined influence of physical training on cognition, mood and QoL

(Cruise et al., 2011). Patients were randomly allocated to exercise or control group. Fifteen patients undertook a program of progressive anabolic and aerobic exercises twice weekly for 12 weeks, while the remaining patients were controls and continued their usual daily routines. Physical activity improved executive functioning in PD patients, but without effects on mood or disease-specific QoL.

A recent study examined various aerobic walking regimes on motor function, cognition, and QoL in PD patients (Uc et al., 2014). The preliminary results showed higher musculoskeletal adverse events in the interval group and absence of difference between interval and continuous group. Because of these findings, further patients were allocated only to continuous training and showed no serious adverse events. Benefits were noticed on gait speed, Unified Parkinson's Disease Rating Scale sections I and III scores, depression, quality of life and executive control.

In a recent review paper, Ahlskog (2011) concluded that there is cumulative evidence that show that constant vigorous exercise may have even neuroprotective effects in PD patients. Large prospective studies documented significant reduction of PD risk in individuals that were engaged in physical activity during their midlives. Also PD patients who exercise improve their cognitive scores. Optimal dopaminergic therapy should be applied to maintain motivation for physical activity among PD patients. Vigorous exercise is defined as aerobic physical activity sufficient to rise heart rate and the need for oxygen. This means that training programs should content minimum 20-30 minutes for each session and maintained for longer periods. Various activities could be applied such as walking, jogging, swimming, tennis etc., as well as home-based activities.

Multiple Sclerosis

Multiple sclerosis (MS) is an incapacitating neurological disorder leading, among other neurological and psychiatric disturbances, to cognitive decline (Pavlović, 2012b). It begins typically in early adulthood leading to disability of various severity.

A randomized controlled study examined effects of physical training on cognition and ambulation in MS patients (Sandroff et al., 2014). The intervention group was engaged in increasing physical activity program delivered via the Internet while control subjects were on the waiting list. After the 6-month period patients with mild disability who were in the training group showed a clinically meaningful improvement in oral Symbol Digit Modalities Test (SDMT) scores and 6-minute walk (6MW) test results.

In a randomized-controlled pilot trial patients with progressive MS and moderate disability were randomized to one of three exercise interventions (arm ergometry, rowing, bicycle ergometry) for 8-10 weeks (Briken et al., 2014). Patients from the control group were only on a waitlist. Significant improvements were seen in several motoric measures: fatigue, depression and cognition (in several domains) and depressive symptoms.

Depression

Depression is probably the most frequent neuropsychiatric condition with patients of all ages. Depression often leads to reduced physical activity and interests, making the state even more severe, leading to vicious circle of mood disorder and inactivity. Even in remission, cognitive decline can be detected with appropriate instruments (Totic-Poznanovic et al., 2005). Physical activity can have beneficent effects on mental health in general and depression in particular.

In a small pilot study ten older adults with major depressive disorder improved cognitively after a single session of moderate exercise (Vasques et al., 2011). A treadmill walking for 30 minutes was used as intervention. Participants showed increase of scores on Digit Span Test (Forward and Backward) and a Stroop Color-Word Test.

Bipolar affective disorder shows also cognitive dysfunction according to meta analysis of relevant studies (Kucyi et al., 2010). There are deficits in verbal working memory, executive function, learning, attention, and processing speed. Authors conclude that there is enough evidence from general population and various disease groups that warrant application of exercise programs in patients with bipolar disorder.

Schizophrenia

Physical health of older adults with schizophrenia is generally poor, and less physical activity is further lowering their capacities. In a cross-sectional study 30 adults with schizophrenia aged more than 55 years were included (Leutwyler et al., 2014). They were assessed with the Extended Positive and Negative Syndrome Scale (PANSS), The Matrics Consensus Cognitive Battery (MCCB), while physical capacities where measured with Sensewear ProArmband, for one week. Participants with more average daily steps done had higher speed-of-processing. Social cognition consists of the Mayer-Salovey-Caruso Emotional Intelligence Test: Managing Emotions. Lower levels of activity correlated with greater severity of schizophrenia and neurocognitive deficits. Patients who led more sedentary lifestyle revealed more severe depressive symptoms.

DIABETES MELLITUS

Diabetes is frequent condition, leading to cognitive decline of various degrees (Salak-Djokić et al., 2014). Diabetes mellitus (DM) is a cause of numerous metabolic disorders that lead to secondary changes in multiple organs and systems. Such ample consequences make diabetes a main cause of morbidity and mortality in the world today (Fauci et al., 2008). DM is often accompanied with cognitive decline. Some authors have named AD a "DM type 3" that underline the connection between DM and severe cognitive impairment (De la Monte, Wands, 2008).

Another risk factor for diabetes and cognitive decline is obesity, increasing probability of dementia, associated with sedentary lifestyle and lack of physical activity. The most consistent cognitive findings in DM are impairments in executive functioning and memory. In a Serbian sample, including 15 patients with adult onset T1DM (age range 19–60 years), 37 patients with T2DM (age range 50–77 years), and 32 healthy controls (28–78 years) comprehensive neuropsychological assessment revealed poorer performance in T2DM subjects than healthy controls (Salak-Djokić et al., 2014). Significant differences were found in global cognitive performance, verbal learning and memory. After correcting for multiple comparisons, significantly poorer performance was found only on Trail Making Test Part B (TMT-B) (Reitan, 1958) in T2DM versus healthy controls. These findings in global cognitive impairment as well as in executive functions and memory poses serious questions about prevention and treatment.

Many studies found exercise to be beneficial for glycoregulation (Anderson-Hanley et al., 2012). Unfortunately only a small number of older adults endure the physical activity of recommended level (American College of Sports Medicine, 2009). In a quasi-experimental exploratory study, older adults with DM and healthy controls were engaged in exercise on stationary bike (Anderson-Hanley et al., 2012). These were 10 patients from larger Cybercycle Study in the state of New York. Subjects had five 45 min sessions per week using a stationary bicycle during 3 months. The results confirm that exercise may increase cognitive capacities in older adult with DM. Physical activity emerges as a promising preventive measure for cognitive decline and dementia. The main problem in exercise implementation remains motivation. Advances in new technologies enabled coupling physical exertion with the computer games, a potential way to increase motivation for exercising.

VASCULAR DISEASES

Vascular risk factors and vascular diseases in general pose serious risk of cognitive decline. A potential protective measure is again physical activity. In the prospective Women's Antioxidant Cardiovascular Study (WACS) a portion of 2809 women with coronary risk factors were assessed for physical activities (Vercambre et al., 2011). Risk factors encompassed were parental history of premature myocardial infarction (MI), diabetes, hypertension, hyperlipidemia, and body mass index $\geq$ 30 kg/m2). Vascular diseases included in the study were myocardial infarction, stroke, symptomatic angina pectoris, transient cerebral ischemia, or revascularization procedures. Questionnaire was given about the length of time of weekly physical activity such as walking, hiking, jogging/running, bicycling (either free or on the machine), including use of stationary machines, aerobic exercises including dance, use of exercise machines, yoga, stretching, tennis, squash and lap-swimming. Also, the intensity of exercise was estimated. Cognitive screening was done on several occasions from 1998 to 2005. There was a significant trend of lower degree of cognitive impairment with increasing energy expenditure, or the equivalent of daily 30-minute rapid walking. The cognitive level of active women was comparable to 5-7 years younger not fit women.

Heart failure leads to brain hypoperfusion and consequent cognitive decline. Heart insufficiency leads to reduced physical activity further decreasing cognition. In 65 patients with heart failure, lower initial step count and less time spent in moderate free-living activity was associated with decreased attention/executive functions and cerebral perfusion 12 months later (Alosco et al., 2014). This longitudinal study used accelerometar to measure level of physical activity during seven days. A calculated number of steps daily classified participants into sedentary if the count was 0-2,499, limited activity if 2,500 to 4,999 and physically active if count of steps was 5,000 to 12,000 daily. Only 23,1% of the participants were classified as active. Many contestants displayed impairments on initial cognitive testing.

CONCLUSION

Association of physical activity and cognition is well documented in animal models and human studies in various healthy populations and medical conditions across the lifespan. Aerobic training has beneficial effects of various important brain structures, mostly frontal and temporal lobes, increasing gray matter volumes and stimulating neurogenesis. The interface of exercise and cognition is the BDNF system that improves synaptic plasticity, neural connectivity and speed of information processing. Physical activity has positive effects on attention, executive functions, cognitive control, memory, learning and other cognitive processes. In today world when sedentary lifestyle, lack of aerobic exercise and obesity prevail, with deleterious effects on human health, there is urgent need for organized programs of exercise both for improvement of mental health and prevention of cognitive decline and dementia.

REFERENCES

Ahlskog, JE. Does vigorous exercise have a neuroprotective effect in Parkinson disease? *Neurology*, 2011, 77(3), 288-94.

Ahlskog, JE; Geda, YE; Graff-Radford, NR; Petersen, RC. Physical exercise as a preventive or disease-modifying treatment of dementia and brain aging. *Mayo Clin Proc*, 2011, 86(9), 876-84.

Alosco, ML; Spitznagel, MB; Cohen, R; Raz, N; Sweet, LH; Josephson, R; et al. Decreased physical activity predicts cognitive dysfunction and reduced cerebral blood flow in heart failure. *J Neurol Sc.*, 2014, 339(1-2), 169-75.

American College of Sports Medicine, Chodzko-Zajko, WJ; Proctor, DN; Fiatarone Singh, MA; Minson, CT; Nigg, CR; Salem, GJ; Skinner, JS. American College of Sports Medicine position stand. Exercise and physical activity for older adults. *Med Sci Sports Exerc.*, 2009, 41(7), 1510–30.

Anderson-Hanley, C; Arciero, PJ; Westen, SC; Nimon, J; Zimmerman, E. Neuropsychological benefits of stationary bike exercise and a cybercycle exergame for older adults with diabetes: an exploratory analysis. *J Diabetes Sci Technol*, 2012, 6(4), 849-57.

Arcoverde, C; Deslandes, A; Moraes, H; Almeida, C; Araujo, NB; Vasques, PE; et al. Treadmill training as an augmentation treatment for Alzheimer's disease: a pilot randomized controlled study. *Arq Neuropsiquiatr*, 2014, 72(3), 190-6.

Ardoy, DN; Fernández-Rodríguez, JM; Jiménez-Pavón, D; Castillo, R; Ruiz, JR; Ortega, FB. A physical education trial improves adolescents' cognitive performance and academic achievement: the EDUFIT study. *Scand J Med Sci Sports*, 2014, 24(1), e52-61.

Arsic, S; Konstantinovic, Lj; Eminovic, F; Pavlovic, D; Popovic, MB; Arsic, V. Correlation between the Quality of Attention and Cognitive Competence with Motor Action in Stroke Patients. *Biomed Res Int.*, 2015, 2015, 823136.

Barrientos, RM; Frank, MG; Crysdale, NY; Chapman, TR; Ahrendsen, JT; Day, HE; Campeau, S; Watkins, LR; Patterson, SL; Maier, SF. Little exercise, big effects:

Reversing aging and infectioninduced memory deficits, and underlying processes. *J Neurosci*, 2011, 31, 11578–11586.

Bherer, L. Cognitive plasticity in older adults: effects of cognitive training and physical exercise. *Ann N Y Acad Sci*, 2015, 1337, 1-6.

Briken, S; Gold, SM; Patra, S; Vettorazzi, E; Harbs, D; Tallner, A; et al. Effects of exercise on fitness and cognition in progressive MS: a randomized, controlled pilot trial. *Mult Scler*, 2014, 20(3), 382-90.

Burkhalter, TM; Hillman, CH. A narrative review of physical activity, nutrition, and obesity to cognition and scholastic performance across the human lifespan. *Adv Nutr*, 2011, 2(2), 201S-6S.

Carvalho, A; Rea, IM; Parimon, T; Cusack, BJ. Physical activity and cognitive function in individuals over 60 years of age: a systematic review. *Clin Interv Aging*, 2014, 12, 9, 661-82.

Casas-Herrero, A; Cadore, EL; Zambom-Ferraresi, F; Idoate, F; Millor, N; Martínez-Ramirez, A; et al. Functional capacity, muscle fat infiltration, power output, and cognitive impairment in institutionalized frail oldest old. *Rejuvenation Res*, 2013, 16(5), 396-403.

Chaddock, L; Erickson, KI; Prakash, RS. A neuroimaging investigation of the association between aerobic fitness, hippocampal volume, and memory performance in preadolescent children. *Brain Res*, 2010, 1358, 172–83.

Chang, M; Jonsson, PV; Snaedal, J; Bjornsson, S; Saczynski, JS; Aspelund, T; et al. The effect of midlife physical activity on cognitive function among older adults: AGES--Reykjavik Study. *J Gerontol A Biol Sci Med Sci*, 2010, 65(12), 1369-74.

Chang, YK; Pan, CY; Chen, FT; Tsai, CL; Huang, CC. Effect of resistance-exercise training on cognitive function in healthy older adults: a review. *J Aging Phys Act*, 2012, 20(4), 497-517.

Clapp, JF. Morphometric and neurodevelopmental outcome at age five years of the offspring of women who continued to exercise regularly throughout pregnancy. *J Pediatr*, 1996, 129, 856–863.

Clapp, JF; Lopez, B; Harcar-Sevcik, R. Neonatal behavioral profile of the offspring of women who continued to exercise regularly throughout pregnancy. *Am J Obstet Gynecol*, 1999, 180, 91–94.

Clapp, JF; Simonian, S; Lopez, B; Appleby-Wineberg, S; Harcar-Sevcik, R. The one-year morphometric and neurodevelopmental outcome of the offspring of women who continued to exercise regularly throughout pregnancy. *Am J Obstet Gynecol*, 1998, 178, 594–599.

Clark, PJ; Brzezinska, WJ; Puchalski, EK; Krone, DA; Rhodes, JS. Functional analysis of neurovascular adaptations to exercise in the dentate gyrus of young adult mice associated with cognitive gain. *Hippocampus*, 2009, 19, 937–950.

Colcombe, SJ; Erickson, KI; Scalf, PE; Kim, JS; Prakash, R; McAuley, E; Elavsky, S; Marquez, DX; Hu, L; Kramer, AF. Aerobic exercise training increases brain volume in aging humans. *J Gerontol A. Biol Sci Med Sci*, 2006, 61, 1166–1170.

Cruise, KE; Bucks, RS; Loftus, AM; Newton, RU; Pegoraro, R; Thomas, MG. Exercise and Parkinson's: benefits for cognition and quality of life. *Acta Neurol Scand*, 2011, 123(1), 13-9.

Curlik, DM; 2nd, Shors, TJ. Training your brain: Do mental and physical (MAP) training enhance cognition through the process of neurogenesis in the hippocampus? *Neuropharmacology*, 2013, 64, 506-14.

Darios, F; Davletov, B. Omega-3 and omega-6 fatty acids stimulate cell membrane expansion by acting on syntaxin 3. *Nature*, 2006, 440, 813–817.

Davis, C; Cooper, S. Fitness, fatness, cognition, behavior, and academic achievement among overweight children: do crosssectional associations correspond to exercise trial outcomes? *Prev Med*, 2011, 52, S65–9.

Davis, CL; Tomporowski, PD; McDowell, JE; Austin, BP; Miller, PH; Yanasak, NE; et al. Exercise improves executive function and achievement and alters brain activation in overweight children: a randomized, controlled trial. *Health Psychol*, 2011, 30(1), 91-8.

De la Monte, SM; Wands, JR. Alzheimer's disease is type 3 diabetes-evidence reviewed. *J Diabetes Sci Technol*, 2008, 2(6), 1101–13.

Deeny, SP; Poeppel, D; Zimmerman, JB; Roth, SM; Brandauer, J; Witkowski, S; Hearn, JW; Ludlow, AT; Contreras-Vidal, JL; Brandt, J; Hatfield, BD. Exercise, APOE, and working memory: MEG and behavioral evidence for benefit of exercise in epsilon4 carriers. *Biol Psychol.*, 2008, 78, 179–187.

Diamond, A. The early development of executive functions. In: Bialystok, E., Craik, F.I. (Eds.), Lifespan Cognition: Mechanisms of Change. Oxford University Press, New York, 2006, pp. 70–95.

Ding, Q; Vaynman, S; Akhavan, M; Ying, Z; Gomez-Pinilla, F. Insulin-like growth factor I interfaces with brain-derived neurotrophic factor-mediated synaptic plasticity to modulate aspects of exercise-induced cognitive function. *Neuroscience*, 2006, 140, 823–833.

Donchin, E. Presidential address, 1980. Surprise!... Surprise? *Psychophysiology.*, 1981, 18, 493–513.

Drollette, ES; Scudder, MR; Raine, LB; Moore, RD; Saliba, BJ; Pontifex, MB; Hillman, CH. Acute exercise facilitates brain function and cognition in children who need it most: an ERP study of individual differences in inhibitory control capacity. *Dev Cogn Neurosci*, 2014, 7, 53-64.

Duncan, M; Johnson, A. The effect of differing intensities of acute cycling on preadolescent academic achievement. *Eur J Sport Sci*, 2014, 14(3), 279-86.

Duncan-Johnson, CC. Young Psychophysiologist Award address, 1980. P300 latency: a new metric of information processing. *Psychophysiology*, 1981, 18, 207–215.

During, MJ; Cao, L. VEGF, a mediator of the effect of experience on hippocampal neurogenesis. *Curr Alzheimer Res*, 2006, 3, 29–33.

Erickson, KI; Raji, CA; Lopez, OL; Becker, JT; Rosano, C; Newman, AB; Gach, HM; Thompson, PM; Ho, AJ; Kuller, LH. Physical activity predicts gray matter volume in late adulthood: The Cardiovascular Health Study. *Neurology*, 2010, 75, 1415–1422.

Fabel, K; Tam, B; Kaufer, D; Baiker, A; Simmons, N; Kuo, CJ; Palmer, TD. VEGF is necessary for exercise-induced adult hippocampal neurogenesis. *Eur J Neurosci*, 2003, 18, 2803–2812.

Fauci, AS; Kasper, DL; Longo, DL; Braunwald, E; Hauser, SL; Jameson, JL; Loscalzo, J. Harrison's principles of internal medicine: Endocrinology (17th ed.). New York, NY: McGraw-Hill Companies, 2008.

Feng, J; Fouse, S; Fan, G. Epigenetic regulation of neural gene expression and neuronal function. *Pediatr Res*, 2007, 61, 58R–63R.

Fisher, A; Boyle, JM; Paton, JY; Tomporowski, P; Watson, C; McColl, JH; Reilly, JJ. Effects of a physical education intervention on cognitive function in young children: randomized controlled pilot study. *BMC Pediatr*, 2011, 11, 97.

Folstein, MF; Folstein, SE; McHugh, PR. "Mini-mental state." A practical method for grading the cognitive state of patients for the clinician. *J Psychiatr Res.*, 1975, 12(3), 189–198.

Forbes, D; Thiessen, EJ; Blake, CM; Forbes, SC; Forbes, S. *Exercise programs for people with dementia Cochrane Database Syst Rev.*, 2013, 12, CD006489.

Garcia-Garcia, FJ; Gutierrez Avila, G; Alfaro-Acha, A; Amor Andres, MS; De Los Angeles De La Torre Lanza, M; Escribano Aparicio, MV; et al. The prevalence of frailty syndrome in an older population from Spain. The Toledo Study for Healthy Aging. *J Nutr Health Aging*, 2011, 15, 852–865.

Gomez-Pinilla, F. Brain foods: The effects of nutrients on brain function. *Nat Rev Neurosci*, 2008, 9, 568–578.

Gomez-Pinilla, F. The combined effects of exercise and foods in preventing neurological and cognitive disorders. *Prev Med*, 2011, 52, S75–80.

Gomez-Pinilla, F; Hillman, C. The influence of exercise on cognitive abilities. *Compr Physiol*, 2013, 3(1), 403-28.

Hardie, DG. AMP-activated protein kinase: A key system mediating metabolic responses to exercise. *Med Sci Sports Exerc*, 2004, 36, 28–34.

Haskell, WL; Lee, IM; Pate, RR; Powell, KE; Blair, SN; Franklin, BA; Macera, CA; Heath, GW; Thompson, PD; Bauman, A. Physical activity and public health: updated recommendation for adults from the American College of Sports Medicine and the American Heart Association. *Med Sci Sports Exerc*, 2007, 39(8), 1423-34.

Hillman, CH; Buck, SM; Themanson, JR; et al. Aerobic fitness and cognitive development: Eventrelated brain potential and task performance indices of executive control in preadolescent children. *Dev Psychol.*, 2009, 45, 114–129.

Hillman, CH; Castelli, DM; Buck, SM. Aerobic fitness and neurocognitive function in healthy preadolescent children. *Med Sci Sports Exerc.*, 2005, 37, 1967–1974.

Hillman, CH; Kamijo, K; Scudder, M. A review of chronic and acute physical activity participation on neuroelectric measures of brain health and cognition during childhood. *Prev Med*, 2011, 52 Suppl 1, S21-8.

Hillman, CH; Pontifex, MB; Castelli, DM; Khan, NA; Raine, LB; Scudder, MR; et al. Effects of the FITKids randomized controlled trial on executive control and brain function. *Pediatrics*, 2014, 134(4), e1063-71.

Ho, AJ; Raji, CA; Becker, JT; Lopez, OL; Kuller, LH; Hua, X; et al. The effects of physical activity, education, and body mass index on the aging brain. *Hum Brain Mapp*, 2011, 32(9), 1371-82.

Hogan, CL; Mata, J; Carstensen, LL. Exercise holds immediate benefits for affect and cognition in younger and older adults. *Psychol Aging*, 2013, 28(2), 587-94.

Hogan, M; Kiefer, M; Kubesch, S; Collins, P; Kilmartin, L; Brosnan, M. The interactive effects of physical fitness and acute aerobic exercise on electrophysiological coherence and cognitive performance in adolescents. *Exp Brain Res*, 2013, 229(1), 85-96.

Hopkins, ME; Davis, FC; Vantieghem, MR; Whalen, PJ; Bucci, DJ. Differential effects of acute and regular physical exercise on cognition and affect. *Neuroscience*, 2012, 215, 59-68.

Hötting, K; Röder, B. Beneficial effects of physical exercise on neuroplasticity and cognition. *Neurosci Biobehav Rev*, 2013, 37(9 Pt B), 2243-57.

Itoh, T; Imano, M; Nishida, S; Tsubaki, M; Hashimoto, S; Ito, A; Satou, T. Exercise increases neural stem cell proliferation surrounding the area of damage following rat traumatic brain injury. *J Neural Transm*, 2011, 118, 193–202.

James, BD; Boyle, PA; Bennett, DA; Buchman, AS. Total daily activity measured with actigraphy and motor function in community-dwelling older persons with and without dementia. *Alzheimer Dis Assoc Disord*, 2012, 26(3), 238-45.

Kluding, PM; Tseng, BY; Billinger, SA. Exercise and executive function in individuals with chronic stroke: a pilot study. *J Neurol Phys Ther*, 2011, 35(1), 11-7.

Kucyi, A; Alsuwaidan, MT; Liauw, SS; McIntyre, RS. Aerobic physical exercise as a possible treatment for neurocognitive dysfunction in bipolar disorder. *Postgrad Med*, 2010, 122(6), 107-16.

Labelle, V; Bosquet, L; Mekary, S; Vu, TT; Smilovitch, M; Bherer, L. Fitness level moderates executive control disruption during exercise regardless of age. *J Sport Exerc Psychol*, 2014, 36(3), 258-70.

Lam, LC; Chau, RC; Wong, BM; Fung, AW; Lui, VW; Tam, CC; et al. Interim follow-up of a randomized controlled trial comparing Chinese style mind body (Tai Chi) and stretching exercises on cognitive function in subjects at risk of progressive cognitive decline. *Int J Geriatr Psychiatry*, 2011, 26(7), 733-40.

Landi, F; Abbatecola, AM; Provinciali, M; Corsonello, A; Bustacchini, S; Manigrasso, L; et al. Moving against frailty: does physical activity matter? *Biogerontology*, 2010, 11(5), 537-45.

Lautenschlager, NT; Cox, K; Cyarto, EV. The influence of exercise on brain aging and dementia. *Biochim Biophys Acta*, 2012, 1822(3), 474-81.

Law, LL; Barnett, F; Yau, MK; Gray, MA. Effects of combined cognitive and exercise interventions on cognition in older adults with and without cognitive impairment: a systematic review. *Ageing Res Rev*, 2014, 15, 61-75.

Lees, C; Hopkins, J. Effect of aerobic exercise on cognition, academic achievement, and psychosocial function in children: a systematic review of randomized control trials. *Prev Chronic Dis*, 2013 Oct 24, 10, E174.

Leutwyler, H; Hubbard, EM; Jeste, DV; Miller, B; Vinogradov, S. Associations of schizophrenia symptoms and neurocognition with physical activity in older adults with schizophrenia. *Biol Res Nurs*, 2014, 16(1), 23-30.

Linde, K; Alfermann, D. Single versus combined cognitive and physical activity effects on fluid cognitive abilities of healthy older adults: a 4-month randomized controlled trial with follow-up. *J Aging Phys Act*, 2014, 22(3), 302-13.

Loprinzi, PDCJ. Exercise and cognitive function: a randomized controlled trial examining acute exercise and free-living physical activity and sedentary effects. *Mayo Clin Proc*, 2015, 90(4), 450-60.

Marosi, K; Mattson, MP. BDNF mediates adaptive brain and body responses to energetic challenges. *Trends Endocrinol Metab*, 2014, 25(2), 89-98.

Marzolini, S; Oh, P; McIlroy, W; Brooks, D. The effects of an aerobic and resistance exercise training program on cognition following stroke. *Neurorehabil Neural Repair*, 2013, 27(5), 392-402.

McKee, AC; Daneshvar, DH; Alvarez, VE; Stein, TD. The neuropathology of sport. *Acta Neuropathol*, 2014, 127(1), 29-51.

McNay, EC. Insulin and ghrelin: Peripheral hormones modulating memory and hippocampal function. *Curr Opin Pharmacol*, 2007, 7, 628–632.

Meeusen, R. Exercise, nutrition and the brain. *Sports Med*, 2014, 44 Suppl 1, S47-56.

Molteni, R; Zheng, JQ; Ying, Z; Gómez-Pinilla, F; Twiss, JL. Voluntary exercise increases axonal regeneration from sensory neurons. *Proc Natl Acad Sci U S A*, 2004, 101, 8473–8478.

Morie, M; Reid, KF; Miciek, R; Lajevardi, N; Choong, K; Krasnoff, JB; Storer, TW; Fielding, RA; Bhasin, S; LeBrausseur, NK. Habitual physical activity levels are associated with performance in measures of physical function and mobility in older men. *J Am Geriatr Soc*, 2010, 58, 1727–1733.

Napoli, N; Shah, K; Waters, DL; Sinacore, DR; Qualls, C; Villareal, DT. Effect of weight loss, exercise, or both on cognition and quality of life in obese older adults. *Am J Clin Nutr*, 2014, 100(1), 189-98.

Nelson, ME; Rejeski, WJ; Blair, SN; Duncan, PW; Judge, JO; King, AC; Macera, CA; Castaneda-Sceppa, C. American College of Sports Medicine; American Heart Association. Physical activity and public health in older adults: recommendation from the American College of Sports Medicine and the American Heart Association. *Circulation*, 2007, 116(9), 1094-105.

Norman, DA; Shallice, T. Attention to action: willed and automatic control of behavior. In: Davidson, R.J., Schwartz, G.E., Shapiro, D. (Eds.), *Consciousness and Self-Regulation: Advances in Research and Theory*, vol. 4. Plenum Press, New York, 1986, pp. 1–18.

Obisesan, TO; Umar, N; Paluvoi, N; Gillum, RF. Association of leisure-time physical activity with cognition by apolipoprotein-E genotype in persons aged 60 years and over: the National Health and Nutrition Examination Survey (NHANES-III). *Clin Interv Aging*, 2012, 7, 35-43.

Pavlović, DM. Omega 3 fatty acids in health and disease. *Belgrade: Orion Art*, 2012a.

Pavlović, DM. Neuropsychology, behavioral neurology and neuropsychiatry. *Belgrade: Orion Art*, 2012b.

Pavlović, DM; Pavlović, AM. Dementia – Neuropsychiatric symptoms. *Belgrade. Orion Art*, 2014.

Pereira, AC; Huddleston, DE; Brickman, AM; Sosunov, AA; Hen, R; McKhann, GM; Sloan, R; Gage, FH; Brown, TR; Small, SA. An *in vivo* correlate of exercise-induced neurogenesis in the adult dentate gyrus. *Proc Natl Acad Sci U S A*, 2007, 104, 5638–5643.

Polich, J. Updating P300: an integrative theory of P3a and P3b. *Clin Neurophysiol.*, 2007, 118, 2128–2148.

Reitan, R. The validity of the trail making test as an indicator of organic brain damage. *Percept Motor Skills*, 1958, 8, 271–276.

Roig, M; Skriver, K; Lundbye-Jensen, J; Kiens, B; Nielsen, JB. A single bout of exercise improves motor memory. *PLoS One*, 2012, 7(9), e44594.

Rossi, A; Gasperi, V; Maccarrone, M. Physical activity and the endocannabinoid system: an overview. *Cell Mol Life Sci*, 2014, 71(14), 2681-98.

Ruscheweyh, R; Willemer, C; Krüger, K; Duning, T; Warnecke, T; Sommer, J; Völker, K; Ho, HV; Mooren, F; Knecht, S; Flöel, A. Physical activity and memory functions: an interventional study. *Neurobiol Aging*, 2011, 32(7), 1304-19.

Salak Djokić, B; Spitznagel, MB; Pavlović, D; Janković, N; Parojčić, A; Ilić, V; Nikolić Djurović, M. Diabetes mellitus and cognitive functioning in a Serbian sample. *J Clin Exp Neuropsychol*, 2014, 18, 1-12.

Sallis, JF. We do not have to sacrifice children's health to achieve academic goals. *J Pediatr.*, 2010, 156, 711–718.

Sandroff, BM; Klaren, RE; Pilutti, LA; Dlugonski, D; Benedict, RH; Motl, RW. Randomized controlled trial of physical activity, cognition, and walking in multiple sclerosis. *J Neurol*, 2014, 261(2), 363-72.

Sibley, BA; Etnier, JL. The relationship between physical activity and cognition in children: A meta-analysis. *Pediatr Exerc Sci*, 2003, 15, 243–256.

Singh, A; Uijtdewilligen, L; Twisk, JW; van Mechelen, W; Chinapaw, MJ. Physical activity and performance at school: a systematic review of the literature including a methodological quality assessment. *Arch Pediatr Adolesc Med*, 2012, 166(1), 49-55.

Strong, WB; Malina, RM; Blimkie, CJR; Daniels, SR; Dishman, RK; Gutin, B; Hergenroeder, AC; Must, A; Nixon, PA; et al. Evidence based physical activity for school-age youth. *J Pediatr.*, 2005, 146, 732–7.

Strout, KA; Howard, EP. The six dimensions of wellness and cognition in aging adults. *J Holist Nurs*, 2012, 30(3), 195-204.

Stubbs, B; Eggermont, L; Soundy, A; Probst, M; Vandenbulcke, M; Vancampfort, D. What are the factors associated with physical activity (PA) participation in community dwelling adults with dementia? A systematic review of PA correlates. *Arch Gerontol Geriatr*, 2014, 59(2), 195-203.

Teague, WE; Fuller, NL; Rand, RP; Gawrisch, K. Polyunsaturated lipids in membrane fusion events. *Cell Mol Biol Lett*, 2002, 7, 262–264.

Tian, Q; Erickson, KI; Simonsick, EM; Aizenstein, HJ; Glynn, NW; Boudreau, RM; et al. Physical activity predicts microstructural integrity in memory-related networks in very old adults. *J Gerontol A Biol Sci Med Sci*, 2014, 69(10), 1284-90.

Totic-Poznanovic, S; Marinkovic, D; Pavlovic, D; Paunovic, VR. Neuropsychological profile of patients with bipolar depression in remission. *Vojnosanit Pregl*, 2005, 62(7-8), 543-50.

Tseng, CN; Gau, BS; Lou, MF. The effectiveness of exercise on improving cognitive function in older people: a systematic review. *J Nurs Res*, 2011, 19(2), 119-31.

Tyndall, AV; Davenport, MH; Wilson, BJ; Burek, GM; Arsenault-Lapierre, G; Haley, E; et al. The brain-in-motion study: effect of a 6-month aerobic exercise intervention on cerebrovascular regulation and cognitive function in older adults *BMC Geriatr*, 2013, 13, 21.

Uc, EY; Doerschug, KC; Magnotta, V; Dawson, JD; Thomsen, TR; Kline, JN; et al. Phase I/II randomized trial of aerobic exercise in Parkinson disease in a community setting. *Neurology*, 2014, 29, 83(5), 413-25.

Uemura, K; Doi, T; Shimada, H; Yoshida, D; Tsutsumimoto, K; Anan, Y; Susuki, T. Effects of exercise intervention on vascular risk factors in olders adults with mild cognitive impairment: A randomized controlled trial. *Dement Geriatr Cogn Disord Extra*, 2012, 2, 445–455.

Vasques, PE; Moraes, H; Silveira, H; Deslandes, AC; Laks, J. Acute exercise improves cognition in the depressed elderly: the effect of dual-tasks. *Clinics (Sao Paulo)*, 2011, 66(9), 1553-7.

Vaynman, S; Ying, Z; Gomez-Pinilla, F. Interplay between brain-derived neurotrophic factor and signal transduction modulators in the regulation of the effects of exercise on synaptic-plasticity. *Neuroscience*, 2003, 122, 647–657.

Vaynman, S; Ying, Z; Gomez-Pinilla, F. Hippocampal BDNF mediates the efficacy of exercise on synaptic plasticity and cognition. *Eur J Neurosci*, 2004, 20, 2580–2590.

Vercambre, MN; Grodstein, F; Manson, JE; Stampfer, MJ; Kang, JH. Physical activity and cognition in women with vascular conditions. *Arch Intern Med*, 2011, 171(14), 1244-50.

Volkers, KM; Scherder, EJ. Physical performance is associated with working memory in older people with mild to severe cognitive impairment. *Biomed Res Int*, 2014, 2014, 762986.

Voss, MW; Prakash, RS; Erickson, KI; Basak, C; Chaddock, L; Kim, JS; Alves, H; Heo, S; Szabo, AN; White, SM; Wójcicki, TR; Mailey, EL; Gothe, N; Olson, EA; McAuley, E; Kramer, AF. Plasticity of brain networks in a randomized intervention trial of exercise training in older adults. *Front Aging Neurosci*, 2010, 2, 1–17.

Vreugdenhil, A; Cannell, J; Davies, A; Razay, G. A community-based exercise programme to improve functional ability in people with Alzheimer's disease: a randomized controlled trial. *Scand J Caring Sci*, 2012, 26(1), 12-9.

Wang, HX; Xu, W; Pei, JJ. Leisure activities, cognition and dementia. *Biochim Biophys Acta*, 2012, 1822(3), 482-91.

Wechsler, DW. Adult Intelligence Scale. *Manual; New York: Psychological Corporation*, 1955.

Winchester, J; Dick, MB; Gillen, D; Reed, B; Miller, B; Tinklenberg, J; et al. Walking stabilizes cognitive functioning in Alzheimer's disease (AD) across one year. *Arch Gerontol Geriatr*, 2013, 56(1), 96-103.

World Health Organisation, World Health Report: *Reducing Risks, Promoting Healthy Life*, WHO, Geneva, 2002.

Yágüez, L; Shaw, KN; Morris, R; Matthews, D. The effects on cognitive functions of a movement-based intervention in patients with Alzheimer's type dementia: a pilot study. *Int J Geriatr Psychiatry*, 2011, 26(2), 173-81.

In: Physical Activity Effects on the Anthropological Status ...   ISBN: 978-1-63484-782-7
Editors: Fadilj Eminović and Milivoj Dopsaj   © 2016 Nova Science Publishers, Inc.

Chapter 15

PHYSICAL ACTIVITY AND QUALITY OF LIFE OF OLDER ADULTS

Evdokia Samouilidu[1], Sanela Pacić[2,], Radmila Nikić[3] and Fadilj Eminović[3]*

[1]Ministry of Education and Culture, Athens, Greece
[2]Regional Care Center Baden, Demenze department, Baden, Switzerland
[3]University of Belgrade, Faculty for Special Education and Rehabilitation,
Belgrade, Serbia

ABSTRACT

Physical activity is considered to be the most important step in improving the health of not only the elderly, but the entire population. Lack of physical activity is a risk factor for chronic diseases (diabetes, depression, cardiovascular disease, and stroke). If we are engaged regularly in physical activity, and even in a minimal amount of, it reduces the risk of many diseases. The main objective of this paper is to examine the opinion of elderly about the impact of physical activity in some segments of the quality of life of people of the third age. The specific objective of this study is to determine whether there were differences in opinion of respondents on the connection between physical exercise and health as an aspect of quality of life among the elderly population in the Republic of Serbia, Switzerland and Greece. The research was conducted on a sample of 410 respondents aged 65 to 70 years. Compared to the half of the respondents were equally represented by men and women. The structure of respondents by country is as follows: Switzerland 134 respondents, 120 respondents Greece and the Republic of Serbia 156 respondents. Data were collected through an anonymous questionnaire consisting of 3 parts. The first part of the questionnaire contained questions on general information of respondents, the second part of the issues are physical exercise and relate to frequency and the type of exercise and the third part of the questionnaire contained statements about the opinion of respondents who are the impacts of physical activity. The third part is divided into four parts. Results of the research suggest that physical activity has a positive influence on a better quality of life of the elderly, that is, it contributes to their better health and functioning in daily life, better mental health and better quality of

* Corresponding Author, Email: sanela.pacic@gmail.com.

interpersonal relationships, regardless of whether the respondents are from Switzerland, Serbia or Greece. The inclusion of the elderly in groups of organized exercise is an important factor in maintaining, preserving and improving the health and also the best way of bringing the body to the physical and the mental shape. An important task of any advanced society is to support elderly to show their age into a more active and productive period of life, which will surely follow and the subjective feeling of complete and qualitative life.

Keywords: physical activity, age, quality of life

INTRODUCTION

Aging is an universal and progressive process which is common for all living organisms and therefore humans. The aging process in humans is comparable with growth, the only difference is in the direction, where in the growth and development all physical, psychological and social abilities range from the start to its maximum value, while the aging of the same values go from their peak towards lower until final disappearance. Development and decline of various abilities happen in a different pace, and each man's ability or characteristic seizes its maximum value at a specific time. Immediately after reaching the maximum the short stagnation emerges, which can be considered as the beginning of aging. What is common to most aspects of this life age, is that in the late years of life natural decline in energy and mental and physical abilities appears. That is why the health of the elderly is often impaired, which results in lower quality of life. In large number of elderly physical ability decreases to a critical level unless they are not engaged in regular physical exercises. In this life age the ability to enjoy in many activities of leisure activities has been reduced, as well as the ability to perform elementary everyday physical activities. One of the most important measures in counseling the elderly is striving to preserve them from falling into complete passivity.

Physical activity is considered to be the most important step in improving the health of not only the elderly, but the entire population. Lack of physical activity is a risk factor for chronic diseases (diabetes, depression, cardiovascular disease, and stroke). If we are engaged in physical activity, even at a minimum, the risk of many diseases is reduced. Accetto (2006) sees the importance of active aging in physical activities that are appropriate for individual according to his age condition. A man should have the ability to quickly adapt to the physical demands faced during the day and in everyday life, as well as the ability recover fast after hard physical work. Any kind of professional or any everyday work and sports activities has specific characteristics, so that the physical ability is not universal in character, nor is a universal phenomenon, but is associated with a specific operation. Also, physical ability represents the condition that depends on the specific physiological, mental and emotional traits that can be inherited and acquired.

Active older people are more satisfied with life, less dependent on others and with better health condition (Weinberg and Gould, 2003). Older persons who care for good health status by maintaining muscle strength, strength of the skeleton and joint mobility and preserve its independence, are able to able to take care of themselves longer, to carry out daily purchases, maintain personal hygiene. The possibility of moving themselves gives a sense of control over their life, allows them to encounter with acquaintances and friends, and reduces feelings of helplessness and abandonment. The inclusion of the elderly in groups organized exercise is an important factor of socialization because this creates the possibility for meeting new friends who have similar problems and equally struggle to overcome. An important task for any advanced society is to support elderly to turn their age into a more active and productive period of life, which will surely follow and the subjective feeling of complete and more qualitative life.

AGING AND AGE

Two concepts that we usually mix, not noticing a difference in their meaning are age and aging. Age is the last period in the life of man. Compared to the previous period, this is when deterioration of the structure and functions of the organism, the characteristics and abilities of human beings came to a certain level (Smolić-Krković, 1974; Defilipis and Havelka, 1984). Defining age is not exclusively a question of one's chronological age and functional abilities, but also the ratio of a person's quality of life, values and characteristics of the environment in which a person lives (Bouillet, 2003). Age is a state which in means disintegration of man as a social being due to physical and mental disorders, defects, malfunctions or defects that age itself causes (Stosljević et al., 1997). On the other side, aging is a natural process in which disorders of homeostatic mechanisms and abilities of loss adjustment over time are fundamental. This is the result: 1. primary aging, which is determined by hereditary factors, 2. secondary aging - associated effects of trauma, acquired diseases, and toxic factors, 3. psychosocial changes - stress, loss of self-esteem, loneliness, prejudice, job losses and 4. physiological deterioration - loss reserves and the strength, mobility, immunity, metabolic changes. Each of the listed components influence each other, and all together lead to aging (Vojvodić et al., 1992).

Rowe and Kahn (1997) divide aging on "normal aging" and "successful aging." Their concept of "normal aging" is associated with the biological process of aging by which capacity is reducing, the weakening associated with diseases and deficiencies in social functioning. They identify three factors of successful aging: optimal physical and cognitive functioning, disease and lack of will to live. According Despot-Lučanin (2003), the age can be seen from different aspects, as biological, psychological and sociological process, therefore we can divide it in: biological, psychological and sociological age. Biological age can be seen as an individual's ability to adapt to environmental factors, usually expressed by endurance, strength, flexibility, coordination and working capacity (Mišigoj-Duraković and Duraković, 1999, according to Hašpl-Jurisić, 2007). Biological theories emphasize that aging is a result of accumulated damage caused by random events of everyday life and can be triggered by internal or external factors (eg, illness, disease, adverse effects). Variety of regressive changes that happen to a person at the biological basis of the aging process, like the permanent loss of a large number of physical abilities, slowing reaction to external influences, reducing resistance and elasticity of the tissue, increasing bone fragility, etc. Such changes weaken the resistance and functionality of the body, by which the danger of illness and injury is increased (Martinčević-Ljumanović 1985 by: Lovrekovic and Leutar, 2010). Biological age is recognizable through a number of external indicators such as gray hair, wrinkled and dehydrated skin, hunched posture, heavy and slow speed, etc. (Schai and Willias, 2001).

Psychological age is the ability to adapt to changes in the environment, and aging refers to the process of change in the mental functions as well as the flow adjustment (Defilipis and Havelka, 1984). During aging, many changes in mental functioning of elderly people occur. Mostly recorded changes in psychological aging in elderly are related to memory and intelligence. Older people often complain about the difficulties in memorizing, poor adapting new content, forgetting data, objects losing etc.

Sociological theories explain changes relating the individual and society that occur during the aging process (changes in social activities, changes in social interactions and social roles in function of aging) as well as the influence of society and culture on aging individuals and aging impacts individuals on society. Social age is closely related to the chronological age, although the biological and psychological are not independent of chronological age, so the age of 65 is the period of life when we move from active phase of labor to the period of retirement, in the social cultural milieu to which we belong. That is the legal standard applied in the large number of countries in Western, developed world. In society there are norms or expectations of the social environment on the behavior of people of certain ages. The company is pressuring a person to act in accordance with his age (Despot-Lučanin, 2003). The newer term that has been in use for active aging, when it is usually thought of in four areas: the presence in the labor market, participation in housework, active participation in community life and leisure activities (Puljiz, 2005). Active, healthy aging involves adapting to new conditions, knowledge and continuous learning and discovering the advantages of aging and age.

Some authors speak of a successful, normal and pathological aging. In "successful" aging there is a positive genetic material, and aging takes place in a positive environment, there are no chronic diseases and functional disorders. The term of "successful aging" as this process is called in gerontology and geriatrics, means striving to find a certain balance between individual needs and desires on the one hand and the objective and subjective circumstances of life, on the other, that is. one has to adapt to the facts and get the most out of them and the best you can for an active life and personal well-being (Tokarski, 2004). In "normal" aging the development of certain diseases and dysfunction is present, but the function of all organs is still at satisfactory level and no major functional limitations. In the "pathological" aging, for genetic reasons or due to poor environmental, major functional limitations with frequent and long-term sick leave, which may result in problems in the functioning of independent (Pospiš, 2001). Besides pathology as a key factor for disability there are physiological aging and disability. Among the relevant aspects of physiological aging, in addition to chronic diseases and biological aging, more loss of muscle mass, balance, strength, movement problems are considered (Stewart, 2003). In addition to these aspects often the psychosocial factors occur (Rockwood et al, 2007) which influence the physiological aging, and among them the most crucial is the personal perception. Also, physical inactivity combined with malnutrition leads to a lowering of physical function, and therefore difficult to move. We can distinguish between primary and secondary aging. Primary aging (physiological aging, or senescence) refers to the normal physiological processes of certain biological factors, and is the result of maturation or the passage of time (eg, menopause), while the secondary aging refers to pathological changes and decline with age, which is caused by external factors including disease and the effects of adverse impacts over the years: the noise, smoking, alcohol and other harmful influences (Despot-Lucanin, 2003).

According to the World Health Organization, old age can be divided into:

- Early (65-74.
- Medium (75-84.)
- Old age (85 and over).

Whereby this division is often applied in gerontological public-health analysis particularly in identifying, studying and monitoring health needs and functional ability of older people (World Health Organization, 2007).

Gerontologists are studying the factors that affect aging and thus have concluded some important facts: 1). the length of a human life can be predicted based on the length of life of the mother and father and grandparents; 2). Nutrition. In describing the diet of long-lived states they mainly eat dairy products, fruits and vegetables, occasionally meat, and they said they drink lots of green tea with every meal (Smiljanjic, 2001); 3). Environmental factors. Studies show that long-lived are more present in the mountains than in the lowlands. In addition to this, one significant factor is engagement in physical activities.

Table 1. Projected population older than 65 years, the case of Serbia (UNITED NATIONS, 2014)

Year	(Thousands)	(%)
2015	1 413	15.0
2020	1 595	17.4
2025	1 705	19.2
2030	1 758	20.5

Demographics of Ageing

In the coming decades, the number of elderly people will increase because of aging of the population. Studies indicate that there is a growing need to care for people aged 65 yrs and older, with an emphasis on people older than 80 yrs (CDC, 2003).

Table 2. The median age of ten demographically oldest countries in the world 2050 (UNITED NATIONS, 2014)

Rank	Country	Median Age
1	Spain	55,2
2	Slovenia	54,1
3	Italy	54,1
4	Austria	53,7
5	Armenia	53,4
6	Japan	52,4
7	Czech Republic	52,4
8	Greece	52,3
9	Serbia (without Kosovo and Metohija)	52,1
10	Switzerland	52,0

**Table 3. The age structure of the population: Greece, Serbia, Switzerland
(The United Nations Population Division's World Population Prospects, 2014)[1]**

	Population	Age	Composition
	Ages 0-14 (%)	Ages 15-64 (%)	Ages 65+ (%)
Greece	15	65	20
Serbia	16	69	15
Switzerland	15	67	18

Demographics of the elderly in western European countries is constantly increasing. These general trends are valid for Serbia (Table 1), accompanied by one characteristic. The Serb population in the first half of the twentieth century was much younger than the European average, but by the end of the century completely leveled with it (Penev, 2006). So it is assumed that Serbia will be in the top 10 European countries with average age of the population of 52.1 years (between Greece and Switzerland) (Table 2).

For the first time in 2000, the population of people over 60 years has surpassed the population of children under 5 years so that the displayed number population The United Nations Population Division's World Population Prospects (2014) shows that the percentage of the population 65 years and older is higher than of children aged 0 to 14 years in Switzerland and, in particular a large difference in Greece, while in Serbia, only 1% are more children than the elderly (Table 3). Depending on the proportion of elderly population in the total population three types of population vary, namely: youth (share of elderly population is less than 4%), mature (share of elderly population ranges between 4% and 7%) and old (the share of persons older than 65 years is above 7%) (Močnik et al., 2015). Therefore we can conclude that all three countries presented in the table belong to the country with old population.

Also, the data obtained showed that the number of "very old," those over 85, is increasing more rapidly than those up to 85 years old, so-called "old." In the next half century the number of people above 85 years of age will increase by six times. This process is sometimes called "aging of the old" (Giddens, 2000).

Characteristics of Older Adults

Age has its own characteristics so that in old age g disorders of systems and functions occur, so-called geriatric syndromes occur such as dementia, falls, incontinence, weight loss, feeling of weakness, severe mobility (Rich, 2005). The process of aging brings with it a large number of physiological changes, such as reduced body weight and body height (Milanović et al., 2011). Loss of muscle mass between 50 and 80 years is probably a result of the aging process in the neuromuscular system, combined with a reduced level of muscle activity. Muscle fibers in the elderly lose elasticity, and speed of response to the stimulus, and such changes may cause negative effect on the muscular system in terms of anatomical damage of various degrees. Second reason for the decrease in muscle strength and endurance is the reduction in the number of muscle fibers during the aging process. Longitudinal studies (Visser et al., 2003) shows that body weight decreased in elderly men and women after age

---

[1] http://wdi.worldbank.org/table/2.1.

60. The research results show that loses about 10% of muscle fibers during each decade after the age of 50 (Lexell et al., 1988).

Obesity is one of the most common health problems that can be acted on preventively (Milanovic et al., 2011) and which is lately a problem that affects the elderly population. Perissinoto et al. (2002) found lower values of BMI between the ages of 65-75 than in the period between 75-80 years of age. The results of these studies have only confirmed the trend of incensement in the number of obese elderly in the last two decades (Misra and Khurana, 2008). Aging is associated with an increase in the proportion of body fat and body fat redistribution. Redistribution of fats mainly from the lower part of the body in the abdominal and visceral part is most common in the elderly. Reduction in BMI occurs due to loss of muscle mass and increase of body fat in the waist and hips. However, although the emergence of obesity is significant for the population of elderly, malnutrition and weight loss occurs more often in older people.

Bones changes and joints are not related only to early aging, but the beginnings of these changes occurring already in many around 50 years of age. During aging there is a loss of bone tissue, which is more pronounced in women than in men. Women in involute period included a lower total bone mass and bone tissue loss begins earlier and more intense as compared to men (about 8% for each decade in women, 3% for men). A well-known loss of bone tissue leading to osteoporosis (Peck et al., 1988). Clinical manifestation of osteoporosis present bone fractures, fractures of the femoral neck, distal part of the forearm... Regressive changes are reflected in the reduction of potassium and phosphorus that provide bone density, which leads to ostheomalacia. Degenerative changes at joints often lead to in the cartilage part. They may lead to losing articular surfaces and in advanced age it may result in considerable difficulties in terms of the mobility of affected joints. Bone fractures due to osteoporosis, in addition to economic effects, are associated with frequent mortality, morbidity, chronic pain, decreased quality of life, long-term problems (Papaioannou et al., 2010).

During the aging process changes in the characteristics of walking also occur, which are emphasized after 70 years. The causes: velocity reduction, reduction of power during the phase of pushing, extension of time in which both feet touch the ground, reduced stride length, increase the width of the steps. Older people also tend to touch the ground all over the surface of the foot. It was also shown that the time of contact with the ground with both feet at the same time extending the 20% of the total runtime prolongs up to 25% in the elderly. It was also found that older people who have experienced a drop in the last 6 months change characteristics walk by slowing gait, reduced stride length and foot turning outward to increase stability (Quail, 1994).

During the aging process the increased risk of falls and injury occurrence in the elderly occurs. Falling is a serious problem for the elderly. Risk factors associated with falls include dementia, visual impairment, neurological and musculoskeletal disabilities, postural hypotension, medication, fear of falling and environmental hazards (Tinetti et al., 1994; Hornbrook et al., 1994). Every year 28-35% of people older than 65 years experienced falling, and the number is growing at 32-42% of people older than 70 years (WHO, 2007). Falling is one of the leading causes of injuries among the elderly and one of the leading causes of death that are the result of injuries. Older people who have experienced falling have the most common violations of hip fractures and head injuries. Older adults who survive injuries after falling may experience chronic effects which will limit their possibilities of movement (Hornbrook et al., 1994). The experienced falling may reduce confidence which will further cause decreasing levels of total movements, which further leads to reduced levels of vital activities and general health, and the final result will be increased number of falls with injuries. A proportion of falls result in fractures. Over 90% of hip fractures result from falls, (Grisso et al., 1991; Parkkari et al., 1999) and in individuals who sustain a hip fracture, the outcome is fatal in 12 to 20% of cases (Riggs and Melton, 1986). In nonfatal cases, long-standing pain, disability and functional impairment often ensue with tremendous socio-economic consequences.

Aging is characterized by emergence of a large number of chronic diseases, as well as atypical clinical features with which these diseases manifest (silent myocardial infarction, lacunar infarctions were asymptomatic, subclinical hypothyroidism, occurrence of metastases of malignant diseases without localization of the primary process) (Božinović, 2006). It is believed that about 80% of persons aged 65 years and above have several chronic diseases. Increased arterial pressure exists in about 40% of elderly people. Insulin-dependent diabetes constitutes one of the most common diseases of older age (Evans, 1995). Heart disease is the main cause of death in people aged 60 years old. One of the two persons from 60 years shows a certain kind of narrowing of the coronary arteries, or about 50% of them will show clinical signs of dysfunction of the coronary arteries (Sedić, 2010). All respiratory function with aging are reduced, vital lung capacity is reduced to about 1 liter, reduced forced expiratory volume and maximum breathing capacity (Duraković et al., 2007).

It is known that aging is a reduction in the sensitivity of sense and it is natural to assume that this can slow down the reaction of the elderly. Hearing problems contribute to 14%, and vision problems to 12% of the health problems (Den Draak, 2010). The weakening of the sense of hearing causes automatic increase in intensity of voice, which can cause ridicule environment. Poor vision makes it difficult to engage in a favorite hobby - reading books, for example, in severe cases, and move outdoors. Due to the weakening of the sense of taste and smell food becomes less palatable, and the sense of touch becomes less sensitive (Tomek-Roksandić and Čulig, 2003).

Among the health problems difficulties in sleeping are also present and could be the cause of relatively easy irritability and nervousness. By regular observation there is a tendency to slow down with the aging overall behavior. The changes are also visible in the mental aspect. There is agreement that in old age a decline in general mental ability. This decline is pretty bland to 65 - 70 years, then the majority of people coming to the rapid deterioration of intellectual abilities (Hrnjica, 2003). The attention visibly weakens, and the same happens with the memory. Memory impairment may be quantitative (amnesia) and qualitative (illusion) (Stosljević et al., 2013). Interesting observation that shows that people of the third age easier to reproduce the experience of youth, than recent experiences.

In certain number of elderly, there are processes of dementia. Dementia is a syndrome (set of symptoms and signs), which consists of cognitive decline and behavioral changes that interferes with daily activities of a person. The most striking sign of this disease is forgetfulness, or any other brain function can be affected, so that can meet the interference of attention, thought, speech, conscience movement, perception, mood, behavior and other functions (Pavlović, 2008). The Mental Health Foundation (2009) has defined dementia as a decline in mental ability that affects memory, thinking, problem solving, concentration and perception. In people with dementia brain functions are more damaged, including memory, ability to solve everyday problems, sensory-motor and social skills, language and communication, and control of emotional reactions, without disturbance of consciousness.

A very important aspect of aging is the possibility of performing everyday activities such as eating, getting up from his chair, brushing teeth, dressing, bathing, and others or instrumental activities of daily living such as cooking, shopping, laundry, medications, walking, solving everyday financial and other ongoing activities. Reduction in functional abilities (strength, endurance, agility and flexibility) caused by the aging process, causing difficulties in their daily life activities and the normal functioning of the elderly. Overall, approximately 18% of persons at or over the age of 65 years are dependent in one or more activities of daily living (ADL) (King et al., 2002). Aniansson et al. (1983) investigated the operation of 70 years persons performing your daily routine: 7% of the overall study population had difficulties in dress and carrying out hygiene. A particular problem was represented by movements such as touching hand-foot work wear socks and shoes. Respondents also had a problem getting up from sitting position and performance of the movements of supination and pronation. Symptoms are included in the framework as they mediate the effects of chronic disease on ADL performance (Bennett et al., 2002). Examples of symptoms in elderly people include musculoskeletal pain, shortness of breath, depression, weakness, and fatigue (Stewart, 2003). The symptoms, rather than the diseases that cause them, may be held responsible for the burden laid on the older person's health. Consequently, physiological fitness together with symptoms determine the way older persons function in their daily life.

Quality of Life in Older Adults

The World Health Organization's definition of quality of life is "an individual's perception of their position in life in the context of the culture and value systems in which they live and in relation to their goals, expectations, standards and concerns" (WHOQOL Group, 1993). It includes physical, social, economic and psychological well-being, a sense of positive social involvement and opportunities to realize their own potential, and includes psychosocial domain (emotional, social) and physical domain or the domain associated with health (Gojčeta et al., 2008; Majnemer et al., 2008; Majnemer et al., 2007 according to Milićević, 2015). Authors in different areas access defining quality of life from the perspective of their interests and their research goals. In mainstream psychology, quality of life is defined as a conscious cognitive judgment of satisfaction with one's life. This construct has an extensive history in cross-cultural research and can be assessed with the Satisfaction With Life Scale (SWU), a five item unidimensional measure with excellent psychometric properties (Pavot and Diener, 1993). Medical researchers have replaced the term "quality of life" with HRQL or health status. This modification was designed to emphasize an interest in the functional effects on patients of an illness and its consequent therapy (Rejeski et al., 1996). Health related quality of life, in one hand, describes difficulties resulting bad health regarding psychological and physical function, partaking in areas of life, but "health status" also (Trgovčević et al., 2011).

By reviewing available literature and also based on research conducted by group interview method Kane et al. (2003) define quality of life as a multidimensional accessment of life experiences and they define 11 major areas in quality of life. These are: certainity, functional competence, relations, comfort, meaningfull activities, dignity, individuality, privacy, autonomy and spiritual wellbeing. Some authors agree that quality of life concept implies combination of objective and subjective factors, thus Krizmanić and Kolesarić (1989) consider quality of life as subjective experience of our own life determined by objective living cicumstances, personal features that affect experience of reality and specific personal life experience. Cummins (1997) agrees that quality of life is both subjective and objective whereby each domain is compound of seven areas: material wellbeing, health, productiveness, intimacy, certainity, communal wellbeing and emotional wellbeing. Objective domains contain culturaly relevant measures of objective wellbeing. Subjective domains contain satisfaction measured by the importaince it has for each individual (according to Podgorelec, 2004.). Sometimes there may be a discrepancy between the level of achievement of life activities (or objective) and the level of satisfaction with life activity (ie subjective) (Nikić et al., 2014). Felce and Perry (1995) define quality of life as general wellbeing that includes descriptors objective and subjective evaluation of physical, material, social and emotional wellbeing, together with personal development and meaningfull activity, all evaluated through individual value system (according to Vuletic, 1999).

The quality of life is the most important indicator of happiness and satisfaction in every society. It is therefore of extreme importance for its follow-up study, because it is the only way to monitor the state of mind and well-being of a nation. The quality of life in some countries is monitored by the index of quality of life. In 2013, Switzerland had the highest quality of life index, which amounted to 215.71, while the lowest was in Venezuela -47.27. Out of 67 countries, which participated in the said survey, Serbia is at the 47th place in the world and in 25th place in Europe, with an index of 63.68. From the southeastern Balkans countries only Greece, Bulgaria and Romania have a lower index of quality of life in the Republic of Serbia (Quality of Life, 2015), however, in 2014 and 2015, Greece had a higher index of quality of life of the Republic of Serbia (Table 4). From the above table it can be seen that Switzerland is at the forefront of a number of years whether it is Europe or the whole world.

Table 4. Europe: Quality of Life Index by Country[2]

Country (Europa)	Year	Rank	Quality of Life Index
	2015	1	222,94
Switzerland	2014	1	206,23
	2013	1	215,71
	2015	24	94,66
Greece	2014	24	77,48
	2013	27	55,51
	2015	30	60,34
Serbia	2014	27	69,31
	2013	25	63,68

The quality of life may depend on many factors, so some authors believe that half (Nikolić et al., 2009; Pacić et al., 2010), age (Nikić et al., 2014), independent living, difficulties in using public transport and poor performance perceived health status may indicate the need for assistance in daily life. Nikolić and associates (2009) found that the type of damage has an impact on quality of life, including, for example, people with quadriparesis harder meet their needs in motion, responsibilities and difficulties in establishing

---

[2] http://www.numbeo.com/quality-of-life/rankings_by_country.jsp.

communication of patients with hemiparesis. The same authors state that the first year of infection is a period when subjects spasticity harder to meet their daily needs and the period when they mostly need help of professional persons in order to facilitate overcoming powerlessness and of better quality of future life (Nikolić et al. 2009).

The activities that elderly can independently perform, or they think they can, are a useful indicator of the health condition of the person and its need for assistance in the case of self-care. Of utmost importance is the ability of seniors to function independently in their own homes. Functional ability is a critical indicator of the quality of life and health among the elderly, sometimes more important than the presence of some disease (Šarić et al., 2014). Studies show that older people adjust their hierarchy of needs state, so that self-esteem, dignity and control over their lives become more important for the quality of life of physical health (Despot-Lučanin et al., 2006). Other authors who have engaged in the research aspects of quality of life in older "more capable" and "less capable" person, they realized that, with "less capable" of older people is the most important aspect of health, while the "more capable" main aspect of the social relationship in life (Puts et al., 2007). Hellstrom et al. (2004, according to Leutar et al., 2007) examined the quality of life in people over 75 years old living at home. The inability to live at home without help, life in single households and fatigue are associated with reduced quality of life in older who receive aid, while the elderly who do not receive help are more frequent sleep problems and reduced the mood 09).

In aging research, quality of life has been used as an umbrella term to describe a number of outcomes that clinicians believe are important in the lives of older adults. Stewart and King (1991) published a study on conceptual options for use in evaluating the efficacy of physical activity on quality of life in older adults. The authors proposed two broad categories of outcomes for quality of life research: functioning and well-being. Under functioning they listed physical abilities and dexterity, cognition, and the ability to perform activities of daily living (ADLs). The well-being category included symptoms and bodily states, emotional well-being, self-concept, and global perceptions related to health and overall life satisfaction (Stewart and King, 1991).

Effects Physical Activity by Older Adults

Numerous studies have enlightened the benefits of daily physical activity and exercise on older adults (Weening et al., 2011). Regular physical activity has been shown to have many health benefits in all age groups. The benefits for older people include improved fitness and quality of life, prevention of osteoporosis and a reduction in the risk of falling. Physical activity also reduces deaths from cardiovascular disease and can improve cardiovascular risk profile. Maintaining health and fitness into old age is a public health priority. However, despite the benefits of physical activity, many older people are much less active than desired (Crombie et al., 2004).

Lepan and Leutar (2012) reported results of the Zagreb City Centre research for health, labor, social welfare and veterans conducted in 2007 among users of gerontological centers, in which 77.08% of them attended Recreational medical gymnastics, and as a result showed that: 1. The use of service centers assisted them in the successful satisfaction of physiological, social and health needs (82.89%), 2. the inclusion of the activities of gerontological centers they feel significantly more useful in the community in which they live (79.4%), 3. that their participation in the activities of the centers improved their health status (82.89%), 4. their social life improved since participating in the activities of the centers (81.40%). The research results of Močnik et al. (2015), on a sample of 38 subjects (28 female and 10 male) aged 65 to 95 years showed that 20 of them (52.6%) believe that physical activity can prevent or control certain diseases while 18 of them (47.4%) believes that it can. From 47.4% of those who know that some diseases can be prevented or controlled physical activity out of 7 (38.9%) stated that it is high blood pressure, 6 (33.3%), diabetes mellitus, 4 (22.2%) states osteoporosis, 3 (16.7%) heart disease, 2 (11.1%) depression, 2 (11.1%), Parkinson's disease and 1 (5.6%) people claimed obesity.

Exercise training programs that are used in recreational activities may have a small, medium or large effects on increasing muscle strength in the elderly. Regular physical activity throughout life may slow down changes, and may even improve muscle function (Nemček, 2011; Tekura et al., 2008; Bates et al., 2009). For older people, there are two different ways to improve muscle strength through exercise. One is by training localized muscle groups. The other is by training functions related to motor activities such as walking, stair climbing, standing up from a chair, rising from the bed, reaching, and bending. These functions are embedded in the daily tasks faced by older institutionalized persons. Exercise programs aimed to improve daily tasks should include functional training items to be as effective as possible (de Vreede et al, 2005). Eyigor et al. (2007) conducted a survey in order to find out the effects of the combined program of exercise on muscle strength, physical performance and quality of life in older women. Twenty women performed an exercise program for 8 weeks, at the rehabilitation unit. Outcome measures included a 4-m and 20-m walk test, a 6-min walk test, stair climbing and chair rise time, timed up and go test, isokinetic muscle testing of the knee and ankle, and the Short Form-36 (SF-36) and geriatric depression scale questionnaires. The mean age of the study group was 70.3 ± 6.5 years. After the completion of the exercise program, all of the physical performance tests and the SF-36 scores for the participants showed statistically significant improvements ($p < 0.05$). In the isokinetic evaluations, most of angular velocities showed a significant increase in the peak torque values for knee extension and flexion, and ankle plantar flexion for ($p < 0.05$). According to the results of their study, the authors concluded that the exercise program implemented successfully contributed to the increase in knee flexor and extensor muscle strength, as well as ankle plantar and dorsal flexions; therefore, it is highly recommendable to older women. In addition to these programs operate primarily on increasing muscle strength and muscle mass, they lead to a reduction in body fat, increase metabolism, reduce blood pressure, reduce the level cholesterol and reduce the risk of osteoporosis (Brown, 2007).

Physical activity is known to prevent a number of chronic diseases including cardiovascular disease, hypertension, type II diabetes, and certain cancers (O'Donovan et al., 2010). It has been proven that regular physical activity reduces blood pressure among middle and late age, especially those who already have high blood pressure. When it comes to the types of physical activity in the prevention of hypertension, aerobic activity, such as briskwalking (crisp uniform walking speed 5-6 km / h), cycling, swimming, jogging, are recommended primarily, ie. these physical activities that are based on stereotyped repetition of movement and that involve large muscle groups and the cardiovascular system (Mujović and Čubrilo, 2012). Physical activity of older people, even in those with previously sedentary lifestyle, can enhance physical fitness and general health. Regular physical activity can help reduce heart rate at rest, as well as systolic and diastolic blood pressure (Živković et al.,

2002). Kida and colleagues (2008) investigated the effects of the program exercise in people who have had a myocardial infarction. Exercise program involved the combination of strength and aerobic exercises. All patients participated in a 12-week exercise training program. Cardiac rehabilitation program combined with resistance and aerobic training improved exercise capacity and increased skeletal muscle not the volume but the skeletal muscle strength in patients with myocardial infarction in their recovery phase. It was presumed that the improvement of exercise capacity was determined by the skeletal muscle strength not by the muscle volume especially in myocardial infarction patients with low muscle volume. Haykowsky et al. (2005) investigated the effects of three different program of exercise on muscle strength, maximum aerobic ability and morphology of the left ventricle in healthy older women. The first experimental group was subjected to aerobic training, which included riding bikes. Another experimentally group was subjected to strength training equipment. The third experimental group was subjected to a combination of aerobic and strength training. Upper and lower extremity strength was significantly higher after 12 weeks of strength training or combined aerobic and strength training with no change after that aerobics or no training. Left ventricular diastolic filling and morphology were not altered significantly after 12 weeks of that aerobics, strength training, combined aerobic and strength training, or no training. Twelve weeks of strength training or combined aerobic and strength training are as effective as 12 weeks of that aerobics for increasing altering relative peak aerobic power, however, strength training and combined aerobic and strength training are more effective than that aerobics for improving overall muscle strength.

Nemoto et al. (2007) investigated whether the high intensity interval walking training has better effects on strength increase, aerobic capacity and reduction in blood pressure, in comparison to the moderate-intensity walking program. From May 2004 to October, 2004 (5-month study period), 60 men and 186 women with a mean ± SD age of 63 ± 6 years were randomly divided into 3 groups: no walking training, moderate-intensity continuous walking training, and high-intensity interval walking training. Participants in the moderate-intensity continuous walking training group were instructed to walk at approximately 50% of their peak aerobic capacity for walking, using a pedometer to verify that they took 8000 steps or more per day for 4 or more days per week. Those in the high-intensity interval walking training group, who were monitored by accelerometry, were instructed to repeat 5 or more sets of 3-minute low-intensity walking at 40% of peak aerobic capacity for walking followed by a 3-minute high-intensity walking above 70% of peak aerobic capacity for walking per day for 4 or more days per week. Isometric knee extension and flexion forces, peak aerobic capacity for cycling, and peak aerobic capacity for walking were all measured both before and after training. The results of this study showed an increase in muscle strength, which were significantly higher in the second than in the first experimental group. The increasement of isometric knee flexion was 17% and 13% extension in the other experimental groups. The authors concluded that high-intensity walking program can be, among other, an effective tool in preventing the decline in muscle strength which is associated with the aging process.

Mavrić et al. (2014) consider walking type "brisk-walking," the easiest, and safest activity that virtually anyone can practice, and almost with no contraindications. Walk with fast pace leads to increased secretion of endorphins and serotonin, which improves mood and are very important for motivation. The main advantage of brisk-walking-and systemic effects on metabolism (basal metabolism speeds), the skeletal system (prevents osteoporosis and, unlike jogging, there is no risk of overloading joints), and in particular the cardio vascular system (strengthens the heart, increasing elasticity of blood vessels, regulates blood pressure, lowers cholesterol) (Mavrić et al., 2014).

Physical activity can favorably influence on some risk factors to the falls, by increasing muscle strength, range of motion, improved balance, walking faster and shorter response time to changes in the environment (Lepan and Leutar, 2012). Exercise intervention can reduce many intrinsic risk factors for falling. Carter et al. (2001) analyzed 13 studies on using exercise as the intervention for fall prevention in the community (n = 12) or institution dwelling (n = 1) older adults. The authors concluded that the studies prior to 1996 did not find that exercise reduced the risk of falling in older adults 9 while the more recent studies confirmed the value of exercise and fall prevention. Five studies demonstrated a significant reduction in falls (Wolf et al., 1996; Campbell et al., 1997; Buchner et al., 1997; Campbell et al., 1999; Lehtola et al., 2000) whilst in the remaining 4, (Rizzo et al, 1996; McMurdo et al., 1997; Steinberg et al, 2000; Rubenstein et al., 2000) some reduction in falls was evident but not statistically significant.

Myers et al. (1996) suggested that strength, flexibility, balance and reaction time, were the factors are most amenable to modification, and thus, provide a rationale for exercise intervention trials measuring the efficacy of exercise in the prevention of falls in the elderly. A literature search from 1976-1994, identified 52 studies examining risk factors for falls, recurrent falls and/or falls resulting in injury. Nine intervention studies were identified with the primary outcome of falls. Physical activity-related risk factors for falls include limitations in general functioning, such as ambulation and mobility problems, difficulty or dependence in activities of daily living, and exposures to the risks of falling as indicated by the nature and frequency of daily activities. Impairments in gait and balance as well as neuromuscular and musculoskeletal impairments frequently underlie changes in physical activity in old age. Reduced activity level may occur as a result of these impairments, leading to further declines in physical functioning and an increased risk of falls. A relatively high level of activity in old age is also associated with risk of falls. Other risk factors for falls, such as cognitive impairment, visual deficits, and medication use, may combine with physical activity-related risk factors that increase the risk of falls. Intervention studies directed at nursing home populations did not prevent falls but had other statistically and clinically significant outcomes. Studies among the community dwelling that targeted potential or current risk factors and included an exercise component reported a significant reduction in falls, prevented the onset of new disabilities and reduced baseline risk factors.

In the study by Campbell et al. (1997) and physiotherapist, individualized program of predominantly lower limb strength and balance exercises for 30 minutes, 3 times per week plus additional walking, resulted in a significantly reduced annual rate of falls among women aged 80 years and older, compared with control women. After 1 year, the relative hazard for the first 4 falls in the exercise group compared with controls was 0.68. The benefit of exercise for the reduction of falls continued in the 2-year follow-up (Campbell et al., 1999). According Vuori (2005) exercise programs for older men and women minimize drops to 19-46%, and injuries due to falls of 28-88%.

Ylinen and al. (2006) examined the effects of strength training to increase muscle strength and decrease neck pain in the neck area in women with chronic pain in the neck. In the first experimental group exercise program has involved a gradual increase in load during the experimental program. In the second experimental group load has not changed during the program. The results showed that both programs significantly contribute to increasing the strength and reducing pain in the neck in the first two months of exercise. But after a year of applied experiment, an exercise program that is administered in the first group gave significantly better results. Based on the results the authors consider the training of the neck muscles and shoulders is effective in increasing muscle strength and reducing pain and limitation of motion in the neck.

A number of studies shows that an active lifestyle and daily physical activity play an important role in the prevention of obesity (Fogelholm et al., 2000; Di Pietro, 1999). Physical activity affects the functional capacity of older people. Lepan and Leutar (2012) in their had a goal to determine whether there are differences in functional abilities (ability to personal hygiene and housekeeping) among older adults who engage in regular leisure-time physical activity and those who do not. The survey was conducted on a sample of 342 people over 65 years, mean age 71 years (SD = 5.20), and range from 65 to 88 years. The sample was 192 persons engaged in recreational exercise and 150 persons who are not engaged in recreational exercise. Results of this study indicate that physical activity positively affects the improvement and maintenance of functional abilities, and thus indirectly to the possibility that prolonged independent living of older people. More often active people in the younger old age which is to be expected because in old age comes from the diminishing functional abilities. But it's cause and effect, because the preservation of functional abilities as possible through active recreational exercise (Lepan and Leutar, 2012).

The researchers also found that the physical activity stimulates and protects the brain function. Physically active people learn better and remember longer, because the physical activity slows the aging degeneration of the brain. Randomized controlled trials have demonstrated that fitness training has a robust effect on improving certain cognitive processes (Colcombe and Kramer, 2003), which may be important for future risk of dementia (Linn et al., 1995; Small et al., 2000).

There is literature that suggests that some cognitive domains are affected by physical activity more than others (Colcombe and Kramer, 2003). Therefore, use of global and composite measures may obscure relationships between physical activity and cognition that differ based upon the cognitive domain. The purpose of study Wilbur et al. (2012) was to explore the relationship between hours spent participating in light- and moderate / vigorous-intensity physical activity and different forms of cognition in older Latinos, controlling for sex and for factors shown to be associated with cognition. Our study extends previous literature because it examines an understudied, at-risk, rapidly growing population and uses accelerometers, innovative, comprehensive means of measuring physical activity. Participants were 174 Latino men (n = 46) and women (n = 128) aged 50-84 years (M = 66 years). After adjusting for control variables (demographics, chronic health problems) and other cognitive measures, regression analyzes revealed that minutes per day of light-intensity physical activity (r = -0.51), moderate / vigorous physical activity (r = -0.56), and counts per minute (r = -0.62) were negatively associated with lower word fluency. Findings suggest that the cognitive benefits of both light-intensity physical activity and moderate / vigorous physical activity may be domain-specific.

Larson et al. (2006) during 6.2 years to examine the effects of exercise on the incidence of dementia in a sample of 1740 persons older than age 65 years without cognitive impairment who scored above the 25th percentile on the Cognitive Ability Screening Instrument (CASI) in the Adult Changes in Thought study and who were followed biennially to identify incident dementia. The results of their study showed that older people who exercise three or more times a week, rarely suffer from Alzheimer's disease and old age dementia. People who regularly practiced, had 30-40% lower risk of developing dementia. It was noted that even light physical activity, such as walking, helps to delay the first symptoms of the disease (Larson et al., 2006). Our results are consistent with earlier observations that modest levels of physical exercise are associated with delayed onset of dementia or Alzheimer's disease (Laurin et al., 2001; Abbott et al., 2004; Weuve et al., 2004).

Hamer and Chida (2009) by reviewing the literature wanted to examine the association between physical activity and risk of neurodegenerative diseases which is not well established. We included 16 prospective studies in the overall analysis, which incorporated 163 797 non-demented participants at baseline with 3219 cases at follow-up. We calculated pooled relative risk using a random effects model. The relative risk of dementia in the highest physical activity category compared with the lowest was 0.72 (95% confidence interval (CI) 0.60-0.86, $p < 0.001$), for Alzheimer's, 0.55 (95% CI 0.36-0.84, $p = 0.006$), and for Parkinson's 0.82 (95% CI: 0:57 to 1:18, $p = 0.28$). Our results suggest that physical activity is inversely associated with risk of dementia. The present meta-analysis of prospective cohort studies suggests that physical activity reduces the risk of dementia and Alzheimer's disease by 28% and 45% respectively. Physical activity was not associated with a significant reduction in risk of Parkinson's disease, although this finding should be viewed in light of limited evidence in this area.

Seidman (2001, by: Andrijašević and Andrijašević, 2006) believe that regular physical activity reduces stress even better than meditation and conventional methods. Also, says that aerobic exercise triggers the release of hormones in the brain that reduce anxiety and depression neutralized. McNeil et al. (1991) is the only other randomized exercise trial in older adults. Their subjects (mean age 72, SD = 6 years) were chosen by self-reported scores of> 12 on the BDI and may or may not have fulfilled diagnostic criteria for depression. Over a 6-week intervention of walking vs. social contact vs wait list, the BDI was reduced approximately 33% in the walking group. Singh et al. (1997), we tested the hypothesis that progressive resistance training would reduce depression while improving physiologic capacity, quality of life, morality, function and self-efficacy without adverse events in an older, significantly depressed population. A total of 32 subjects aged 60-84, mean age 71.3 ± 1.2 yr., were randomized and completed the study. We conducted a 10-week randomized controlled trial of volunteers aged 60 and above with major or minor depression or dysthymia. Subjects were randomized for 10 weeks to either a supervised program of progressive resistance training three times a week or an attention control group. The results of this study are progressive resistance training program significantly reduced all measures depression (Beck Depression Inventory and exercisers 21.3 ± 1.8 to 9.8 ± 2.4 versus 18.4 ± 1.7 controls to 13.8 ± 2, $p = 0.002$; Hamilton Rating Scale of Depression and exercisers 0.9to5.3 12.3 ± ± 1.3 versus 11.4 ± controls 1.0 to 8.9 ± 1.3, $p = 0.008$). Quality of life Subscales of bodily pain ($p = 0.001$), vitality ($p = 0.002$), social functioning (p -0.008), and emotional role ($p = 0.02$) were all significantly improved by exercise compared to controls. Strength increased a mean of 33% ± 4% in exercisers and decreased 2% ± 2% in controls ($p < 0.0001$). In a stepwise multiple regression model, the intensity of training was a significant independent predictor of decrease in depression scores ($R^2 = 0.617$, $p = 0.0002$).

METHODS

Physical activity is one of the key factors in maintaining, preserving and improving health. The best way for body to gain the physical and mental shape. Extensive exercise slows aging and preventively influences our body, organs and tissues. Physical activity affects the ability of elderly to maintain an independent lifestyle, to keep the old job if they want to and to maintain a high level of quality of life. Psychophysical engagement through sports and physical exercise have positive influence on physical abilities and resistance of human body, preservation of health and better regeneration of motor functions (Eminović et al., 2009). Physical activity increases the level of remained physical abilities, reduces the potential complications of underlying disease and prolongs life expectancy, encourages self-evaluation, self-realization and the level of social contacts. However, it is dependent on both the individual as well as the participation of the community (Trgovčević et al., 2011).

Starting from the aforementioned facts, and based on the literature review, the objective of this paper is to examine the opinion of elderly about the impact of physical activity in some segments of the quality of life of people of the third age. In other words, you will see the contribution of physical exercise in reducing anxiety and stress, and increasing the health status of the individual as well as the relationship between physical exercise and self-esteem, as well as to try to explain the impact of physical exercise on socialization and psychosomatic state of the individual. The specific objective of this study is to determine whether there are differences in attitudes about the connection between physical exercise and health as an aspect of quality of life among the elderly population in the Republic of Serbia, Switzerland and Greece.

Table 5. Structure of respondents by country and gender

	Male	Female	Σ
Switzerland	69 (51.5%)	65 (48.5%)	134
Greece	51 (42.5%)	69 (57.5%)	120
Serbia	85 (54.5%)	71 (45.5%)	156
Total	205	205	410

Participants

The research was conducted on a sample of 410 respondents aged 65 to 70 years. Compared to the half of the respondents were equally represented by men and women. The structure of respondents by country is as follows: Switzerland 134 respondents, 120 respondents Greece and the Republic of Serbia 156 subjects (Table 5).

Instruments

The data were collected through an anonymous questionnaire consisting of 3 parts. The first part of the questionnaire contains questions on general information of respondents, the second part of the issues are physical exercise and relate to frequency and the type of exercise and the third part of the questionnaire contains statements about the opinion of respondents who are the impacts of physical activity. The third part is divided into four parts. The first part examines the opinion of respondents on the impact of physical activity on health and general condition. The second part examines the respondents' opinion on the impact of physical activity on functional abilities. In the third part examines opinion of respondents on the impact of physical activity on some psychological indicators. And a fourth section examines the respondents` opinion on the impact of physical activity on interpersonal relationships. The respondents for each item could choose one score between 1 and 3 (1-false, 2-partially true and 3-true).

Statistics

The values were expressed as mean and SDs. All statistical procedures were conducted with the SPSS 17.0 statistical package (SPSS Inc., Chicago, IL, USA). The level of significance was set at $p < 0.05$ for all analyses.

RESULTS

Examining the frequency of application of physical activity among participants we have obtained data that the elderly from the Swiss practice physical activity daily to 48.8%, from 2 to 3 times a week 34.3% while only 17.2% of respondents didn`t engage in any physical activity. In the case of Greece it is also the highest percentage of those who engage in physical activity every day 42.5%, 35.8% of respondents, who exercise 2 to 3 times a week while 21.7% of respondents were not engaged in some form of physical activity. As for Serbia, most of the respondents are in the category of those who do not engage in physical activity, the 35.9%, slightly less number is involved 2 to 3 times per week and the least are those who exercise every day (Table 6).

Table 6. Structure of respondents according to the frequency of dealing with some form of physical activity and country

	Every day	2 to 3 times per week	Never
Switzerland	48.5%	34.3%	17.2%
Greece	42.5%	35.8%	21.7%
Serbia	28.8%	35.3%	35.9%

In examining the types of physical activities the respondents engaged in these three countries found that in Switzerland the most represented walking and jogging (primarily Nordic), as well as walking and hiking for a few days, which is especially popular among respondents in Switzerland. Then elderly from Switzerland alleged swimming and aqua fitness, tennis and badminton, folk dances and cycling. In the lowest percentage winter sports are present (especially skiing), yoga, Tai Chi and other sports. In Greece, the elderly are engaged in the following types of physical activity: walking, dancing, yoga, and aerobics exercise and leisure activities such as social gatherings, cultural activities, and leisure trips are offered. In Serbia the most present are Nordic hiking or walking, embossing, chess, bike rides, swimming, fishing and yoga.

The respondents` opinion about the impact of physical activities on health and general condition was examined through an opinion on whether physical exercise affects them to feel healthier and that their health care system problems can be reduced if they engage in physical activity. In the case of respondents from Serbia, as many as 58.4% said it was true that physical activity affects health, 35.9% of them considered that it is partially true, while 5.7% of them consider that it is incorrect. In Switzerland it is also the highest percentage of those who agree that this is exactly 56.6%, partly true declares 40% of respondents in for incorrectly answered only 3.4% of respondents. In Greece, the percentage of those who believe that it is incorrect 6.6%, partly true 39.3%, while 54.2% of respondents considered that physical activity contributes to better health state as accurate (Table 7).

Respondents' opinions on the impact of physical activity on functional abilities were tested through impact of physical activity to feel stronger and more able to easily move around the apartment and easier to perform daily activities (activities related to nutrition, personal hygiene). The 73.3% of respondents from Greece considers that this is true, 20.8% partially true, while only 5.9% considered incorrect. A somewhat smaller percentage of respondents from Serbia believes that this is exactly 60.9%, partly true, 35.3% and 3.8% not true. When it comes to respondents from Switzerland is a smaller percentage of those who believe that this is exactly 38.1% compared to those who think that this is partly true and untrue 53.7% of them 8.2% (Table 8).

Table 7. Respondents' opinions on the impact of physical activity on health and general condition

	True	Partially true	False
Switzerland	56.6%	40%	3.4%
Greece	54.2%	39.3%	6.6%
Serbia	58.4%	35.9%	5.7%

Table 8. Respondents' opinions on the impact of physical activity on functional abilities

	True	Partially true	False
Switzerland	38.1%	53.7%	8.2%
Greece	73.3%	20.8%	5.9%
Serbia	60.9%	35.3%	3.8%

Table 9. Respondents' opinions on the impact of physical activity on some psychological indicators

	True	Partially true	False
Switzerland	56%	39.6%	4.4%
Greece	45%	45.8%	9.2%
Serbia	43.6%	41%	15.4%

Table 10. The respondents` on the impact of physical activity on interpersonal relationships

	True	Partially true	False
Switzerland	29.%	41.8%	29.2%
Greece	60.8%	19.2%	20%
Serbia	70.5%	17.9%	11.6%

We examined the effect of physical activity on psychological indicators the opinion of respondents whether engaging in physical activities may make them feel happier, less nervous and that if their engagement in physical activity can increase self-confidence. With this fact, most respondents agree from Switzerland - 56% believe this is true, 39.6% believe that this is partly true, while only 4.4% considered incorrect. As for respondents from Greece almost the same percentage believe that this is true 45% as well as partially true 45.8%, while 9.2% of them considered incorrect. In respondents from Serbia more participants than in Greece and Switzerland consider that this is true - 15.4%, partially true 41% of them, while the largest number considered this fact true 43.6% (Table 9).

The impact of physical activities on interpersonal relationships is examined through an opinion on whether physical exercise might affect them feel less lonely and whether engaging in physical activities may affect to meet new people and make new friends. The respondents from Serbia in the highest percentage, 70.5% believe that this is true, 19.2% are considered partially correct, while 11.6% is considered incorrect. Respondents in Greece show a similar opinion and in 60.8% considered exact, 19.2% partly true and 20% not true. Somewhat different results can be seen in participants from Switzerland to the same percentage considered accurate 29% as well as inaccurate 29.2%, while 41.8% considered them partly true (Table 10).

DISCUSSION

The frequency of practicing physical activity among respondents in the three countries where the research was undertaken show that when it comes to practice every day participants from Switzerland are present in the highest percentage while the respondents from Greece are present to a lesser level, while respondents from Serbia are at a minority when it comes to exercising daily. When it comes to frequency of exercise 2 to 3 times a week, respondents in all three countries are represented in relatively the same percentage. In the category where they do not exercise at all, respondents from Serbia are represented twice as much comparing to those from Switzerland, while Greece is between the two countries by those who do not exercise (Table 6). In Canada, percentages of older women in comparison to older men were lower for participation: in vigorous physical activity (20% women, 24% men), in moderate intensity physical activity (26% women, 27% men), as well as in low intensity physical activity (19% women and 20% men) (Craig et al., 1997). Mestheneou and Antoniadou (2004) reported the following characteristics of sport in ancient Greece: the physical activity of the elderly is moderate to low; the income factor is considered to be the main contributing factor; the limited physical activity for the Greek elderly is due to the prevailing socio-educational conditions according to which a "way of life" is being established, which does not encourage physical activity; the elderly women markedly prefer watching TV, visiting friends, or going to church; contrary to what happens internationally, the Greek elderly women are more active than men as far as overall activity is concerned, especially regarding activities having to do with running the household; housework helps Greek women remain more active than men, even past the age of 80. It is, therefore, more urgent to find ways of motivating men of the same age group to become active: in all recreational activities Greek men hold higher degrees of participation then women and all forms of physical activity become significantly limited with age, especially after the age of 80 (Mestheneou and Antoniadou, 2004).

Sun et al. (2013) based on a review of the literature on physical activity in older 20 studies excluded household work with physical activity reported prevalence ranging from 23.06% to 67.51%, while 14 included household work with reported physical activity prevalence of 10.86% to 66.7%. Seventeen studies measured all domains of physical activity (including occupational, household, transportation and recreational physical activity) with reported physical activity prevalence of 11.67% to 77.22%, and two studies reported that 31.7% and 62.4% of older people achieved sufficient physical activity through walking.

Harahousou and Kabitsis (1993) reported that the vast majority of older individuals are engaged in passive rather than active recreation. The same author suggested a variety of reasons for older individuals' low participation rates in active recreation. The low rates could stem from cultural reasons related to the role of older individuals in society and the family (especially the role of women). Furthermore, environmental problems related to lack of spaces for recreation in big cities or problems related to lack of time, health problems, and limited opportunities for participation might influence older adults' physical activity participation.

If we compare Switzerland, Greece and Serbia in relation to the type of physical activity they are engaged respondents we can conclude that in the first place in all three countries are walking as a form of physical activity while the sequence of other activities differs from country to country. Mestheneou and Antoniadou (2004) reported that in Greece the most popular activities among the elderly are walking, gardening, swimming, dancing. Much time is spent in sedentary activities, especially watching TV the elderly having a family, especially the women, constitute the percentage of Greek population with the lowest participation in recreational athletic activities. It is likely that the choice of sports influence has bid so when analyzing various offers and categories of the population in Switzerland can conclude that in the first place with 58% in the offer represented walking and jogging, Nordic walking and then 9%, water sports (swimming, Aqua Fitness, 8%), hiking (6%), tennis and badminton (4%), dances (4%), cycling (4%) and at the end of winter sports, Tai Chi, Qi Gong and team sports with a total of 7% representation among offers (Lamprecht et al., 2014). Qualitative research indicates that older people participate in a diverse range of activities including:

- Club, team or group activities (dancing, golf, bowls etc.).
- Activities that require infrastructure support e.g., swimming, weights, and gym.
- Individual activities such as walking, cycling.
- Work around the home and yard.
- Community activities or other, such as community service or playing with grandchildren (Brown et al., 1999).

The impact of the physical activity is often associated with health (physical inactivity was also estimated to be responsible for 10-16% of cases of breast, colon and rectal cancers and diabetes mellitus, and about 22% of cases of ischemic heart disease) which was confirmed by the subjects in which slightly more than half of respondents in all three countries said it was true while slightly less than half of the respondents as partially true. The reason why a relatively large number of respondents have chosen the answer partly true rather than precisely we seek in their uncertainty or perhaps fear that during physical activities can happen to a fall and injury. Illness and frailty are barriers to participation, as is the expectation that exercising could result in physical harm – "supposed health risks and the perceived inevitability of physical decline are used to justify non participation." Previous major health problems can pose a barrier to activity (Crombie et al., 2004) amongst older people. According to Harahousou and Kambitsis (1993) limited participation in physical activity reported by Greek older adults is related to social and educational factors that exclude participation in sports and physical activity from their lifestyle.

An important risk factor that contributes to decreased ADL performance is low levels of physical activity. One way to improve physical fitness is to exercise (Weening-Dijksterhuis et al., 2011). Our research shows minimal differences when it comes to comparing the results whether physical exercise affects the functional abilities needed for activities of daily living. The respondents from Switzerland pleaded to a higher percentage that's partly true, but absolutely true what was not the case in the other two countries especially in Greece where as many as 73.3% of respondents (Table 8) gave the answer that it is true. The percentage of those who believe that it is incorrect in all three countries is small. In support of these results, saying the claims of other authors. The elderly involved in some of the recreational activities assess their functional ability better than the ones who are not involved in any of the activities. This result is also an incentive to all persons older age to engage in group recreational exercise and thus contributing to the improvement and maintenance of their functional state, which is an important element of quality of life (Lepan and Leutar, 2012).

About half of our respondents from all three countries see the benefit of physical activities on the psychological aspect. In most percentage is present in respondents from Switzerland and Greece, while Serbia is on the third place (Table 9). The primary motivation for exercising is to gain psychological and emotional rewards. Achievement ethic plays a part in motivation to continue (attain a goal – walk right up to that road one day). For older people exercise is often related to self-esteem and self image (feeling good) and physical appearance (looking good) (Brown et al., 1999). McAuley and Katula (1998) recently published a review on physical activity interventions in elderly individuals. They provided a compelling argument for the favorable effect that physical activity has on self-efficacy beliefs in older adults and the possible mediational role of self-efficacy on both physical and psychological outcomes that have been found to be associated with physical activity. They emphasized that if a goal of physical activity programs is to increase sense of control in aging individuals, it is necessary to provide information specific to the domain of interest.

One of the most important perceived rewards associated with physical activity is social: meeting new people, maintaining friendships and generally getting out are some of the main incentives to participate. Opportunities to socialize, combat social isolation and mental stagnation were considered important, with the exercise considered incidental. There is a preference for all age groups to do activities with people with similar age, ability and outlook (individuals feel more comfortable in a homogenous group). Social contact is a primary motive, both as a prerequisite (no one to go with is a barrier to participation), and as a desired outcome (meeting new friends). In relation to social support, people identified as important for encouraging activity were partners and other family members, service providers, including practitioners and fitness leaders (Brown et al., 1999). In examining the effects of physical activity on interpersonal relationships, we can conclude that there are different opinions among our respondents in relation to their country of origin, especially between respondents from Switzerland in relation to the other two countries. The respondents from Serbia and Greece consider that a high percentage of participation in physical activity can affect interpersonal compacting while only a third of respondents in Switzerland is considered to be true. The same number of respondents believe it is not true (Table 10). Alexandris and Carroll (1997) reported that older individuals reported higher levels of intrapersonal constraints than did other age groups; the same authors suggested that intrapersonal constraints seem to be, in large degree, responsible for the inactivity of older adults. Promoting active recreation among older individuals in Greece is important today, because demographic statistics indicate that the older population is getting larger. This trend is more pronounced in rural areas.

CONCLUSION

Today, there are studies examining the need for physical exercise and sports, such as in persons with disabilities, the impact on quality of life, as well as researches that include finding solutions in order to assess motor abilities and body composition (Kljajić et al., 2013). Such studies also exists among the population of elderly because it is believed that physical activity is one of the most important step in improving health for people with chronic diseases of any age, especially among members of the elderly population. Regular physical activity improves quality of life at different ages and in different states. Evidence supports the positive relationship between physical activity and quality of life as it is the case with the population of elderly. Numerous studies have examined the relationship between physical activity and overall quality of life, and the effects of physical activity on individual areas that make up the quality of life. This study showed that opinions on the impact of elderly that physical activity has on the quality of life does not differ much although they are three very different countries, primarily in economic terms as well as geographical location. So we can conclude that physical activity has a positive impact on a better quality of life for the elderly, ie to contribute much better health, functioning in daily life, better mental health and better quality interpersonal relationships, regardless of whether the respondents from Switzerland, Serbia or Greece. All this leads us to that, due to the rapid aging of the population worldwide, it is necessary to establish that greater international cooperation among professionals who deal with this population in order to create conditions for the promotion of a greater number of programs related to the impact of physical activity for elderly population.

Of great importance are also international comparative researches and reviews as well, where they compare the results of different authors and conclusions, but such studies make sense only if there are concrete actions. Weening - Dijksterhuis et al. (2011) published a systematic review of 27 studies, where they discussed the influence of the applied training on physical fitness, daily activity and quality of life of institutionalized people aged over 70 years. The aim of the study was to propose criteria for the exercise protocols, which improve physical fitness, daily activity and quality of life for poor institutionalized elderly people, based on evidence. They summarized the recommendations from various studies in a proposal on the method and type of physical exercise in the elderly depending on what we want to influence, and so the following characteristics exercises for developing strength, balance, endurance, functional performance, activities of daily living and increase the quality of life. As for the quality of life it is proposed the following: types of exercise: a combination of progressive resistance training and progressive functional training; intensity: 40 - 80% of 1 RM; volume: increase of one series of repetitions of the eight, and three series of eight replications; frequency: three times a week; duration per session: 60 min.; the total length of 6 months.

Of particular importance are the current problems which certain countries face, as well as ways to overcome them. The problems faced by people with disabilities are similar with elderly population, especially in the case of the Republic of Serbia where the fact stands out that the media do not often cover these issues. They do not have the information, first of all, where, to whom and when to turn to if they want to engage in sporting activities. It takes more to propagate different activities for the elderly, through the media and with the help of experts in various fields as well as offer more diverse content. Permanent physical activity should be an essential measure of primary health care of older persons (Lepan and Leutar, 2012). In Switzerland the promotion of physical activities is present at all levels and in age and thus related to the elderly population. There are numerous projects related to the promotion of sports. Also, municipal organizations, which are registered for the sport and recreation of these persons, in most cases do not have a specialist trained professional person whose task is to organize, create and implement a plan of their work. In addition to this, a common problem is to provide sports grounds on which they conducted the daily sports and recreational activities, as well as lack of customized equipment for each activity, which a direct consequence of insufficient material is issuing from the budget. Architectural barriers are a particular significance. Approaches to public facilities, buildings, hospitals, elevators, renovated jobs, adapted residential buildings, buses, parking lots make the social life of the people impossible. Primarily, this section refers to the investment of the government and state institutions. Without the architectural problem being solved it is hard to think of any form of social integration of people who have sustained a spinal cord injury, and who are determined to move in a wheelchair (Trgovčević et al., 2011). Recreational sports area is important for all other people because with this activity they achieve better psychological and physical stability. Recreational sports activity is organized according to the wishes and abilities of the elderly. Some individuals can engage in hunting and fishing, some can visit the swimming pools and sports centres where they can swim and perform light physical exercises, others can walk etc. (Stošljević et al., 1997). Inclusion in organized exercises of various groups, participation in field trips and other events organized in the framework of gerontology centres helps older people to make new contacts, to create a new social network. Socializing among people of their generation gives them the opportunity to compare their life and life's problems to other people's problems. The very awareness to exercise regular and do something for their health increases the self-esteem and sense of responsibility for their own health and functional capacity. All this with the support of the social environment creates a feeling of greater satisfaction with oneself and a stronger sense of life satisfaction (Lepan and Leutar, 2012).

Limitations

Research related to the impact of physical activity on the elderly population is significant when we take into account the fact that the number of elderly increases from year to year, which creates a need to include a growing number of experts from various fields in order to offer opportunities for the elderly to live better and more qualitative and comprehensive life.

Comparative studies between different countries are very important in all segments and also when it comes to the elderly persons. Limitations of this study are reflected in a relatively small sample and the questionnaire. However, if one takes into account that this is the beginning of the comparative study which will be conducted over the next 3 years in order to collect and compare the results from very different countries and geographic and economic.

REFERENCES

Abbott, R.D., White, L.R., Ross, G.W., Masaki, K.H., Curb, J.D. and Petrovitch, H. (2004). Walking and dementia in physically capable elderly men. *JAMA*, 292, 1447-1453.

Acetto, B. (2006). *Between doctors and patients*. Ljubljana: Anton Trstenjak Institute.

Adamović, M., Eminović, F., Mentus, T. and Stošljević, M. (2014). *Determining functional abilities of lower extremities in elderly as a predictor of falls in relation to the expected norms*. In M., Kulić et al. (eds.), International thematic collection "Education and rehabilitation of adult persons with disabilities," (pp. 75-86). Belgrade: University of East Sarajevo, Faculty of Medicine, Foča; University of Belgrade, Faculty of Special Education and Rehabilitation.

Andrijašević, M. and Andrijašević, M. (2006). *Sports recreation – life factor quality in the elderly population*. http://www.hrks.hr/skole/15_ljetna_skola/45.pdf.

Aniansson, A., Sperling, L., Rundgren, A. and Lehnberg, E. (1983). Muscle funtion in 75-zear old men and women. *Scandinavian Journal of Rehabilitation Medicine*: 9, 92-102.

Alexandris, K. and Carroll, B. (1997). Demographic differences in the perception of constraints on recreational sport participation: Results from a study in Greece. *Leisure Studies*, 16, 107-125.

Bates, A., Donaldson, A., Lloyd, B., Castell, S., Krolik, P. and Coleman, R. (2009). Staying active, staying strong: pilot evaluation of a onceweekly, community-based strength-training program for older adults. *Health Promotion Journal of Australia*, 20(1), 42 – 47.

Bennett, J.A., Stewart, A.L., Kayser-Jone, J. and Glaser, D. (2002.) The mediating effect of pain and fatigue on level of functioning in older adults. *Nursing Research*, 51, 252-265.

Božinović, S. (2006). *Cardiovascular diseases in patients with cerebrovascular insult of the elderly over 60 years of age*. Sub-specialist thesis. Belgrade. Faculty of Medicine

Brown, L.E. (2007). *Strength Training*. Champaign: Human Kinetics.

Brown, W., Fuller, B., Lee, C., Cockburn, J. and Adamson, L. (1999). Never too late: Older people's perceptions of physical activity. *Health Promotion Journal of Australia*, 9(1), 55–63.

Bouillet, D. (2003). Possibilities of out-of-institutional care of the elderly. *Social Policy Review*, 10 (3), 321-333.

Buchner, D., Cress, M., de Lauteur B., et al. (1997). The effect of strength and endurance training on gait, balance, fall risk and health services use in community-living older adults. *The Journals of Gerontology Series A: Biological Sciences and Medical Sciences*, 52(4), 218-224.

Campbell, A., Robertson, M., Gardner, M., et al. (1999). Falls prevention over 2 years: a randomized controlled trial in women 80 years and older. *Age Ageing*, 28, 513-518.

Campbell, A., Roberton, M., Gardner, M., et al. (1997). Randomized controlled trial of a general practice programme of home based exercise to prevent falls in elderly women. *BMJ. 315,* 1065-1069.

Carter, N., Kannus, P. and Khan, K. (2001). Exercise in the prevention of falls in older people: a systematic literature review examining the rationale and the evidence. *Sports Medicine, 31,* 427–438.

Center for Disease Control and Prevention (CDC) (2003). *Public health and aging: Trends in aging V United States and worldwide.* MMWR Morbidity and Mortality Weekly Report, 52, 101Y6.

Colcombe, S. and Kramer, A. (2003). Fitness effects on the cognitive function of older adults: a meta-analytic study. *Psychological Science, 14,* 125–130.

Council of Europe. (2004). *Recent Demographic Developments in Europe.* Strasbourg: Council of Europe Publishing.

Craig, C. L., Russell, S. J., Cameron, C. and Beaulieu, A. (1997). *Foundation for Joint Action. Reducing Inactivity Report.* Canadian Fitness and Lifestyle Research Institute.

Crombie, I., Irvine, L., Williams, B., McGinnis, A., Slane, P., Alder, E. and McMurdo, M. (2004). Why older people do not participate in leisure time physical activity: a survey of activity levels, beliefs and deterrents. *Age and Aging, 33,* 287–292.

Cummins, R.A. (2005). Moving from the quality of life concept to a theory. *Journal of Intellectual Disability Research, 49,* 699-706.

Defilipis, B. and Havelka, M. (1984). *The Elderly.* Zagreb: Stvarnost.

Despot-Lučanin, J. (2003). The experience of aging. Jastrebarsko: Naklada Slap.

Despot-Lučanin, J., Lučanin, D. and Havelka, M. (2006). The quality of growing old, self-evaluation of health and care services requirements. *Social Explorations* 15 (4-5), 84-85.

Despot-Lučanin, J. (1997). A longitudinal study of the correlation of psychological, social and functional factors in the process of aging. Doctoral dissertation. Zagreb. Faculty of Philosophy Zagreb. Department of Psychology.

Di Pietro, L. (1999). Physical activity in the prevention of obesity. Medicine and Science in *Sports and Exercise, 31,* 542-548.

Dowling, S., McConkey, R., Hass, D., Menke, S., Eminović, F.,Wilski, M., Nadolska, A., Kogut, I., Goncharenko, E., Pochstein, F., Bethge, M., Viranyi, A., Regenyi, E., Felegyhazi, J. and Pasztor, S. (2010). *Unified gives us a chance- Anevaluation of Special Olympics Youth Unified Sports® Programme in Europe/Eurasia,* Belfast: University of Ulster, Special Olympics, (pp. 96). On line: http://www.science.ulster.ac.uk/ unifiedsportsunder 'Unified Gives Us a Chance' - Unified Sport - Final Report Sept 2010.pdf.

Dragon, the M. (2010). SCP. The Hague: Elderly nursing home residents.

Duraković, Z. i sar. (2007). Geriatrics. Zagreb: Poslovne informacije Ltd.

Eminović, F. (2014). *Motor learning and exercise adaptations for athletes with intelectual disabilities.* In: D. Hassan, et al. (eds.). Sport, coaching and intellectual disability, (pp 195-210). London: Routledge.

Eminović, F. and Arsić, S., (2014). Corelation between executive and motor function in patients after a stroke. In: K. Bennett (Ed.). Executive Functioning Role in Early Learning Processes, Impairments in Neurological Disorders and Impact of Cognitive Behavior Therapy (CTB), (pp. 323-358). NewYork: Nova Publishers.

Eminović, F., Čanović, D. and Nikić, R. (2011). Physical education 1 - Physical education of children with disabilities - scientific monographs. Belgrade: Faculty for Special Education and Rehabilitation.

Eminović, F., Nikić, R., Stojković, I. and Pacić, S. (2009). Attitudes toward inclusion of persons with disabilities in sport activities. *Sport Science*, 2(1), 72 – 77.

Eyigor, S., Karapolat, H. and Durmaz, B. (2007). Effects of a group-based exercise program on the physical performance, muscle strength and quality of life in older women. *Archives of Gerontology and Geriatrics, 45,* 259–271.

Evans, W.J. (1995). Effects of exercise on body composition and functional capacity of the elderly. *The Journals of Gerontology Series A: Biological Sciences and Medical Sciences, 50,* 147-50.

Fogelholm, M., Kukkonen-Harjula, K., Nenonen, A. and Pasanen, M. (2000). Effects of walking training on weight maintenance after a very low-energy diet in premenopausal obese women: a randomized controlled trial. *Archives of Internal Medicine, 160*(14), 2177-2184.

Gidens, E. (2000). *Sociologija.* Beograd: Nolit.

Grisso, J.A., Kelsey, J.L., Strom, BL, et al. (1991). Risk factors for falls as a cause of hip fractures in women. *Lancet, 324,* 1326-31.

Hamer, M. and Chida, Y. (2009). Physical activity and risk of neurodegenerative disease: A systematic review of prospective evidence. *Psychological Medicine, 39,* 3–11.

Harahousou, Y.S. and Kabitsis, C.N. (1993). Important reasons that motivate Greek women into participation in physical recreation. In: Bell, F. I., Van Gyn, G. H. (Eds), *Proceedings for the 10th Commonwealth and International scientific congress: access to active living* (pp. 113 118). Victoria BC: University of Victoria.

Hašpl-Jurišić, H. (2007). *Active aging of the retired.* Master's Thesis. Zagreb: Faculty of Law – Study centre of social work.

Haykowsky, M., McGavock, J., Muhll, I. V., Koller, M., Mandić, S., Welsh, R. and Taylor, D. (2005). Effect of exercise training on peak aerobic power, left ventricular morphology, and muscle strength in healthy older women. *The Journals of Gerontology, 60*(3), 307-311.

Hornbrook, M.C., Stevens, V.J. and Wingfield, D.J. (1994). Preventing falls among community dwelling older persons: results from a randomized trial. *Gerontologist, 34,* 16-23.

Hrnjica, S. (2003). General psychology and personality psychology. Belgrade: Naučna knjiga.

Kane, R.A., Kling, K.C., Bershadsky, B., Kane, R.L., Giles, K., Degenholtz, H.B. et al. (2003). Quality of life measures for nursing home residents. *Journal of Gerontology, 58,* 240-248.

Kida, K., Osada, H., Akashi, Y.J., Sekizuka, H., Omiya, K. and Miyake, F. (2008). The exercise training effects of skeletal muscle strength and muscle volume to improve functional capacity in patients with myocardial infarction. *International Journal of Cardiology, 129,* 180–186.

King, M.B., Whipple, R.H., Gruman, C.A., Judge, J.O., Schmidt, J.A. and Wolfson, L.I., (2002). The performance enhancement project: improving physical performance in older persons. *Archives of Physical Medicine and Rehabilitation, 83,* 1060–1069.

Kljajić, D., Dopsaj, M., Eminović, F. And Kasum, G. (2013). Sport in the rehabilitation of individuals with disability. *Health Care* 42(3), 58-66.

Krizmanić, M. and Kolersarić, V. (1989). An attempt of conceptualisation of the notion of "quality of life". *Applied Psychology*, 10, 5-11.

Lamprecht, M., Fischer, A. and Stamm, H.P. (2014). *Sport Schweiz 2014: Sportaktivität und Sportinteresse der Schweizer Bevölkerung.* Magglingen: Bundesamt für Sport BASPO.

Larson, E., Wang, L., Bowen, J., McCormick, W., Teri, L., Crane, P. and Kukull, W. (2006). Exercise is associated with reduced risk for incident dementia among persons 65 years of age and older. *Annals of Internal Medicine, 144,* 73–81.

Laurin, D., Verreault, R., Lindsay, J., MacPherson, K. and Rockwood, K. (2001). Physical activity and risk of cognitive impairment and dementia in elderly persons. *Archives of Neurology, 58,* 498-504.

Lehtola, S., Hanninen, L. and Paatalo, M. (2000). The incidence of falls during a six-month exercise trial and four-month followup among home dwelling persons aged 70-75 years. *Liikunta Tiede, 6,* 41-47.

Lepan, Ž. And Leutar , Z. (2012). The importance of physical activities at an elderly age. *Social ecology: Journal for ecological thought and sociological research of the environment,* 21(2), 203-224.

Leutar, Z. Štambuk, A, and Rusac, S. (2007). Social policy and quality of life of the elderly with physical disability. *Social Policy Review* 3-4(14), 327-346.

Lexell, J., Taylor, C. C. and Sjöström, M. (1988). What is the cause of the ageing atrophy? Total number, size and proportion of different fiber types studied in whole vastus lateralis muscle from 15- to 83-year-old men. *Journal of the Neurological Sciences, 84*(2-3), 275–294.

Linn, R.T., Wolf, P.A., Bachman, D.L., Knoefel, J.E., Cobb, J.L., Belanger, A.J., Kaplan, E.F. and D'Agostino, R.B. (1995). The 'preclinical phase' of probable Alzheimer's disease. A 13-year prospective study of the Framingham cohort. *Archives of Neurology, 52,* 485–490.

Lovreković, M. and Leutar, Z. (2010). The quality of life of individuals in elderly foster care homes in Zagreb. *Social ecology: Review for ecological thought and sociological research I* (1), 55-79.

Mavrić, F., Kahrović, I., Muric, B. and Radenkovic, O. (2014). The effects of regular physical exercise on the human body. *Physical Culture, 68*(1), 29-38.

McAuley, E. and Katula, J. (1998). Physical activity interventions in the elderly: influence on physical health and psychological function. In: Shulz R., Maddox G., Lawton M.P., (eds.), *Annual Review of Gerontology and Geriatrics* (pp. 111–154). New York: Springer.

McNeil, K., LeBlanc, E. and Joyce, M. (1991). The effect of exercise on depressive symptoms in the moderately depressed elderly. *Psychology and Aging, 3,* 487-488.

McMurdo, E., Mole, P. and Paterson, C. (1997). Controlled trial of weight bearing exercise in older women in relation to bone density and falls. *BMJ, 314,* 569.

Mental Health Foundation (2009). Dementia. Available from: http://tiny.cc/a-z-dementia.

Michalopoulos, M., Zisi, V., Malliou, P. and Godolias, G. (2004). Habitual activity and motor function in an urban Greek Elderly Population. *Journal of Human Movement Studies, 46,* 519-530.

Μεσθεναίου Ελ., Κ. Αντωνιάδου (Mestheneou El., Antoniadou K) (2004). Εθνική Αναφορά της Ελλάδας για το πρόγραμμα MERI, (National Report of Greece for the MERI Project), Αθήνα 2004.

Milanović, Z., Pantelić, S., Trajković, N. and Sporiš, G. (2011). Basic anthropometric and body composition characteristics in elderly population: A Systematic Review. *Facta Universitatis: Series Physical Education and Sport, 9*(2), 173−182.

Milićević, M. (2015). Evaluation of the quality of life of children and adolescents with cerebral palsy in the Republic of Serbia. *Belgrade School of Defectology,* 21(1), 9-22.

Misra, A. and Khurana, L. (2008). Obesity and the metabolic syndrome in developing countries. *The Journal of Clinical Endocrinology and Metabolism*, *93*, S9–S30.

Močnik, A., Neuberg, M. and Canjuga, I. (2015). Physical activity of the elderly in stationary institutions. *Technical Gazette* 9(1), 112-119.

Mujović, V. and Čubrilo. D. (2012). The role of physical activity in the prevention and treatment of diseases. *Physical Culture* 66(1), 40-47.

Myers, A., Young, Y. and Langlois, J. (1996). Prevention of falls in the elderly. *Bone*, *18*(1 Suppl.), 87-101.

Nemček, D. (2011). The status of motor performances in elderly women in Slovakia. Physical Culture 65(2), 79-86.

Nemoto, K., Gen-no, H., Masuki, S., Okazaki, K. and Nose, H. (2007). Effects of high-intensity interval walking training on physical fitness and blood pressure in middle-aged and older people. *Mayo Clinic Proccedings*, *82*, 803–812.

Nikić, R., Pacić, S., Gavrilović, M., Zolnjan, M. (2014): Quality of life in patients with stomas. In: M. Kulić and D. Ilić-Stosović, (Eds.), *Internacional thematic collection of papers "Education and rehabilitation of adult persons with disabilities,"* (pp. 261-274). Belgrade: Faculty of Special Education and Rehabilitation and Foca: University of East Sarajevo, Faculty of Medicine.

Nikolić, S., Ilić, D., Pacić, S. and Zolnjan, M. (2009). Quality of life of individuals with spasticity. *Belgrade School of Defectology*, 15(3), 157-168.

O'Donovan, G., Blazevich, A.J., Boreham, C., Cooper, A.R., Crank, H., Ekelund, U. et al. (2010). The ABC of Physical Activity for Health: a consensus statement from the British Association of Sport and Exercise Sciences. *Journal of Sports Science, 28*, 573–591.

Pacić, S., Zolnjan, M., Đorđević, M. and Potić, S. (2010). Daily activities of individuals with spasticity with regard to gender. In V. Bumbaširević, (Ed.), *Proceedings from the 51st congress of biomedical students of Serbia with international participation* (383). Belgrade: Faculty of Medicine, University of Belgrade.

Parkkari, J., Kannus, P., Palvanen, M., Natri, A., Vainio, J., Aho, H. and Jarvinen, M. (1999). Majority of hip fractures occur as a result of a fall and impact on the greater trochanter of the femur: a prospective controlled hip fracture study with 206 consecutive patients. *Calcified Tissue International, 65*, 183–187.

Pavlović, D.M. and Pavlović, A.M. (2014). *Dementia – Neuropsychiatric symptoms*. Belgrade: Orion Art.

Pavlović, D. (2008). *Dementias, neurological and psychological problem.* Belgrade: Kaligraf.

Papaioannou, A., Morin, S., Cheung, A.M., Atkinson, S., Brown, J.P., Feldman, S., Hanley, D.A., Hodsman, A., Jamal, S.A., Kaiser, S.M., Kvern, B., Siminoski, K. and Leslie W.D. (2010). Scientific Advisory Council of Osteoporosis Canada. 2010 clinical practice guidelines for the diagnosis and management of osteoporosis in Canada: Summary. *Canadian Medical Association Journal, 182*, 1829– 1830.

Pavot, W. and Diener, E. (1993). Review of the satisfaction with life scale. *Psychological Assessment, 5*, 164–172.

Peck, W.A., Riggs, B.L., Bell, N.H., et al. (1988). Research directions in osteoporosis. *New England Journal of Medicine, 85*, 275-82.

Penev, G. (2006). Population structure by gender and age. In G. Penev (Ed.), *The population and households in Serbia according to the 2002 population census* (109-138). Belgrade:

Republic Institute for Statistics, Serbia - Social Science Institute, Centre for Demographic Research, Demographic Society of Serbia.

Perissinotto, E., Pisent, C., Sergi, G. and Grigoletto, F. (2002). Anthropometric measurements in the elderly, age and gender differences. *British Journal of Nutrition*, 87(2): 177-86.

Podgorelec, S. (2004). *The quality of life of the elderly in isolated areas – the example of Croatian islands*. Doctoral dissertation. Zagreb: Faculty of Philosophy Zagreb, Department of Sociology.

Pospiš, M. (2001). *Cerebral palsy and aging. Aging and cerebral palsy*. Zagreb: Croatian Union of Associations of Cerebral Palsy and Poliomyelitis.

Puljiz, V. (2005). Documentation. *Social Policy Review* 12(2). 263-271.

Puts, M.T., Shekary, N., Widdershoven, G., Heldens, J., Lips, P. and Deeg, D.J. (2007). What does quality of life mean to older frail and non-frail community-dwelling adults in the Netherlands? *Quality of Life Research*, *16*, 263-277.

Quail, G.C. (1994). An approach to the assessment of falls in the elderly. *Australian Family Physician*, *23*, 876-82.

Rejeski, W.J., Brawley, L.R. and Shumaker, S.A. (1996). Physical activity and healthrelated quality of life. *Exercise and Sport Science Review*, *24*, 71–108.

Rich, M.W. (2005). Heart failure in the oldest patients: The Impact of Comorbid Conditions. *American Journal of Geriatric Cardiology*, *14*(3), 134-141.

Riggs, B.L., Melton, L.J. (1986). Involutional osteoporosis. *New England Journal of Medicine*, *314*, 1676-1686.

Rizzo, J., Baker, D., McAvay, G., et al. (1996). The cost-effectiveness of a multifactorial target prevention program for falls among the community elderly persons. *Medical Care*, *34*, 954-69.

Rockwood, K., Andrew, M. and Mitnitski, A., (2007). A comparison of two approaches to measuring frailty in elderly people. *Journal of Gerontology*, 62, 738–743.

Rowe, J. W. and Kahn, R. L. (1997). Successful Aging. *The Gerontologist*, *37*(4), 433–440.

Rubenstein, L. (2006). Falls in older people: epidemiology, risk factors and strategies for prevention. *Age and Ageing*, *35*(2), 37–41.

Rubenstein, L., Josephson, K., Trueblood, P., et al. (2000). Effects of a group exercise programon strength, mobility, and falls among fall-prone elderly men. *The Journals of Gerontology Series A: Biological Sciences and Medical Sciences*, *55*(6), M317-M21.

Šarić, E. (2014). The third age. Tuzla: Bosanska riječ.

Schaie, K.W. and Willis, S.L. (2001). The psychology of the adult age and aging. Jastrebarsko: Naklada Slap.

Singh, N.A., Clements, K.M. and Fiatarone, M.A. (1997). A randomized controlled trial of progressive resistance training in depressed elders. *The Journals of Gerontology Series A: Biological Sciences and Medical Sciences*, *52*, 27-35.

Small, B.J., Fratiglioni, L., Viitanen, M., Winblad, B. and Backman, L. (2000). The course of cognitive impairment in preclinical Alzheimer disease: 3- and 6-year follow-up of a population-based sample. *Archives of Neurology*, *57*, 839–844.

Smiljanjić, V. (2001). *The psychology of aging*. Belgrade: Nolit.

Smolić-Krković, N. (1974). *Gerontology*. Zagreb: Association of Social Workers Societies of the Socialist Republic of Croatia.

Štambuk, A, Žganec, N. and Nižić, M. (2012). Some dimensions of the quality of life of the elderly with disability. *Croatian Review for Rehabilitation Research* 48(1), 84-95.

Steinberg, M., Cartwright, C., Peel, N., et al. (2000). A sustainable programme to prevent falls and near falls in community dwelling older people: results of a randomised trial. *Journal of Epidemiology and Community Health*, *54,* 227-232.

Stewart, A.L. (2003). Conceptual challenges in linking physical activity and disability research. *American Journal of Preventive Medicine*, *25*(3), 137-140.

Stewart, A.L. and King, A.C. (1991). Evaluating the efficacy of physical activity for influencing quality-of-life outcomes in older adults. *Annals of Behavioral Medicine*, *13,* 108–116.

Stošljević, L. Rapaić, D., Stošljević, M. and Nikolić, S. (1997). Somatopedy. Belgrade: Naučna knjiga.

Stošljević, M. Nikić, R., Eminović, F. and Pacić, S. (2013). *Psychophysical impairments of children and youth.* Belgrade: The Society of Defectologists of Serbia.

Sun, F., Norman, I.J. and While, A.E. (2013). Physical activity in older people: A systematic review. *BMC Public Health*, *13,* 1–17.

The World Bank. (2014). The United Nations Population Division's World Population Prospects. Available from: http://wdi.worldbank.org/table/2.1#

The United Nations Population Division's World Population Prospects. 2014.

Tekur, P., Nagendra, H.R. and Raghuram, N. (2008). Effect of short-term intensive yoga program on pain, functional disability and spinal flexibility in chronic low back pain: a randomised control study. *Journal of Alternative and Complementary Medicine*, *14*(6), 637– 644.

Tinetti, M.E., Baker, D.I., McAvay, G., Clans, E.B., Garrett, P., Gottschalk, M., Koch, M.L., Trainor, K. and Horwitz, R.I. (1994). A multifactorial intervention to reduce the risk of falling among elderly people living in the community. *New England Journal of Medicine*, *33,* 821–827.

Tokarski, W. (2004). Sports in the elderly population. *Kinesiology* 36(1), 98-103.

Tomek-Roksandić, S., Perko, G, Mihok, D, Radašević, H. and Puljak, A. (2004). A guide to aging. The Centre for Gerontology of the Institute for Public Health of the City of Zagreb – Reference Centre of the Ministry of Health for the protection of health of the elderly.

Tomek-Roksandić, S. and Čulig, J. (2003). *Living a healthy active aging.* Zagreb: CZG ZZJZ City of Zagreb.

Trgovčević, S. Kljajić, D. and Nedović, G. (2011). Social integration as a determinant of the quality of life of individuals with traumatic paraplegia. *Social policy and social work*, 6, 493-505.

United Nations. (2014). World Population Prospects: The 2010 Revision. Available from: http://esa.un.org/.

Visser, M., Pahor, M., Tylavsky, F., Kritchevsky, S. B., Cauley, J. A., Newman, A. and Harris, T.B. (2003). One- and two-year change in body composition as measured by DXA in a population-based cohort of older men and women. *Journal of Applied Physiology*, *94*(6), 2368-2374.

Vreede, de P.L., Samson, M.M., Meeteren, van N.L., Duursma, S.A. and Verhaar, H.J. (2005). Functional task exercise versus resistance strength exercise to improve daily function in older women: a randomized controlled trial. *Journal of American Geriatric Society*, *53,* 2-10.

Vojvodić, N. Bojović, D. and Božinović, S. (1992). *Elementary psychophysical features and functional ability of the elderly.* Gerontology Developments Journal (9-27). Belgrade.

Vuletić, G. (1999). *Sociopsychological factors of personal life quality.* Master's Thesis. Zagreb: Faculty of Medicine.

Vuori, I. (2005). Physical activity as an efficient means against non-favourable health effect of physical inactivity. *Gazette of the Croatian Union of sports recreation Sports for All,* 3-12.

Weening-Dijksterhuis, E., de Greef, M.H., Scherder, E.J., Slaets, J.P. and van der Schans, C.P. (2011). Frail institutionalized older persons: A comprehensive review on physical exercise, physical fitness, activities of daily living, and quality-of-life. *American Journal of Physical Medicine and Rehabilitation/Association of Academic Physiatrists, 90,* 156–168.

Weinberg, R. and Gould, D. (2003). *Foundations of sport and exercise psychology.* Champaign, IL: Human Kinetics.

Weuve, J., Kang, J.H., Manson, J.E., Breteler, M.M., Ware, J.H. and Grodstein, F. (2004). Physical activity, including walking, and cognitive function in older women. *JAMA, 292,* 1454-461.

WHOQOL group. (1993) Measuring quality of life: the development of the World health organization Quality of Life Instrument (WHOQOL). Geneva: WHO.

Wilbur, J., Marquez, D. X., Fogg, L. et al. (2012). The relationship between physical activity and cognition in older Latinos. *The Journals of Gerontology Series B: Psychological Sciences and Social Sciences, 67,* 525-534.

Wolf, S., Barnhart, M., Kutner, N. et al. (1996). Reducing frailty and falls in older persons: an investigation of Tai-Chi and computerized training. *Journal of the American Geriatric Society, 44,* 489-497.

World Health Organisation Global recommendations on physical activity for health, WHO Library Cataloguing-in-Publication Data, Printed in Switzerland 2010. Available from: http://whqlibdoc.who.int/publications/2010/9789241599979_eng.pdf.

World Health Organisation Working together for health-The World Health Report 2006, WHO Library Cataloguing-in-Publication Data, Printed in Switzerland 2006. Available from: http://www.who.int/whr/2006/whr06_en.pdf.

World Health Organisation Health and Development Through Physical Activity and Spor, Library Cataloguing-in-Publication Data, Printed in Switzerland 2003. Available from: http://whqlibdoc.who.int/hq/2003/WHO_NMH_ NPH_PAH_03.2.pdf.

World Health Organization. World Health Report on Reducing Risks and Promoting Healthy Life [Internet]. 2002. Available from: http://www. who.int/whr/2002/en/whr02_en.pdf.

World Health Organization. (2007). Global report on falls prevention in older age. Geneva: WHO.

Ylinen, J., Takala, E., Nykanen, M., Kautiainen, H. et al. (2006). Effects of twelve-month strength training subsequent to twelve-month stretching exercise in treatment of chronic neck pain. *Journal of Strength and Conditioning Research, 20*(2), 304-308.

Živković, M., Jakovljević, V. Mujović, V.M. (2002). Use of hyperbaric oxygenation in the treatment of ischemic heart diseases. *Acta Biologica Medicine Exp.,* 27(2), 41-45.

EDITORS' CONTACT INFORMATION

Dr. Fadilj Eminović,
Faculty for Special Education and Rehabilitation,
University of Belgrade, Serbia,
Associate Professor,
Secretary of Department for People with Motor Disabilities
Email: eminovic73@gmail.com

Dr. Milivoj Dopsaj,
Faculty of Sport and Physical Education,
University of Belgrade, Serbia
Associate Professor,
Vice Dean for Science

INDEX

D

I

Q

R

S

T